STEM CELL CULTURE
Three Dimensional

Kruger Brentt
Publishers

STEM CELL CULTURE
Three Dimensional

Peter Adler
Victor Betancourt

Kruger Brentt
Publishers
2025

Kruger Brentt Publishers UK. LTD.
Company Number 9728962

Regd. Office: 68 St Margarets Road, Edgware, Middlesex HA8 9UU

ISBN: 978-1-78715-336-3

For information on all our publications visit our website at http://krugerbrentt.com/

PREFACE

"Stem Cell Culture: Three Dimensional" ventures into the innovative realm of three-dimensional (3D) stem cell culture, offering readers a comprehensive exploration of the principles, techniques, and applications that define this cutting-edge field. This book serves as an essential resource for researchers, scientists, clinicians, and students seeking to understand the intricacies of 3D stem cell culture and its potential for advancing regenerative medicine, drug discovery, and tissue engineering.

Stem cells hold immense promise for regenerative therapies and disease modeling due to their unique ability to self-renew and differentiate into various cell types. Traditional two-dimensional (2D) cell culture systems have limitations in mimicking the complex microenvironment of living tissues, prompting the development of 3D culture techniques that better recapitulate in vivo conditions and cellular interactions.

The primary objective of this book is to provide readers with a comprehensive overview of 3D stem cell culture techniques, covering key topics such as scaffold-based and scaffold-free culture systems, microfluidic platforms, bioreactor systems, cell-matrix interactions, and tissue engineering applications. Each chapter offers insights, methodological approaches, and case studies to help readers understand the fundamental principles and practical considerations of 3D stem cell culture.

Contributions from leading experts in the field explore various aspects of 3D stem cell culture, including advances in biomaterials, biofabrication techniques, imaging technologies, and high-throughput screening methods. Special emphasis is placed on the diverse applications of 3D stem cell culture in regenerative medicine, disease modeling, drug screening, personalized medicine, and organ-on-a-chip platforms.

As we strive to harness the potential of stem cells for therapeutic and research purposes, it is essential to explore innovative approaches that more accurately replicate the complexity of human tissues and organs. By embracing 3D stem cell culture techniques and interdisciplinary collaborations, we can accelerate discoveries, improve treatment outcomes, and ultimately enhance human health and well-being.

We extend our sincere gratitude to the contributors whose expertise and dedication have enriched this book. It is our hope that "Stem Cell Culture: Three Dimensional" will serve as a valuable resource and inspiration for researchers and practitioners at the forefront of regenerative medicine and tissue engineering.

Peter Adler
Victor Betancourt

CONTENTS

PREFACE V

1. THREE-DIMENSIONAL STEM CELL CULTURE 1

1. Introduction: An overview 1

2. Applications of three-dimensional stem cell culture 3

3. At a Glance 5

References 5

2. CARDIAC FIBROBLASTS REGULATE THE CONTRACTION OF HUMAN FIBROTIC CARDIAC MICROTISSUES BY A MECHANISM THAT DEPENDS ON Β-ADRENORECEPTORS 7

1. Introduction: An overview 7

2. Material and Methods 9

3. Results 13

4. Discussion 23

5. At a Glance 26

References 27

3. 3D-NEUROSPHERES DERIVED FROM HUMAN INDUCED PLURIPOTENT STEM CELLS ARE APPROPRIATE FOR SCREENING NEUROTOXICITY 33

1. Introduction: An Overview

2. Methods 34

3. Results 39

4. Discussion 52

6. At a Glance 59

References 59

4. VERTICAL FUNCTIONALIZED SILICON MICROPILLARS FOR THREE-DIMENSIONAL CULTIVATION OF HUMAN PLURIPOTENT STEM CELL-DERIVED CORTICAL PROGENITORS 69

1. Introduction 69

2. Materials and Methods 70

3. Results and Discussion 74

4. Concise Summary 84

5. At a Glance 85

References 85

5. HUMAN BONE MARROW MESENCHYMAL STEM CELLS EXPRESS TENDON AND CYTOKINE MARKERS IN A HYALURONATE/POLY-LACTIC-CO-GLYCOLIC ACID (PLGA)/FIBRIN THREE-DIMENSIONAL (3D) SCAFFOLD **93**

1. Introduction: An Overview 93

2. Materials and Methods 95

3. Results 100

4. Discussion 109

5. Concise Summary 112

6. At a Glance 113

References 113

6. SELF-ASSEMBLING SCAFFOLDS FACILITATED EXTENDED GROWTH OF HUMAN PRIMED EMBRYONIC STEM CELLS AND INCREASED THE EXPRESSION OF CORE AND NAÏVE PLURIPOTENT MARKERS **123**

1. Introduction: An Overview 123

2. Materials and Methods 125

3. Results 130

4. Discussion 139

5. At a Glance 143

References 143

7. REATING SPECIALIZED AND LONG-LASTING INTESTINAL STRUCTURES THAT MIRROR THE VARIED CELL TYPES FOUND IN THE CANINE INTESTINE **153**

1. Introduction: An Overview 153

2. Materials and Methods 155

3. Results 158

4. Discussion 165

5. Concise Summary 168

6. At a Glance 168

References 169

8. PP2A DEFICIENCY ENHANCES CARCINOGENESIS OF LGR5⁺ INTESTINAL STEM CELLS BOTH IN ORGANOIDS AND IN VIVO 175

1. Introduction: An Overview 175

2. Materials and Methods 177

3. Results 181

4. Discussion 193

5. Concise Summary 194

6. At a Glance 195

References 195

9. MOUSE EMBRYONIC STEM CELL-DERIVED URETERIC BUD PROGENITORS STIMULATE NEPHROGENESIS 201

1. Introduction: An Overview 201

2. Materials and Methods 202

3. Results 204

4. Discussion 213

5. At a Glance 214

References 215

10. COMPARING TRADITIONAL AND ADVANCED CELL CULTURES IN HEMATOPOIETIC STEM CELL RESEARCH 221

1. Introduction: An Overview 221

2. Hematopoietic Stem Cells 221

3. Stem Cell Culture Methods 224

4. 3D Hematopoietic Stem Cell Culture 227

5. Concise Summary 231

6. At A Glance 232

References 232

INDEX 241

01 THREE-DIMENSIONAL STEM CELL CULTURE

1. INTRODUCTION: AN OVERVIEW

Three-dimensional stem cell culture represents a paradigm shift in biomedical research and therapeutic development. Unlike conventional two-dimensional cell culture methods, which often oversimplify the complex cellular interactions and tissue architectures found in living organisms, 3D stem cell culture offers a more physiologically relevant environment for studying cell behavior, differentiation, and tissue development. By allowing cells to grow and interact within three-dimensional matrices that mimic the native extracellular matrix, researchers can better replicate the intricate microenvironments found within the human body. This technology holds tremendous promise across various fields, including regenerative medicine, disease modeling, drug discovery, and toxicology testing. Through the precise control of cellular environments and the recreation of tissue-specific conditions, 3D stem cell culture has the potential to unlock new insights into disease mechanisms, accelerate the development of novel therapeutics, and ultimately pave the way for more personalized and effective treatment strategies. As researchers continue to refine and innovate in this rapidly evolving field, the impact of three-dimensional stem cell culture on healthcare and biomedical science is poised to be profound and far-reaching.

Stem cells possess the capacity for self-renewal and differentiation. Various stem cells can be extracted from embryonic or adult tissues, with different levels of potency ranging from pluripotent to unipotent based on the kind of stem cell. Cells are commonly located in certain areas inside the human body, creating a supportive environment for stem cells to grow and develop. Stem cells are commonly grown on 2D tissue culture plastic to allow for convenient and maximum expansion, as a significant quantity is usually required for translational research and medicines. 2D preparations do not accurately mimic the natural milieu of stem cells in the body. The advantageous characteristics of stem cells may be diminished or compromised in 2D preparations. Thus, the utilization of 3D culture methods has become increasingly prevalent in fundamental and translational studies. 3D cultures offer enhanced cell-to-cell and cell-to-matrix interactions, closely resembling the natural environment of stem cells compared to 2D cultures. Moreover, numerous preferred cellular traits are preserved or enhanced in 3D cultures, which reinforces their utility in fundamental and translational studies. This Special Issue focuses on the latest developments in the 3D cultivation of stem cells, with a compilation of articles that showcase different types of stem cells and their attributes in 3D settings. This book includes chapter highlighting the effective use of induced pluripotent stem cells (iPSCs) to develop cardiac microtissue [**1**], neurospheres [**2**], and cortical progenitors [**3**]. In addition, this Special Issue contains work on scaffolds with mesenchymal stem cells (MSCs) [**4**] and embryonic stem cells (ESCs) [**5**]. Furthermore, research on generating intestinal organoids from stem cells [**6**,**7**] and nephrogenesis studies utilizing ESCs [**8**] are included in thisbook, along with a comprehensive review on the 3D culture of hematopoietic stem cells (HSCs) [**9**].

A very relevant problem in cardiology is cardiac fibrosis. In the work by Blyszczuk et al., a model of fibrotic cardiac microtissue was generated using iPSC-derived cardiomyocytes and cardiac fibroblasts by treatment with transforming growth factor β1 (TGF- β1) or by use of cardiac fibroblasts from heart failure patients [**1**]. The authors demonstrated that activated cardiac fibroblasts could, via direct stimulation of β-adrenoreceptor signaling, promote cardiac contraction rate. Furthermore, the generated model could be used as a high-throughput model for drug testing or general studies of cardiac fibrosis [**1**].

A 3D in vitro model utilizing iPSCs was generated by Kobolak et al. to study neurotoxicity [**2**]. In this work, iPSC-derived, 3D, free-floating neurospheres, exhibiting the various cells of the nervous system, were developed and tested in neurotoxicity studies. Furthermore, these neurospheres could open some further opportunities for the detection of developmental neurotoxicity, and hence support the existing animal models [**2**].

The work by Cutarelli et al. employed iPSC-derived cortical progenitors and scaffolds to mimic the radially oriented cortical radial glia fibers that play an important role in the development of the cerebral cortex [**3**]. The authors used silicon vertical micropillar arrays to promote the expansion and preservation of stemness of the cortical progenitors. Furthermore, the described model of iPSC-derived cortical progenitors and silicon micropillars could be used in cortical tissue engineering [**3**].

Another in vitro 3D model was generated by Ciardulli et al. for the study of MSCs and their tenogenic differentiation [**4**]. This work employed a hyoluronate/poly-lactic-co-glycolic acid (PLGA)/fibrin 3D scaffold with MSCs that were studied under static and cyclic-strain conditions. The research demonstrated that MSCs grown in this scaffold increased their tenogenic marker and pro-repair cytokine expression, supporting the notion of this model as a potential predictive system to be used in future studies employing the sustained release of biochemicals [**4**].

To circumvent some of the challenges with the 2D culture expansion of ESCs, McKee et al. developed a 3D scaffold to mimic in vivo stem cell niches [5]. The authors used polyethylene glycol (PEG) polymers with thiol and acrylate end-groups to guide the self-assembly of the scaffolds. ESCs grown in these scaffolds were able to maintain their viability, self-renewal, and differentiation potential. ESCs in the scaffolds also exhibited a high expression of pluripotency markers and some mechanosensitive genes, supporting the notion of these scaffolds as potentially helpful for many ESC studies [5].

To aid in the study of intestinal disorders, Kramer et al. developed intestinal organoids from stem cells obtained from various parts of the intestine [6]. These intestinal organoids showed long-term expansion of the cells while inhibiting cell differentiation when cultured in expansion media, while differentiation into goblet and enteroendocrine cells was promoted with culture in differentiation media. These organoids could possibly be employed in various in vitro models of functional intestinal disorders [6].

Another study utilizing intestinal stem cell organoids explored the cellular origin of carcinogenesis [7]. In this study, Yen et al. developed a tumorigenesis model based on carcinogenesis and genetically engineered mice. The authors were able to demonstrate the interplay between extrinsic carcinogen and intrinsic genetic modification and their contribution towards transformation while elucidating the involvement of molecular factors, such as protein phosphatase 2A (PP2A), in this process [7].

A study by Tan et al. utilized ESCs to generate ureteric bud progenitor cells [8]. The authors then used these progenitor cells to induce nephrogenesis in co-culture with primary metanephric mesenchyme. These kidney organoids exhibited nephron structures with collecting ducts connected to nephron tubules. This study demonstrated a relatively simple and reproducible way of generating ureteric bud progenitors [8].

This book also highlighting recent discoveries in 3D stem cell cultures using MSCs [4], ESCs [5,8], iPSCs [1,2,3], and intestinal stem cells [6,7]. This Special Issue also includes a review article by Ribeiro-Filho et al. that discusses the 2D and 3D culture of hematopoietic stem cells (HSCs) as a relevant model to study both normal and abnormal hematopoiesis [9]. Furthermore, this Special Issue includes articles that utilize various scaffolds together with stem cells from various sources to study 3D cultures [3,4,5].

2. APPLICATIONS OF THREE-DIMENSIONAL STEM CELL CULTURE

Three-dimensional stem cell culture holds immense promise across a wide range of applications in biomedical research and therapeutic development. Some of the key applications include:

- **Regenerative Medicine:** 3D stem cell culture enables the generation of tissue constructs that closely mimic the native architecture of organs and tissues. These constructs can be used for tissue engineering and regenerative medicine purposes, including the repair and replacement of damaged or diseased tissues.
- **Disease Modeling:** Researchers can use 3D stem cell culture to create disease models that better recapitulate the complex microenvironment of human tissues. This allows for the study of disease mechanisms, the screening of potential therapeutics, and the identification of novel drug targets.
- **Srug Discovery and Development:** Three-dimensional stem cell culture provides a more physiologically relevant platform for drug screening and toxicity testing compared to traditional two-dimensional cultures. By culturing cells in 3D environments, researchers can better predict drug responses and assess potential adverse effects, leading to more accurate preclinical evaluation of drug candidates.
- **Cancer Research:** 3D stem cell culture systems have been instrumental in studying cancer biology, tumor formation, and metastasis. These models allow researchers to investigate tumor-stroma interactions, drug resistance mechanisms, and the development of more effective cancer therapies.
- **Organ-on-a-Chip Technology:** Integration of stem cells into organ-on-a-chip platforms enables the creation of microscale models of human organs. These systems can replicate organ-level functions and responses, offering a valuable tool for studying organ physiology, disease pathology, and drug effects in vitro.
- **Personalized Medicine:** With advancements in induced pluripotent stem cell (iPSC) technology, patient-specific stem cells can be generated and incorporated into 3D culture systems. This allows for the development of personalized disease models and drug screening assays tailored to individual patients, facilitating precision medicine approaches.
- **Bioprinting:** Stem cells cultured in three dimensions can be incorporated into bioprinting technologies to create complex tissue constructs layer by layer. Bioprinted tissues and organs have the potential to be used for transplantation, drug testing, and disease modeling, advancing the field of regenerative medicine.

Overall, the applications of three-dimensional stem cell culture are vast and continually expanding, driving innovation in biomedical research and paving the way for the development of novel therapies and treatments for a wide range of diseases and conditions.

3. AT A GLANCE

Stem cells have garnered significant attention in both fundamental and translational research with the purpose of comprehending basic stem cell biology and creating novel treatments for various illnesses. Stem cells are typically cultivated easily, although the most frequent procedures include employing plastic in 2D techniques. These cultures inadequately depict the stem cell niches in the body, which are complex microenvironments consisting of stem cells, supportive stromal cells, extracellular matrix, and growth factors. Researchers and clinicians are looking for the best stem cell preparations for fundamental research and therapeutic use, which could be achieved by growing stem cells in a 3D culture. 3D cultures mimic in vivo cell-to-cell and cell-to-matrix interactions more accurately, resulting in cells with distinct and favorable traits. Stem cell cultivation in 3D utilizes different matrices or scaffolds, together with cells, to aid complicated constructions. This Special Issue aims to consolidate contemporary research on 3D cultures of different stem cells to enhance the fundamental knowledge of stem cells and culture methods, as well as to showcase stem cell preparations for potential innovative therapeutic uses.

REFERENCES

1. Błyszczuk, P.; Zuppinger, C.; Costa, A.; Nurzynska, D.; Di Meglio, F.D.; Stellato, M.; Agarkova, I.; Smith, G.L.; Distler, O.; Kania, G. Activated Cardiac Fibroblasts Control Contraction of Human Fibrotic Cardiac Microtissues by a β-Adrenoreceptor-Dependent Mechanism. *Cells* 2020, *9*, 1270. [Google Scholar] [CrossRef]

2. Kobolak, J.; Teglasi, A.; Bellak, T.; Janstova, Z.; Molnar, K.; Zana, M.; Bock, I.; Laszlo, L.; Dinnyes, A. Human Induced Pluripotent Stem Cell-Derived 3D-Neurospheres are Suitable for Neurotoxicity Screening. *Cells* 2020, *9*, 1122. [Google Scholar] [CrossRef] [PubMed]

3. Cutarelli, A.; Ghio, S.; Zasso, J.; Speccher, A.; Scarduelli, G.; Roccuzzo, M.; Crivellari, M.; Maria Pugno, N.; Casarosa, S.; Boscardin, M.; et al. Vertically-Aligned Functionalized Silicon Micropillars for 3D Culture of Human Pluripotent Stem Cell-Derived Cortical Progenitors. *Cells* 2019, *9*, 88. [Google Scholar] [CrossRef] [PubMed] [Green Version]

4. Ciardulli, M.C.; Marino, L.; Lovecchio, J.; Giordano, E.; Forsyth, N.R.; Selleri, C.; Maffulli, N.; Porta, G.D. Tendon and Cytokine Marker Expression by Human

Bone Marrow Mesenchymal Stem Cells in a Hyaluronate/Poly-Lactic-Co-Glycolic Acid (PLGA)/Fibrin Three-Dimensional (3D) Scaffold. *Cells* 2020, *9*, 1268. [Google Scholar] [CrossRef] [PubMed]

5. McKee, C.; Brown, C.; Chaudhry, G.R. Self-Assembling Scaffolds Supported Long-Term Growth of Human Primed Embryonic Stem Cells and Upregulated Core and Naïve Pluripotent Markers. *Cells* 2019, *8*, 1650. [Google Scholar] [CrossRef] [PubMed] [Green Version]
6. Kramer, N.; Pratscher, B.; Meneses, A.M.C.; Tschulenk, W.; Walter, I.; Swoboda, A.; Kruitwagen, H.S.; Schneeberger, K.; Penning, L.C.; Spee, B.; et al. Generation of Differentiating and Long-Living Intestinal Organoids Reflecting the Cellular Diversity of Canine Intestine. *Cells* 2020, *9*, 822. [Google Scholar] [CrossRef] [PubMed] [Green Version]
7. Yen, Y.T.; Chien, M.; Lai, Y.C.; Chen, D.P.; Chuong, C.M.; Hung, M.C.; Hung, S.C. PP2A Deficiency Enhances Carcinogenesis of Lgr5. *Cells* 2019, *9*, 90. [Google Scholar] [CrossRef] [PubMed] [Green Version]
8. Tan, Z.; Rak-Raszewska, A.; Skovorodkin, I.; Vainio, S.J. Mouse Embryonic Stem Cell-Derived Ureteric Bud Progenitors Induce Nephrogenesis. *Cells* 2020, *9*, 329. [Google Scholar] [CrossRef] [PubMed] [Green Version]
9. Ribeiro-Filho, A.C.; Levy, D.; Ruiz, J.L.M.; Mantovani, M.D.C.; Bydlowski, S.P. Traditional and Advanced Cell Cultures in Hematopoietic Stem Cell Studies. *Cells* 2019, *8*, 1628. [Google Scholar] [CrossRef] [PubMed] [Green Version]

02 CARDIAC FIBROBLASTS REGULATE THE CONTRACTION OF HUMAN FIBROTIC CARDIAC MICROTISSUES BY A MECHANISM THAT DEPENDS ON β-ADRENORECEPTORS

1. INTRODUCTION: AN OVERVIEW

Cardiac fibrosis is the abnormal buildup of stromal cells and extracellular matrix proteins in the heart muscle, which is a common issue in various heart conditions like heart attacks, high blood pressure, heart inflammation, and certain types of heart muscle diseases. Cardiac fibroblasts and myofibroblasts are the most thoroughly studied forms of stromal cells that have a role in fibrotic processes in the heart. According to the traditional perspective, local cardiac fibroblasts get activated and create an excess of ECM proteins such collagen type I and III and fibronectin. Fibrogenesis is controlled by many pro-fibrotic stimuli that trigger a sophisticated signaling network. Transforming growth factor β (TGF-β) is identified as the primary profibrotic cytokine that triggers dormant cardiac fibroblasts in cardiac fibrosis. Continuous high levels of TGF-β caused interstitial cardiac fibrosis and cardiac hypertrophy in transgenic mice. In contrast, inhibiting TGF-β or its downstream components effectively decreased or stopped cardiac fibrosis in several animal models. Progressive fibrosis leads to tissue becoming rigid and can impact the heart's rhythm. Clinical data links fibrotic heart condition to higher resting heart rate [7] and an increased likelihood of developing life-threatening arrhythmias [8,9]. The underlying mechanisms remain unclear.

Pacemaker cells in the sinoatrial node of the heart establish the heart rhythm, which is mostly regulated by the autonomic nervous system. Sympathetic stimulation elevates the rate, while parasympathetic stimulation reduces it. Sympathetic neurons release the neurotransmitter noradrenaline, which increases heart rate by stimulating β-adrenergic receptors on cardiomyocytes. During stress, β-adrenoreceptors are additionally stimulated by adrenaline, a catecholamine secreted by the adrenal glands and discharged into the bloodstream. Agonists binding to β-adrenergic receptors triggers the production of cyclic adenosine monophosphate and activates protein kinase A, which phosphorylates various proteins such as myosin light chains(10). This process enhances the relaxation capability of cardiomyocytes after excitation-contraction coupling. Enhanced relaxation in the heart is linked to heightened rate and intensity of contraction.

Studying the intracardiac mechanisms of cardiac contractility using in vivo systems alone is challenging due to the significant influence of extracardiac stimuli on heart rhythm regulation. Information from ex vivo and in vitro cardiac models can provide further insight into particular features of intracardiac rhythm control. Utilizing human cells in disease models presents an inherent advantage over animal models due to the accurate genetic and cellular environment they give. Challenges in acquiring and cultivating contractile primary human cardiomyocytes hindered the progress of creating in vitro human models in cardiovascular research for an extended period. Human induced pluripotent stem cell (iPSC) technology has provided a readily available and abundant source of spontaneously contracting heart muscle cells for applications in regenerative medicine, medication development, and toxicity testing (11).

Many in vitro models lack a physiologically realistic experimental context. Traditional two-dimensional (2D) cell culture techniques typically do not accurately replicate the biomechanical and metabolic conditions seen in actual tissue microenvironments. Three-dimensional (3D) cell culture technologies more accurately depict organ complexity and offer a compelling alternative to the frequently employed 2D models. 3D cell culture systems, known as microtissues or organoids, consist of cellular models on different bioscaffolds, as well as scaffold-free spheroids made up of one or more cell types. In recent years, various types of cardiac microtissues have been successfully used predominantly in regenerative medicine, but also as platforms for drug screening or as disease models [**12**]. Self-aggregating, scaffold-free cardiac microtissues consisting of human iPSC-derived cardiomyocytes and human primary cardiac fibroblasts cultured in nonadherent plates represent a high-throughput in vitro model of human cardiac tissue. These spontaneously beating cardiac microtissues show typical structures including well-developed myofibrils and recapitulate cardiac functionality including responsiveness to electrical stimulation [**13**]. In this work, we aimed to address how fibrotic changes affect contractility of human cardiac microtissues. We discovered that a situation promoting fibrosis, specifically the activation of cardiac fibroblasts, enhances the beating rate of cardiac microtissues. This action is partly facilitated by the natural activation of β-adrenergic receptors. Moreover, we showed that human cardiac microtissues are a simple, consistent, and efficient approach for doing small molecule screening in large quantities.

2. MATERIAL AND METHODS

2.1. Cellular Sources

Frozen human iPSC-derived cardiomyocytes (>99% troponin-positive) were purchased from Cellular Dynamics International, and were used directly upon thawing. Foetal human cardiac fibroblasts were purchased from Sigma (Cell Applications) and cells from passages 10–15 (>99% vimentin-positive, >99% collagen I-positive and <5% positive for filamentous form of α-SMA) were used. Adult cardiac fibroblasts were isolated from cardiac tissue samples obtained from the left atria of hearts from the patients with end-stage heart failure due to ischemic heart disease undergoing heart transplantation and from the waste fragments of donor normal hearts that were trimmed off while adjusting atrium size and shape during transplantation. Specimens were collected without patient identifiers according to the protocol revised by the Ethics Committee of the University of Naples Federico II (approval number 79/18) and in conformity with the principles outlined in the Declaration of Helsinki.

2.2. Isolation of Human Adult Cardiac Fibroblasts

Adult cardiac fibroblasts were isolated as described previously [**14**]. Briefly, cardiac tissue samples were minced and then enzymatically disaggregated by incubation in 0.25% trypsin and 0.1% (w/v) collagenase II (both Sigma-Aldrich, Basel, Switzerland) for 30 min at 37 °C. The digestion was stopped by adding Hanks' Balanced Salt solution supplemented with 10% foetal bovine serum (FBS, Gibco, Paislay, UK). The tissue was further disaggregated by pipetting; noncardiomyocyte cells were separated from debris and cardiomyocytes by sequential centrifugation and passage through 20 μm cell sieve. Fibroblasts were isolated from cell suspension by immunomagnetic cell sorting through positive selection with anti-fibroblast MicroBeads (MiltenyiBiotec, Bergisch Gladbach, Germany). Following selection, fibroblasts were cultured in Dulbecco's Modified Eagle's Medium (DMEM, Sigma, Basel, Switzerland) supplemented with 10% FBS, penicillin 10,000 U, and streptomycin 10 mg/mL (all from Sigma, Basel, Switzerland) at 37 °C in 5% CO_2. The aCFs from patients with heart failure and unaffected donors were used individually. Cells from passages 4–6 were used.

2.3. Fabrication and Culture of Microtissues

Three types of microtissues containing: (1) iPSC-derived cardiomyocytes and fibroblasts mixed in ratio 4:1, (2) fibroblasts only, and (3) iPSC-derived cardiomyocytes only were generated by self-assembling in 96-well GravityTRAP plates (InSphero, Schlieren, Switzerland), and cultured as one microtissue per well. Accordingly, for generation of one microtissue, 5000 cells suspended in 70 μL maintenance medium were placed in the GravityTRAP plates for three days in the slanted position. Maintenance medium contained 2% FBS (Gibco, Paislay, UK), 50 μM phenylephrine hydrochloride (Sigma), 0.3 μM L-ascorbic acid (Sigma), 50 μM 2-mercaptoethanol (Gibco, Paislay, UK), 50 U/mL penicillin/streptomycin (Gibco, Paislay, UK) in high glucose DMEM (Sigma). Upon self-assembly, microtissues were further cultured in the GravityTRAP plates in the maintenance medium for 10 days. Microtissues were cultured under standard culture conditions (at 37 °C, 5% CO_2 in a humidified incubator). Medium was changed at days 0, 2, 4, and 7. Fibrotic differentiation of cardiac microtissues was induced at day 0 with 10 ng/mL recombinant human TGF-β1 (Peprotech, London, UK) and TGF-βR1 was blocked with 10^{-8}–10^{-5} g/mL SD208 (Tocris, Zug, Switzerland). To address β-adrenoceptor-dependent mechanisms, microtissues were treated with 10 nM isoproterenol (Tocris) and/or 1 μM nadolol (Sigma) 15–90 min prior to video recording. Controls received solvents only.

2.4. Live Imaging and Video Analysis

Randomly chosen live microtissues were analysed using microscopes equipped with a humidified chamber at 37 °C and 5% CO_2. Pictures of microtissues were captured using the Live Cell Imaging System (Olympus, Shinjuku, Japan) and size of microtissues was measured with the Xcellence Pro software (Olympus) as area in pixels. Increase in size was calculated as the size of microtissue at day 10/size of microtissue at day 0. Videos of contracting microtissues were recorded using the AxioObserver Z1 (Zeiss, Hombrechtikon, Switzerland) and the ZEN software. Videos were processed using Fiji software and custom-made macro. Contraction analysis was performed using Fiji software and MUSCLEMOTION macro [**15**].

2.5. FluoVolt Measurements

Voltage experiments were conducted on day 11. The microtissues were washed in serum-free medium consisting of DMEM (Gibco, Paislay, UK) supplemented with 10 mM D-Galactose (Sigma) and 1 mM sodium pyruvate (Sigma). The microtissues were loaded with voltage-sensitive dye: 0.1% FluoVolt and 1% PowerLoad (ThermoFisher, Waltham, WA, USA) in the above listed serum-free medium for 25 min at 37 °C 5% CO_2. The voltage-sensitive dye was removed by washing in serum-free medium, and the multiwell plate was placed in an environmentally controlled stage incubator (37 °C, 5% CO_2, >75% humidity) in the CellOPTIQ® platform (Clyde Biosciences, BioCity Scotland) 30 min before experimentation. The fluorescent signal was recorded with an excitation at 470 nm, and emitted light was collected from the entire microtissue using a 10× Fluor objective and the intensity recorded by a photomultiplier tube at 510–560 nm at 10 kHz. A 15 s recording was taken of each microtissue. Offline analysis was performed using CellOPTIQ®.

2.6. Electrical Pacing

Prior to experiment, microtissues were transferred into a glass bottom cell culture dish. Electrical field pacing of microtissues was performed using a modified glass bottom culture dish with inserted platinum wires attached to a MyoPacer (IonOptix, Westwood, MA, USA) set to a frequency of 3 Hz. Microtissues were recorded using the Eclipse TE2000-U microscope (Nikon, Tokyo, Japan) equipped with heating chamber, temperature controller (Ibidi, Graefelfing, Germany) and HeroBlack6 GoPro camera (Back-Bone Gear, Ontario, Canada).

2.7. Quantitative RT-PCR

For one sample, 12 microtissues were pooled. Total RNA was isolated using the Quick RNA Micro Kit (Zymo Research, Irvine, CA, USA). cDNAs were amplified using the cDNA Synthesis Kit (Roche). Gene expression was detected using oligonucleotides complementary to transcripts of the analysed genes and the GoTaq qPCR Master Mix (Promega, Dubendorf, Switzerland) using the 7500 Fast Real-Time PCR System (Applied Biosystems, Waltham, MA, USA). Transcript levels of human RPLP0 were used as endogenous reference, and relative gene expression was analysed using the $2^{-\Delta\Delta Ct}$ method.

2.8. Immunocytochemistry

A total of 25-30 microtissues were combined, then fixed overnight using 4% paraformaldehyde, and finally embedded in 2% agarose and paraffin. Sections of microtissues of 3–5 μm were cut using a Sophistolab machine in Muttenz, Switzerland, and then deparaffinized using conventional procedures. Sections were blocked with 10% goat serum (Vector Laboratories, Burlingame, CA, USA) and stained with primary/secondary antibodies: rabbit anti-human α-SMA (Sigma, dilution 1:750)/goat anti-mouse AP (Dako, Glostrup, Denmark, dilution 1:50), rabbit anti-human vimentin (Abcam, Cambridge, UK, dilution 1:250)/goat anti-rabbit (Vector Laboratories, Burlingame, CA, USA, dilution 1:200), rabbit anti-human periostin (Abcam, dilution 1:250)/Polymer anti-rabbit (Histofine, Nichirei Biosciences Inc. Tokyo, Japan), rabbit anti-human fibronectin (Abcam, dilution 1:100)/Polymer anti-rabbit (Histofine), rabbit anti-human Ki67 (Abcam, dilution 1:100)/goat anti-rabbit (Vector Laboratories, dilution 1:200), rabbit anti-human connexin 43 (Abcam, dilution 1:200)/goat anti-rabbit (Vector Laboratories, dilution 1:500), and rabbit anti-human troponin T (Origene Technologies, Rockville, Maryland, USA, dilution 1:2000)/Polymer anti-rabbit (Histofine). Detection was performed with the Bond Polymer HRP Refine Detection kit (Leica, Heerbrugg, Switzerland) according to the manufacturer's guidelines for troponin T, and with DAB or Vector Red (Vector Laboratories) for all other antibodies. Nuclei were counterstained with haematoxylin (J.T.Backer, Gliwice, Poland). Direct Red Sirius Red (Sigma-Aldrich, Basel, Switzerland) staining was used to detect collagen deposition. Stained sections were analysed using the Olympus DP80 microscope and the cellSens Standard imaging software (Olympus, Shinjuku, Japan). The ImageJ program was used to quantify the intensity of immunopositive signals and nuclei counterstaining for each region. The staining intensity is expressed in arbitrary units (AU) which indicate the intensity of the immunopositive signal adjusted by the value of the counterstained nuclei.

2.9. Procollagen Type I and IL-6 ELISA

Supernatants from individual microtissues were collected at day 10 and stored at -80 °C. Undiluted supernatants were analysed with the human Procollagen I alpha 1 DuoSet ELISA (R&D Systems, Abingdon, UK) and the human IL-6 DuoSet ELISA (R&D Systems) following manufacturer's protocol. Optical density was measured with the Synergy microplate reader (Biotek, Winooski, Vermont, USA) and the Gen5 software.

2.10. Caspase 3/7 Activity

Supernatants containing one microtissue each were collected at day 10 and immediately measured for apoptosis with the Caspase-Glo 3/7 Assay (Promega, Dubendorf, Switzerland) following the manufacturer's protocol. Luminescence was measured with the Synergy microplate reader (Biotek, Winooski, Vermont, USA) and the Gen5 software.

2.11. Western Blotting

Proteins from fetal human cardiac fibroblasts were extracted using RIPA buffer (Sigma-Aldrich) with a protease inhibitor cocktail (Complete ULTRA Tablets, Roche) and phosphatase inhibitors (PhosphoStop, Roche) from cultured cells. Protein content was determined using a colorimetric bicinchoninic acid assay following the manufacturer's instructions (Thermo Fisher Scientific). SDS-PAGE electrophoresis and wet-transfer method were used to separate and transfer proteins on nitrocellulose membranes, followed by 45 min incubation in blocking solution (tris buffered saline, Tween-20 (TBST, Thermo Fisher Scientific) containing 5% skim milk powder (Becton Dickinson AG, Allschwil, Swizterland). Membranes were incubated overnight with the following primary antibodies: anti-αSMA (1:1000, A2547, clone 1A4, Sigma-Aldrich), anti-Fibronectin (1:2000, Abcam: ab2413) or GAPDH (1:10,000, clone 14C10, #2118, Cell Signalling). HRP-conjugated secondary antibodies at a dilution of 1:5000 were utilized for detection using ECL substrate (SuperSignal West Pico Plus, Thermo Fisher Scientific) and processed on the Fusion Fx system (Vilber, Collegien, France). Densitometric analyses were conducted using ImageJ 1.47t. Fold changes were calculated following normalization to GAPDH.

2.12. Cell Contraction Assay

To assess the contractile properties of foetal human cardiac fibroblasts, the Contraction Assay Kit (Cell Biolabs, San Diego, CA, USA) was used following the manufacturer's protocol. Cells were cultivated with or without 10 ng/mL TGF-β for 72 h and reseeded in collagen gels for a further 72 h. Each condition was analysed in triplicates or quadruplicates. Images were taken at time 0, 24, 48 and 72 h after reseeding in a collagen gel. Areas of the gels were measured by ImageJ. Percentage of contraction of all conditions was measured compared to the average of unstimulated cells at day 0.

2.13. Statistics

The analysis used normally distributed data using two-tailed unpaired or paired Student's t-test and unpaired two-tailed ANOVA with uncorrected Fisher's LSD post-hoc test. The studies were performed using GraphPad Prism 8 software. Differences were considered as statistically significant for $p < 0.05$.

3. RESULTS

3.1. Cardiac Fibroblasts Improve Integrity and Contractility of Human Cardiac Microtissues

We created a high-throughput in vitro model of human cardiac tissue using human iPSC-derived cardiomyocytes (iCMs) and human fetal cardiac fibroblasts (fCFs)(16). Cardiac microtissues, each composed of 5000 cells, were created through self-assembly (Figure S1). iCMs assembling without fibroblasts, however, formed loose cell aggregates. Addition of fCFs to iCMs in a ratio of 1:4 (fCFs:iCMs) allowed for formation of compact, spontaneously contracting cardiac microtissues In the next step, we performed transcriptional profiling of microtissues by qPCR for genes characteristic for cardiomyocytes and fibroblasts. Seven genes characteristic for cardiomyocytes were detected in microtissues containing iCMs (iCM and iCM:fCF microtissues), but not in those generated with fCFs only. In contrast, nine out of twelve genes associated with fibroblasts and fibrosis were consistently detected in all types of microtissues (**Figure** 1C). However, expression levels of most of fibroblastic genes were substantially higher in fCFs than in iCMs microtissues. As expected, the expression profile of iCMs:fCFs microtissues showed high levels of all cardiac and fibroblastic genes (**Figure** 1C).

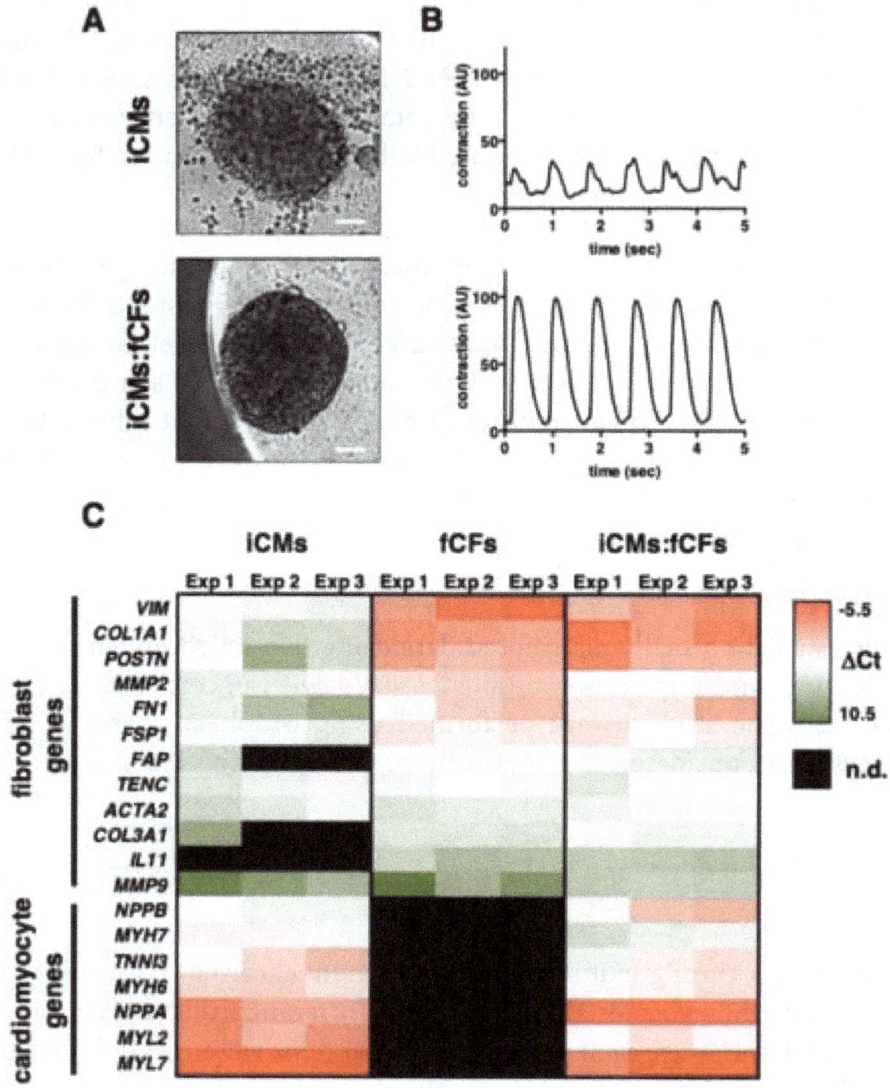

Figure 1. Characteristics of cardiac microtissues. Panel (A) illustrates typical morphologies (bar = 50 μm) and panel (B) shows typical contraction patterns of cardiac microtissues generated using iPSC-derived cardiomyocytes (iCMs) only (top) or iCMs mixed with foetal cardiac fibroblasts (fCFs) in a ratio of 4:1 (iCMs:fCFs, bottom). Representative contractions are available in the Supplementary Materials (Videos S1 and S2). A heat map in panel (C) indicates expression of cardiomyocyte and fibroblast genes in microtissues containing iCMs only (left), fCFs only (center) or iCMs:fCFs (right). Each segment indicates the average (n = 3–5) expression of one experiment. Lower -Δ C_t values indicate higher relative expression. n.d.—not detected.

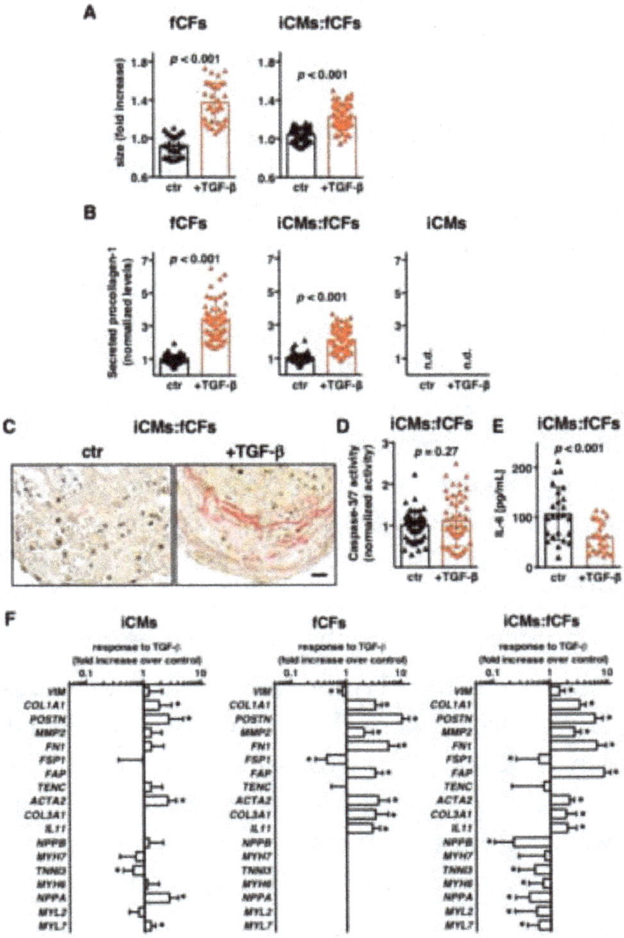

Figure 2. **TGF-β1 activates foetal cardiac fibroblasts in microtissues. Panel (A) demonstrates changes in size of microtissues generated with fCFs only (fCFs, left) and iCMs mixed with fCFs in ratio 4:1 (iCMs:fCFs, right) cultured in the presence (red) or absence (black) of TGF-β1 (10 ng/mL) for 10 days. Panel (B) shows relative levels of procollagen I (measured by ELISA), at day 10 in supernatants of all three microtissue types: fCFs (left), iCMs:fCFs (middle) and iCMs (right). Graphs show cumulative data of 2–5 independent experiments. Each dot represents data of one microtissue. Panel (C) illustrates representative picrosirius red staining in iCMs:fCFs microtissues at day 10 (bar = 10 μm). Panel (D) shows caspase 3/7 activity measured at day 10 in iCMs:fCFs microtissues. Graphs show cumulative data of 3 independent experiments. Panel (E) shows IL-6 levels measured by ELISA, at day 10 in supernatants of iCMs:fCFs microtissues. Graphs show cumulative data of 3 independent experiments. Each triangle represents data of one microtissue. Panel (F) summarizes fold changes in gene expression in indicated microtissues in the presence of TGF-β1 (in relation to expression in the absence of TGF-β1). * $p < 0.05$. Graphs show cumulative data of 3–4 independent experiments, n = 11–20. For all graphs, p values were calculated with the Student's t-test. n.d.—not detected.**

3.2. TGF-β1 Induces Fibrotic Changes in Human Cardiac Microtissues

TGF-β1 is a strong stimulator of fibrotic alterations in cardiac fibroblasts. We exposed microtissues to TGF-β1 for 10 days in the initial stage. In the presence of TGF-β1, both fCFs and iCMs:fCFs microtissues significantly increased their size (**Figure 2**A). In the next step, we measured procollagen type I secretion, which is an important hallmark of the ongoing fibrotic processes. As expected, fCFs microtissues produced markedly more collagen I upon TGF-β1 stimulation. Under this stimulatory condition, significant increase in procollagen type I production was also observed for iCMs:fCFs microtissues). Importantly, iCMs microtissues did not produce detectable levels of procollagen I (**Figure 2**B) pointing to fibroblasts as the main source of collagen I in cardiac microtissues. Increased collagen production in iCMs:fCFs microtissues treated with TGF-β1 was confirmed by picrosirius red staining (**Figure 2**C). To address whether treatment with TGF-β1 induced apoptosis in this model, we measured caspase 3/7 activity in iCMs:fCFs microtissues. We observed similar caspase 3/7 activity in iCMs:fCFs microtissues treated with and without TGF-β1 (**Figure 2**D). Additionally, iCMs:fCFs microtissues treated with TGF-β1 produced significantly less IL-6 (**Figure 2**E).

Cardiac fibrogenesis is a transcriptionally regulated process. Upon TGF-β1 stimulation, genes characteristic for cardiomyocytes were only slightly dysregulated in iCMs microtissues. In iCMs:fCFs microtissues, instead, cardiomyocyte-specific genes were downregulated following TGF-β1 treatment (**Figure 2**F). Analysis of fibrotic genes showed that most of them were strongly upregulated in fCFs and iCMs:fCFs microtissues in response to TGF-β1 (**Figure 2**F).

TGF-β1-induced changes in gene expression was followed by the analysis of the respective proteins in cardiac microtissues. To this aim, selected markers were analysed by immunohistochemistry in iCMs:fCFs microtissues cultured with or without TGF-β1. We found significantly less expression of the cardiac cell marker troponin T and gap junction protein connexin 43 in iCMs:fCFs microtissues exposed to TGF-β1. Instead, proteins produced by quiescent (vimentin, fibronectin) or activated (α-SMA, periostin) fibroblasts were more abundant in TGF-β1-treated cardiac microtissues. The number of proliferative (Ki67-positive) cells was also higher in iCMs:fCFs microtissues cultured with TGF-β1 (**Figure 3**). In conclusion, our results indicate that TGF-β1 effectively induced fibrogenesis in cardiac microtissues.

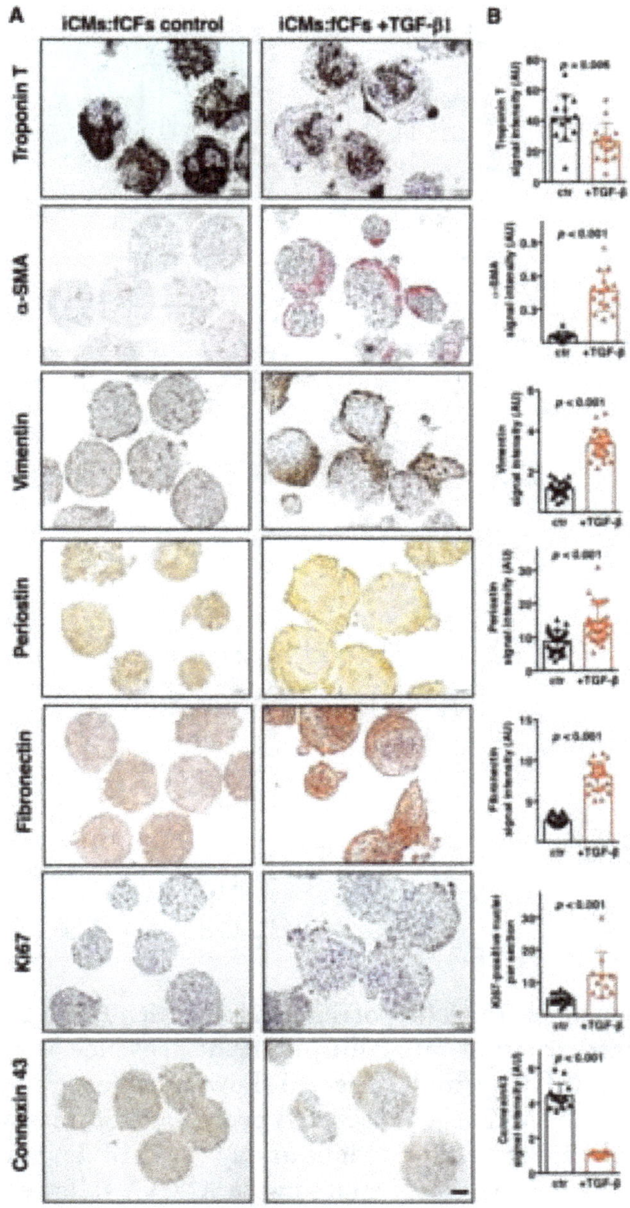

Figure 3. TGF-β1 induces fibrotic phenotype in cardiac microtissues. Immunohistochemistry of iCMs:fCFs microtissues cultured in the presence or absence of TGF-β1 (10 ng/mL) at day 10. Panel (A) illustrates representative staining for the indicated proteins at the indicated condition (bar = 50 μm). Higher magnification pictures are available in the Supplementary Materials (Figure S3). Panel (B) shows quantification of the respective staining for microtissues cultured in the presence (red) or absence (black) of TGF-β1. Graphs show cumulative data of 3 independent experiments. Each triangle represents data for one microtissue. p values were calculated with the Student's t-test.

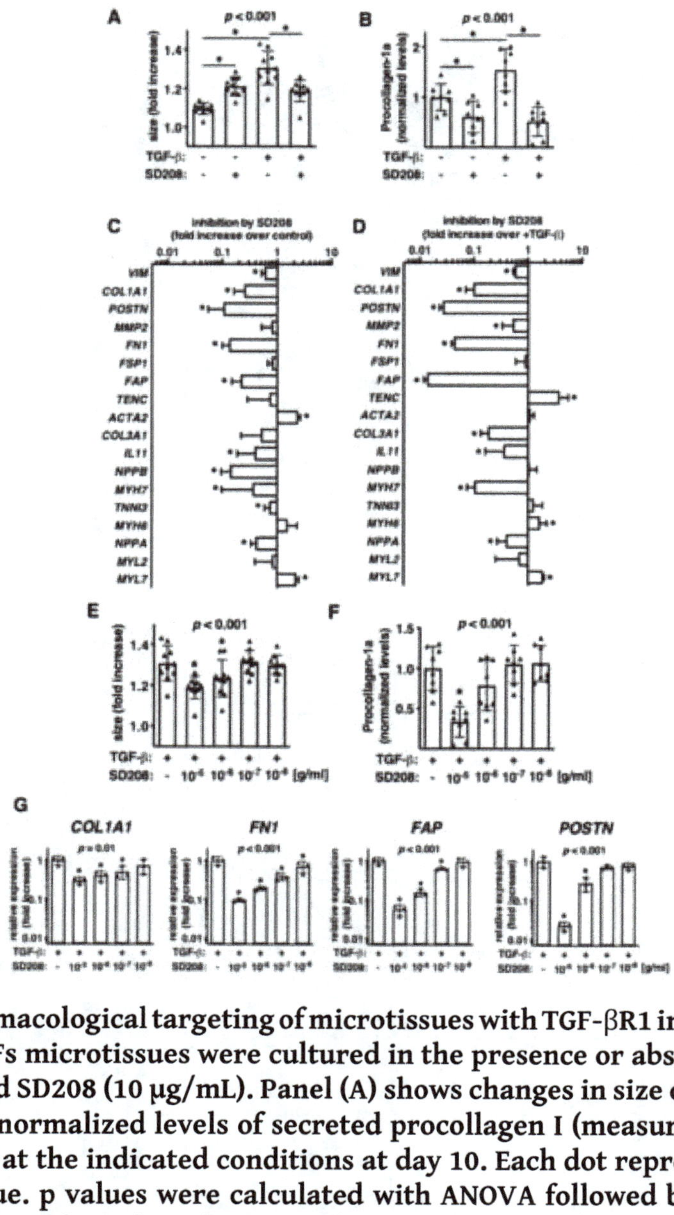

Figure 4. Pharmacological targeting of microtissues with TGF-βR1 inhibitor SD208. (A–D) iCMs:fCFs microtissues were cultured in the presence or absence of TGF-β1 (10 ng/mL) and SD208 (10 μg/mL). Panel (A) shows changes in size of microtissues and panel (B) normalized levels of secreted procollagen I (measured by ELISA in supernatants) at the indicated conditions at day 10. Each dot represents data for one microtissue. p values were calculated with ANOVA followed by uncorrected Fisher's LSD tests for selected groups, * $p < 0.05$. Panels (C,D) show changes in gene expression in response to treatment with SD208 of microtissues cultured in the absence (C) or presence (D) of TGF-β1. n = 6, p values were calculated with the Student's t-test, * $p < 0.05$. (E–G) iCMs:fCFs microtissues were cultured in the presence of TGF-β1 (10 ng/mL) and serial dilutions of SD208. Panel (E) shows changes in microtissue size, panel (F) normalized levels of secreted procollagen I and panel (G) relative expression of selected genes at the indicated conditions at day 10. Each dot represents data for one microtissue. Each triangle represents data for one microtissue. p values were calculated with ANOVA followed by uncorrected Fisher's LSD tests versus +TGF-β group, * $p < 0.05$.

3.3. Pharmacological Targeting of TGF-βR1 Signalling Prevents from Fibrotic Changes in Human Cardiac Microtissues

In the next step, we asked whether the fibrotic cardiac microtissue model is relevant to test anti-fibrotic compounds. To this aim, we used the TGF-βR1 inhibitor SD208 and tested it in the iCMs:fCFs microtissues cultured in the presence or absence of TGF-β. We observed that SD208 inhibitor effectively blocked TGF-β1-mediated microtissue growth (**Figure** 4A).

Furthermore, we found that SD208 suppressed procollagen type I production in iCMs:fCFs microtissues cultured not only with, but also without TGF-β1 (**Figure** 4B). Given the effect of the inhibitor in the absence of exogenous TGF-β1, we analysed gene expression in iCMs:fCFs microtissues cultured with and without SD208. Expression of 12 out of 18 analysed genes were significantly changed in response to SD208 treatment (**Figure** 4C). Similar results were obtained for treatment of iCMs:fCFs microtissues with SD208 in the presence of TGF-β1 (**Figure** 4D). Next, we analysed dose-dependent responses of microtissues to SD208. In these experiments, iCMs:fCFs microtissues were cultured in the presence of TGF-β1 and serial dilutions of SD208. Our results showed dose-dependent responses of iCMs:fCFs microtissues to SD208 in terms of microtissue size (**Figure** 4E), collagen type I secretion (**Figure** 4F) and expression of profibrotic genes (**Figure** 4G). Taken together, these data suggest that cardiac microtissues represent a useful model for pharmacological studies.

3.4. Cardiac fibroblasts that are Activated Enhance the Rate of Contraction in Cardiac Microtissues

Contractility represents the main functional feature of cardiomyocytes. Using high-speed movies and motion-tracking analysis, we examined contractile properties of iCMs:fCFs microtissues at day 10. Fibrotic changes triggered by TGF-β1 substantially deteriorated the contraction pattern of iCMs:fCFs microtissues. We consistently observed significantly increased contraction rate and reduced contraction amplitudes of fibrotic microtissues in all experiments. A more detailed analysis of contraction pointed mainly to the shortening of relaxation phase in iCMs:fCFs microtissues upon treatment with TGF-β1.

We hypothesized that TGF-β1 affected the contractility of iCMs:fCFs microtissues by activation of fCFs, rather than by a direct effect on iCMs. To validate this hypothesis, we generated cardiac microtissues using fCFs pretreated with TGF-β1 for three days (prior microtissue formation) and analysed their contractility in the absence of exogenous TGF-β1 at day 10. Pretreatment with TGF-β1 effectively activated fCFs as indicated by increased production of collagen, α-SMA and fibronectin in 2D cultures. We observed that iCMs:fCFs microtissues containing activated fCFs displayed increased size and secreted significantly more procollagen I, showed increased contraction rate, reduced contraction amplitudes and shortened relaxation phase, and successfully reproduced the contraction pattern observed in fibrotic (+TGF-β1) cardiac microtissues.

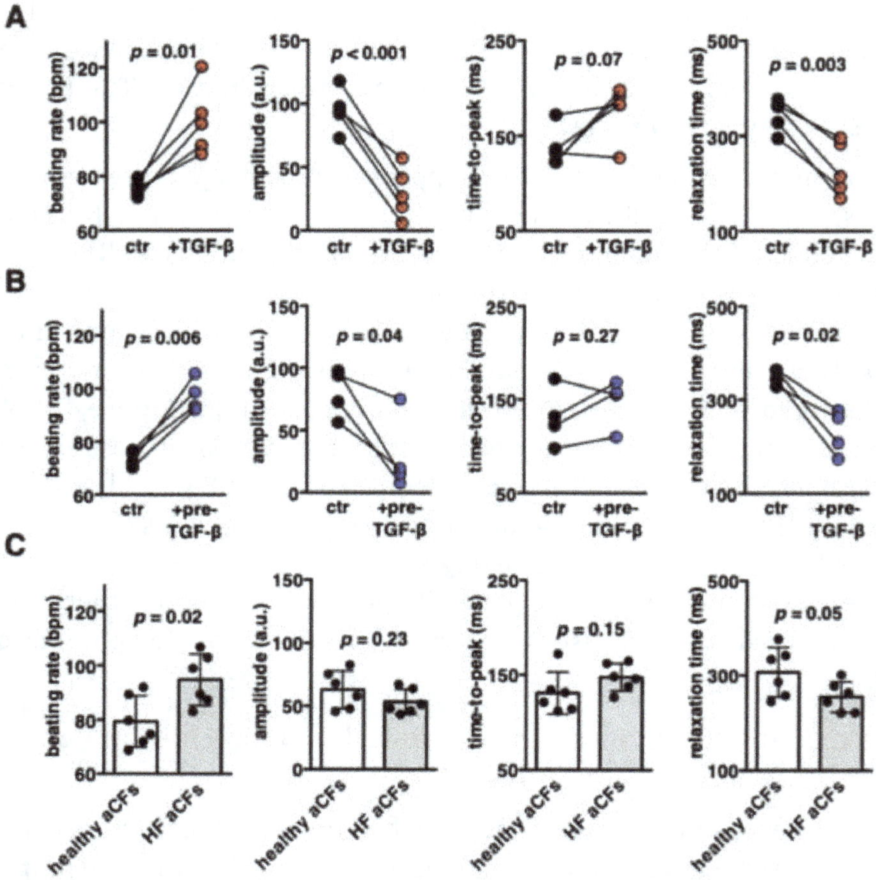

Figure 5. Contractile properties of cardiac microtissues containing foetal or adult cardiac fibroblasts. Panel (A) shows quantification of contraction parameters of iCMs:fCFs microtissues cultured in the presence (red) or absence (black) of TGF-β1 (10 ng/mL) at day 10. Quantification of contraction parameters of microtissues containing fCFs pretreated with TGF-β1 for 3 days prior microtissue formation (blue) or untreated fCFs (black) recorded at day 10 are shown in panel (B). Each dot represents average data of one experiment. Data of individual experiments are available in the Supplementary Materials (Figures S5 and S8). p values were calculated with the paired Student's t-test. Panel (C) shows quantification of contraction parameters of cardiac microtissues containing aCFs from unaffected hearts (white) or heart failure (HF) patients (grey). Each dot represents average data of one experiment (n = 14–18). p values were calculated with the Student's t-test. Representative contraction records are available in the Supplementary Materials (Figures S5, S10B and S11 and Videos S2–S6).

To further address the relevance of CFs to cardiac microtissue contractility, we compared cardiac microtissues containing adult CFs (aCFs) obtained from unaffected hearts of mostly young individuals (healthy aCFs) to aCFs from patients with heart failure (HF aCFs). Cardiac microtissues containing healthy aCFs and HF aCFs showed similar sizes at day 10. We found that iCMs:aCFs microtissues with HF aCFs showed increased contraction rate and shortened relaxation phase in comparison to cardiac microtissues containing healthy aCFs (**Figure 5c**). Of note, microtissues containing healthy iCMs:aCFs more often responded to TGF-β1 stimulation by increasing contraction rate than those with HF aCFs (four of six vs. one of six). All these data indicate that contractile properties of cardiac microtissues depend on the activation status of CFs.

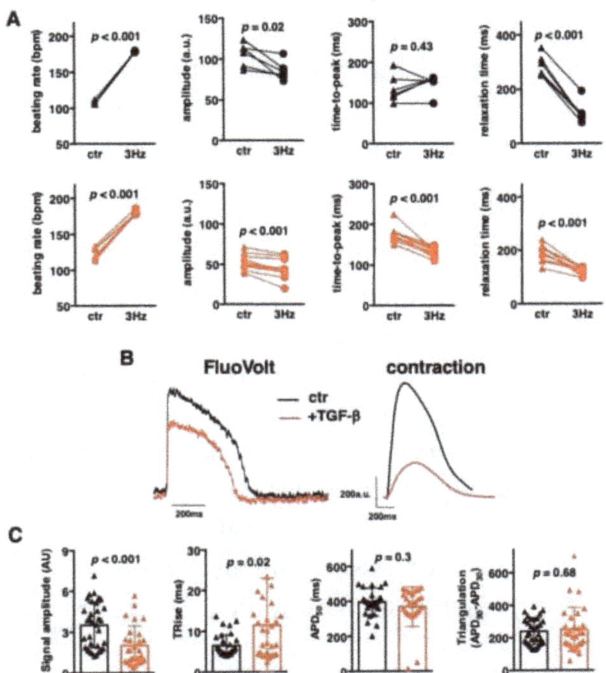

Figure 6. Cardiac microtissue electrophysiology. iCMs:fCFs microtissues were cultured in the presence (red) or absence (black) of TGF-β1 (10 ng/mL) for 10 days. Panel (A) shows quantifications of the contraction parameters recorded during spontaneous contractile activity (triangles, ctr) and then upon electrical stimulation with 3 Hz (circles, 3 Hz). Each dot represents data for one microtissue at the indicated condition, lines match data obtained from the same microtissue. p values were calculated with the paired Student's t-test. Panel (B) illustrates representative action potentials recorded with FluoVolt probe (left) and the respective contractions (right). Quantifications of action potential parameters are shown in panel (C). Graphs show cumulative data of 3 independent experiments. Each dot represents data for one microtissue. p values were calculated with the Student's t-test. APD—action potential duration, TRise—depolarisation phase.

3.5. Unaltered Repolarization Phase in Fibrotic Cardiac Microtissues

Cardiomyocytes initiate mechanical contraction in response to electrical excitation. We then examined how external electrical stimulation affected cardiac microtissues. Stimulation at 3 Hz induced a beating rate of 178–179 bpm in responsive microtissues, reduced contraction amplitude and substantially shortened contraction duration in both control and TGF-β1-treated iCMs:fCFs microtissues (**Figure 6**A), pointing to their full electrical responsiveness. Next, we analysed changes in membrane potential of control and fibrotic iCMs:fCFs microtissues using the relevant fluorescent probe (**Figure 6**B).

We found significantly lower action potential amplitudes in TGF-β1-treated iCMs:fCFs microtissues in comparison to controls (**Figure 6**C), suggesting reduced number of electrically active cells in fibrotic microtissues. Instead, there was no difference in the action potential duration, although treatment with TGF-β1 slightly prolonged the depolarization phase (**Figure 6**C). It seems that electrical activity of iCMs in cardiac microtissues was not significantly affected by profibrotic changes.

3.6. Endogenous signaling of β-adrenergic receptors controls Enhanced Contraction Frequency in Fibrotic Cardiac Microtissues

Action potential triggers cardiomyocyte contraction, but β-adrenoceptor-coupled mechanisms can modulate it. First, we used iCMs:fCFs and iCMs:aCFs microtissues and treated them with β-adrenoceptor agonist isoproterenol. As expected, stimulated microtissues showed increased contraction rate (**Figure 7**A). Isoproterenol significantly shortened both the contraction and relaxation phases of spontaneously contracting microtissues. In contrast, contraction amplitude remained unaffected. Nadolol, a β-adrenergic receptor blocker, successfully reversed the alterations in microtissue contraction generated by isoproterenol. The data validated the presence of functioning β-adrenoceptors in our cardiac microtissues.

We then discussed the importance of endogenous β-adrenoceptor signaling in cardiac microtissues. We examined the contractile ability of iCMs:fCFs and iCMs:aCFs microtissues with and without nadolol. Nadolol treatment minimally decreased contraction of iCMs:fCFs microtissues (Figure 7B). In the following experiment, we utilized iCMs:aCFs microtissues that exhibited a high spontaneous contraction rate. In this model, nadolol decreased the pace of contraction considerably, although the amplitude of contraction stayed the same (Figure 7C). Nadolol was discovered to have a particular impact on the relaxation phase, without affecting the contraction phase. The results indicate the activation of natural β-adrenoceptor signaling in iCMs:aCFs microtissues., we addressed the relevance of endogenous β-adrenoceptor signalling in cardiac microtissues. To this aim, we analysed the contractility of iCMs:fCFs and iCMs:aCFs microtissues in the presence and absence of nadolol. Treatment with nadolol only slightly reduced contraction of iCMs:fCFs microtissues (**Figure** 7B). In the next experiment, we used iCMs:aCFs microtissues showing high spontaneous contraction rate. In this model, nadolol significantly reduced contraction rate, whereas contraction amplitude remained unchanged (**Figure** 7C). We found that nadolol specifically affected relaxation, but not contraction phase. These results suggest activation of endogenous β-adrenoceptor signalling in iCMs:aCFs microtissues.

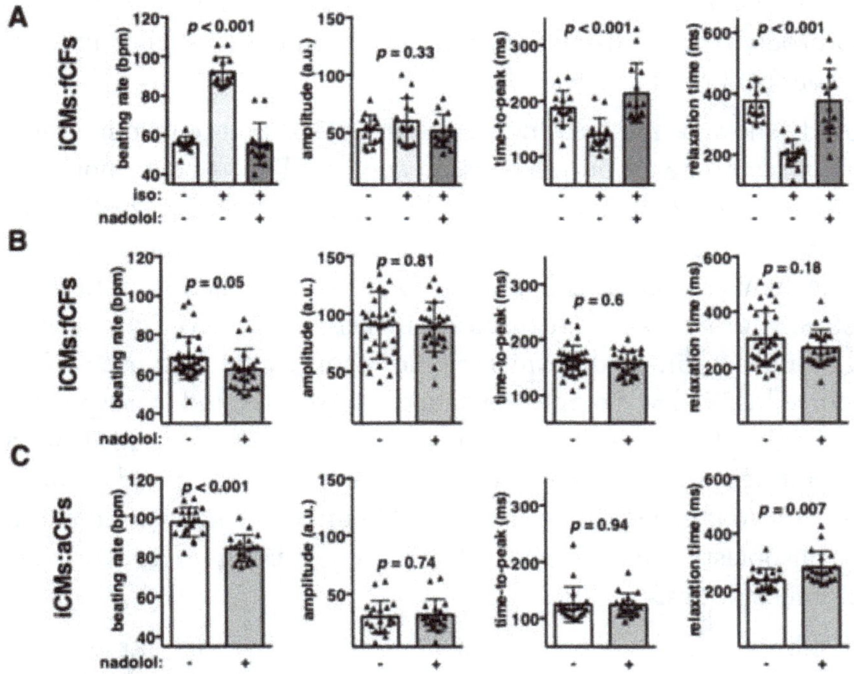

Figure 7. β-adrenergic receptor signalling in cardiac microtissues. Panel (A) shows quantification of contraction parameters of iCMs:fCFs microtissues stimulated with β-adrenoceptor agonist isoproterenol (iso, 10 nM) in the presence or absence of β-adrenoceptor blocker nadolol (1 μM). Unstimulated microtissues were used as controls. Graphs in panels (B,C) show contraction parameters of iCMs:fCFs (B) and iCMs:aCFs (C) microtissues treated with vehicle or 1 μM nadolol in the absence of isoproterenol. Each triangle represents data for one microtissue. p values were calculated with ANOVA for (A) and with the Student's t-test for (B,C).

4. DISCUSSION

Fibroblasts in 3D microtissue models enhance microtissue structure and dynamics by supplying appropriate ECM. We confirm that CFs notably enhanced the coherence and coordinated contraction of human cardiac microtissues. Recent research has shown that utilizing a 4:1 ratio of induced cardiomyocytes to cardiac fibroblasts produces cardiac microtissues that maintain a consistent phenotypic and beating characteristics for a duration of one month. Our research showed that the contractility of cardiac microtissues was significantly impacted when exposed to a profibrotic environment, namely in the presence of TGF-β1. TGF-β1 is a cytokine that promotes fibrosis by increasing the growth of fibroblasts and the synthesis of extracellular matrix proteins. In our model, TGF-β1 caused a fibrotic phenotype in cardiac microtissues, demonstrated by increased expression of fibrotic genes, production of procollagen I, and proliferation of fibroblasts. Exogenous TGF-β1 has previously been demonstrated to cause fibrosis in rat or human cardiac microtissue models. Furthermore, fibrotic phenotypes in cardiac microtissues or in biowire were also produced by collagen/fibroblast enrichment [20,21] or by constitutive activation of profibrotic pathways [22].

Our study showed that treating fCFs with TGF-β1 before forming microtissues had a comparable impact on microtissue contractility as continuously exposing them to TGF-β1. This outcome indicated that the activation of cardiac fibroblasts, rather than a direct impact of TGF-β1 on induced cardiomyocytes, was the primary mechanism accountable for the impaired contraction of fibrotic cardiac microtissues. The fact that aCFs caused a contraction pattern (high contraction rate with low amplitude) in cardiac microtissues comparable to those with activated fCFs supported this idea. Complement factors are activated in response to heart failure and aging (23) . Cardiac microtissues with aCFs from aged heart failure patients exhibited a markedly increased beating rate compared to microtissues with aCFs from young, healthy hearts. The data indicated that the activation status of cardiac fibroblasts played a crucial role in determining the contraction pattern of cardiac microtissues.

Heart fibrosis is linked to irregular heart rhythms. Research findings demonstrated that activated rodent cardiac fibroblasts can lead to irregular contraction and provoke potentially dangerous alterations in heart muscle cells by influencing their electrical activity (22, 24). In our model, fibrotic microtissues showed arrhythmic contractions only occasionally and their action potential profile remained unaffected. Instead, the fibrotic condition was associated with reduced action potential signal amplitude, suggesting a lower number of electrically active iCMs in these microtissues. Impaired conduction and contraction of these microtissues might be a consequence of iCMs decoupling and coupling of iCMs with CFs, reduced levels of gap junction protein connexin 43 and/or overproduction of cytokines and ECM by activated CFs. Secreted factors by activated CFs, biomechanical signalling through excessive ECM deposition and remodelling of mechanical junctions are known factors disturbing proper propagation of electrical impulses [**25**]. Signal conduction abnormalities, such as re-entry, can cause cardiac arrhythmias and may have serious clinical implications for patients with fibrotic hearts [**9**].

Clinical evidence indicates that ventricular fibrosis is a significant indicator of life-threatening ventricular arrhythmia and sudden cardiac death in both ischemic and nonischemic heart conditions. [**8**].

Our model consistently showed that a profibrotic condition led to an enhanced beating rate of cardiac microtissues. Similar data were obtained in human cardiac microtissues containing mesenchymal stem cells instead of CFs following treatment with TGF-β1 [**19**]. Physiologically, increased beating rate of the heart is achieved by activation of β-adrenoreceptors. In normal adult cardiomyocytes, β1-adrenoreceptors are dominant, whereas iCMs contractility can be regulated by both β1- and β2-adrenoreceptors [**26**]. Previous data showed that the beating rate of human iCMs could be increased by treatment with the β-adrenergic agonist isoproterenol [**26,27**]. In line with these data, we could demonstrate the responsiveness of human cardiac microtissues containing iCMs to isoproterenol. In case of cardiac microtissues showing high beating rate (due to presence of activated aCFs), blockade of β-adrenergic receptors in the absence of exogenous agonists significantly decreased frequency. This finding indicated that activated CFs triggered endogenous β-adrenoreceptor signalling in cardiac microtissues. Mechanistically, stimulation of β-adrenoreceptors increases beating rate by enhancing cardiomyocyte relaxation [**10**]. Indeed, we observed that the reduced beating rate observed in the presence of β-adrenoreceptor blockers was associated with longer relaxation time. Accordingly, increased contraction rate of fibrotic cardiac microtissues correlated with shortened relaxation time. These results may suggest that activated CFs produce β-adrenergic agonists. Alternatively, fibrotic condition may sensitize β-adrenoreceptors. Cellular response to β-adrenergic stimulations is further modulated by multiple factors, such as cell surface receptor density, activity of the downstream signalling pathway, or by specific costimulations [**28**]. For example, fibrotic hearts of TGF-β-overexpressing mice showed increased density of β-adrenoreceptors on cardiomyocytes and altered β-adrenergic signalling [**3**]. Furthermore, collagen receptor β_1-integrin [**29**], connective tissue growth factor [**30**] or tissue stiffness [**31**] have also been shown to regulate β-adrenergic signalling. A successful preclinical platform has to combine physiological-like relevance with the high-throughput processing. Our fibrotic cardiac microtissue model is established in a 96-well format and certain parameters, such as size, contractile properties, changes in membrane potential, procollagen-I production or apoptosis can be measured for individual microtissues. In particular, recently developed software measuring the contractile activity of the whole microtissue allows for quick and easy analysis of the key properties of beating cardiac microtissues [**15**]. We gathered transcriptome data from 10–12 pooled microtissues and analyzed gene expression using basic RT-PCR in our investigations. Utilizing next-generation sequencing technologies can provide transcriptome data from a single microtissue. This model can serve as a high-throughput platform for pharmacological screening for a period of at least 10 days. Experiments using the TGF-βR1 inhibitor SD208 shown that fibrotic cardiac microtissues are a reliable model for drug screening.

Our human cardiac microtissue-based fibrotic platform offers technological ease, high throughput, reproducibility, and physiological relevance, but its limits must also be considered. iCMs are defined by their fetal developmental stage. [**32**]. Currently, there is no satisfactory alternative to iCMs. The usefulness of adult primary human cardiomyocytes is limited, as these cells contract upon chemical or electrical stimulation only [**33**]. Despite recent advances in the maturation of iCMs through improved biomechanics and cocultures with other cell types, so far, their maturation status does not reflect adult cardiomyocytes [**13,34,35,36**]. Another limitation of our model is the heterogeneity of iCMs. Conventional differentiation of iPSCs into iCMs results in populations of pacemaker, ventricular-like, atrial-like cells as well as nonbeating progenitors. Utilizing specific types of distinct cardiomyocytes could enhance the significance of the cardiac microtissue model. Furthermore, including additional cell types like endothelial cells or macrophages into induced cardiomyocytes (iCMs) and cardiac fibroblasts (fCFs) could lead to the development of microtissues that more accurately replicate the shape and function of human heart tissue.

5. AT A GLANCE

Cardiac fibrosis is a significant clinical issue. Novel therapeutic techniques are limited by the absence of appropriate experimental models in a human genetic environment. This study involved creating self-aggregating, scaffold-free, 3D cardiac microtissues utilizing human inducible pluripotent stem cell (iPSC)-derived cardiomyocytes and human cardiac fibroblasts. Fibrotic state was induced in cardiac microtissues by treating them with the profibrotic cytokine transforming growth factor β1 (TGF-β1), preactivating fetal cardiac fibroblasts with TGF-β1, or using cardiac fibroblasts derived from heart failure patients. TGF-β1 efficiently triggered fibrotic alterations in cardiac fibroblasts and cardiac microtissues in our model. The fibrotic characteristics of cardiac microtissues were suppressed by SD208, a TGF-β-receptor type 1 inhibitor, in a way that depended on the dosage. We noticed that fibrotic cardiac microtissues significantly raised the spontaneous beating rate by reducing the relaxation phase and exhibited a decreased contraction amplitude. No alterations in the action potential profile were observed. We showed that human cardiac microtissues' contraction may be controlled by direct electrical stimulation or therapy with the β-adrenergic receptor agonist isoproterenol. In the absence of external stimulants, the β-adrenoreceptor antagonist nadolol reduced the beating rate of fibrotic cardiac microtissues by extending relaxation time.

Our observations indicate that in fibrosis, active cardiac fibroblasts may enhance ventricular contraction rate through direct activation of β-adrenoreceptor signaling. Ultimately, a fibrotic cardiac microtissue model can serve as an efficient model for drug testing and investigating the cellular and molecular processes involved in cardiac fibrosis.

REFERENCES

1. Kong, P.; Christia, P.; Frangogiannis, N.G. The pathogenesis of cardiac fibrosis. Cell. Mol. Life Sci. 2014, 71, 549–574. [Google Scholar] [CrossRef] [Green Version]
2. Travers, J.G.; Kamal, F.A.; Robbins, J.; Yutzey, K.E.; Blaxall, B.C. Cardiac fibrosis: The fibroblast awakens. Circ. Res. 2016, 118, 1021–1040. [Google Scholar] [CrossRef] [Green Version]
3. Rosenkranz, S.; Flesch, M.; Amann, K.; Haeuseler, C.; Kilter, H.; Seeland, U.; Schluter, K.D.; Bohm, M. Alterations of beta-adrenergic signaling and cardiac hypertrophy in transgenic mice overexpressing TGF-beta(1). Am. J. Physiol. Heart Circ. Physiol. 2002, 283, H1253–H1262. [Google Scholar] [CrossRef] [PubMed]
4. Ikeuchi, M.; Tsutsui, H.; Shiomi, T.; Matsusaka, H.; Matsushima, S.; Wen, J.; Kubota, T.; Takeshita, A. Inhibition of TGF-beta signaling exacerbates early cardiac dysfunction but prevents late remodeling after infarction. Cardiovasc. Res. 2004, 64, 526–535. [Google Scholar] [CrossRef] [PubMed] [Green Version]
5. Kuwahara, F.; Kai, H.; Tokuda, K.; Kai, M.; Takeshita, A.; Egashira, K.; Imaizumi, T. Transforming growth factor-beta function blocking prevents myocardial fibrosis and diastolic dysfunction in pressure-overloaded rats. Circulation 2002, 106, 130–135. [Google Scholar] [CrossRef] [PubMed] [Green Version]
6. Kania, G.; Blyszczuk, P.; Stein, S.; Valaperti, A.; Germano, D.; Dirnhofer, S.; Hunziker, L.; Matter, C.M.; Eriksson, U. Heart-infiltrating prominin-1^+/$CD133^+$ progenitor cells represent the cellular source of transforming growth factor beta-mediated cardiac fibrosis in experimental autoimmune myocarditis. Circ. Res. 2009, 105, 462–470. [Google Scholar] [CrossRef] [Green Version]
7. Clements, I.P.; Miller, W.L.; Olson, L.J. Resting heart rate and cardiac function in dilated cardiomyopathy. Int. J. Cardiol. 1999, 72, 27–37. [Google Scholar] [CrossRef]
8. Disertori, M.; Mase, M.; Ravelli, F. Myocardial fibrosis predicts ventricular tachyarrhythmias. Trends Cardiovasc. Med. 2017, 27, 363–372. [Google Scholar] [CrossRef]

9. Nguyen, T.P.; Qu, Z.; Weiss, J.N. Cardiac fibrosis and arrhythmogenesis: The road to repair is paved with perils. J. Mol. Cell. Cardiol. 2014, 70, 83–91. [Google Scholar] [CrossRef] [Green Version]

10. Najafi, A.; Sequeira, V.; Kuster, D.W.; Van der Velden, J. Beta-adrenergic receptor signalling and its functional consequences in the diseased heart. Eur. J. Clin. Investig. 2016, 46, 362–374. [Google Scholar] [CrossRef] [Green Version]

11. Karakikes, I.; Ameen, M.; Termglinchan, V.; Wu, J.C. Human induced pluripotent stem cell-derived cardiomyocytes: Insights into molecular, cellular, and functional phenotypes. Circ. Res. 2015, 117, 80–88. [Google Scholar] [CrossRef] [PubMed] [Green Version]

12. Zuppinger, C. 3D culture for cardiac cells. Biochim. Biophys. Acta 2016, 1863, 1873–1881. [Google Scholar] [CrossRef] [PubMed]

13. Beauchamp, P.; Moritz, W.; Kelm, J.M.; Ullrich, N.D.; Agarkova, I.; Anson, B.D.; Suter, T.M.; Zuppinger, C. Development and characterization of a scaffold-free 3D spheroid model of induced pluripotent stem cell-derived human cardiomyocytes. Tissue Eng. Part C Methods 2015, 21, 852–861. [Google Scholar] [CrossRef] [PubMed] [Green Version]

14. Castaldo, C.; Di Meglio, F.; Miraglia, R.; Sacco, A.M.; Romano, V.; Bancone, C.; Della Corte, A.; Montagnani, S.; Nurzynska, D. Cardiac fibroblast-derived extracellular matrix (biomatrix) as a model for the studies of cardiac primitive cell biological properties in normal and pathological adult human heart. Biomed. Res. Int. 2013, 2013, 352370. [Google Scholar] [CrossRef] [PubMed]

15. Sala, L.; van Meer, B.J.; Tertoolen, L.G.J.; Bakkers, J.; Bellin, M.; Davis, R.P.; Denning, C.; Dieben, M.A.E.; Eschenhagen, T.; Giacomelli, E.; et al. MUSCLEMOTION: A versatile open software tool to quantify cardiomyocyte and cardiac muscle contraction in vitro and in vivo. Circ. Res. 2018, 122, e5–e16. [Google Scholar] [CrossRef]

16. Beauchamp, P.; Jackson, C.B.; Ozhathil, L.C.; Agarkova, I.; Galindo, C.L.; Sawyer, D.B.; Suter, T.M.; Zuppinger, C. 3D co-culture of hiPSC-derived cardiomyocytes with cardiac fibroblasts improves tissue-like features of cardiac spheroids. Front. Mol. Biosci. 2020, 7, 14. [Google Scholar] [CrossRef]

17. Figtree, G.A.; Bubb, K.J.; Tang, O.; Kizana, E.; Gentile, C. Vascularized cardiac spheroids as novel 3D in vitro models to study cardiac fibrosis. Cells Tissues Organs 2017, 204, 191–198. [Google Scholar] [CrossRef]

18. Sadeghi, A.H.; Shin, S.R.; Deddens, J.C.; Fratta, G.; Mandla, S.; Yazdi, I.K.; Prakash, G.; Antona, S.; Demarchi, D.; Buijsrogge, M.P.; et al. Engineered 3D cardiac fibrotic tissue to study fibrotic remodeling. Adv. Healthc. Mater. 2017, 6. [Google Scholar] [CrossRef]

19. Lee, M.O.; Jung, K.B.; Jo, S.J.; Hyun, S.A.; Moon, K.S.; Seo, J.W.; Kim, S.H.; Son, M.Y. Modelling cardiac fibrosis using three-dimensional cardiac microtissues derived from human embryonic stem cells. J. Biol. Eng. 2019, 13, 15. [Google Scholar] [CrossRef]

20. Van Spreeuwel, A.C.C.; Bax, N.A.M.; Van Nierop, B.J.; Aartsma-Rus, A.; Goumans, M.T.H.; Bouten, C.V.C. Mimicking cardiac fibrosis in a dish: Fibroblast density rather than collagen density weakens cardiomyocyte function. J. Cardiovasc. Transl. Res. 2017, 10, 116–127. [Google Scholar] [CrossRef] [Green Version]

21. Wang, E.Y.; Rafatian, N.; Zhao, Y.; Lee, A.; Lai, B.F.L.; Lu, R.X.; Jekic, D.; Davenport Huyer, L.; Knee-Walden, E.J.; Bhattacharya, S.; et al. Biowire model of interstitial and focal cardiac fibrosis. ACS Cent. Sci. 2019, 5, 1146–1158. [Google Scholar] [CrossRef] [PubMed] [Green Version]

22. Kofron, C.M.; Kim, T.Y.; King, M.E.; Xie, A.; Feng, F.; Park, E.; Qu, Z.; Choi, B.R.; Mende, U. Gq-activated fibroblasts induce cardiomyocyte action potential prolongation and automaticity in a three-dimensional microtissue environment. Am. J. Physiol. Heart Circ. Physiol. 2017, 313, H810–H827. [Google Scholar] [CrossRef] [PubMed] [Green Version]

23. Nurzynska, D.; Di Meglio, F.; Romano, V.; Miraglia, R.; Sacco, A.M.; Latino, F.; Bancone, C.; Della Corte, A.; Maiello, C.; Amarelli, C.; et al. Cardiac primitive cells become committed to a cardiac fate in adult human heart with chronic ischemic disease but fail to acquire mature phenotype: Genetic and phenotypic study. Basic Res. Cardiol. 2013, 108, 320. [Google Scholar] [CrossRef] [PubMed]

24. Trieschmann, J.; Bettin, D.; Haustein, M.; Koster, A.; Molcanyi, M.; Halbach, M.; Hanna, M.; Fouad, M.; Brockmeier, K.; Hescheler, J.; et al. The interaction between adult cardiac fibroblasts and embryonic stem cell-derived cardiomyocytes leads to proarrhythmic changes in in vitro cocultures. Stem Cells Int. 2016, 2016, 2936126. [Google Scholar] [CrossRef] [Green Version]

25. Pellman, J.; Zhang, J.; Sheikh, F. Myocyte-fibroblast communication in cardiac fibrosis and arrhythmias: Mechanisms and model systems. J. Mol. Cell. Cardiol. 2016, 94, 22–31. [Google Scholar] [CrossRef] [Green Version]

26. Wu, H.; Lee, J.; Vincent, L.G.; Wang, Q.; Gu, M.; Lan, F.; Churko, J.M.; Sallam, K.I.; Matsa, E.; Sharma, A.; et al. Epigenetic regulation of phosphodiesterases 2A and 3A underlies compromised beta-adrenergic signaling in an iPSC model of dilated cardiomyopathy. Cell Stem Cell 2015, 17, 89–100. [Google Scholar] [CrossRef] [Green Version]

27. Preininger, M.K.; Jha, R.; Maxwell, J.T.; Wu, Q.; Singh, M.; Wang, B.; Dalal, A.; McEachin, Z.T.; Rossoll, W.; Hales, C.M.; et al. A human pluripotent stem cell model of catecholaminergic polymorphic ventricular tachycardia recapitulates patient-specific drug responses. Dis. Models Mech. 2016, 9, 927–939. [Google Scholar] [CrossRef] [Green Version]

28. Ferrara, N.; Komici, K.; Corbi, G.; Pagano, G.; Furgi, G.; Rengo, C.; Femminella, G.D.; Leosco, D.; Bonaduce, D. Beta-adrenergic receptor responsiveness in aging heart and clinical implications. Front. Physiol. 2014, 4, 396. [Google Scholar] [CrossRef] [Green Version]

29. Krishnamurthy, P.; Subramanian, V.; Singh, M.; Singh, K. Beta1 integrins modulate beta-adrenergic receptor-stimulated cardiac myocyte apoptosis and myocardial remodeling. Hypertension 2007, 49, 865–872. [Google Scholar] [CrossRef] [Green Version]

30. Gravning, J.; Ahmed, M.S.; Qvigstad, E.; Krobert, K.; Edvardsen, T.; Moe, I.T.; Hagelin, E.M.; Sagave, J.; Valen, G.; Levy, F.O.; et al. Connective tissue growth factor/CCN2 attenuates beta-adrenergic receptor responsiveness and cardiotoxicity by induction of G protein-coupled receptor kinase-5 in cardiomyocytes. Mol. Pharmacol. 2013, 84, 372–383. [Google Scholar] [CrossRef]

31. Kim, T.J.; Sun, J.; Lu, S.; Zhang, J.; Wang, Y. The regulation of beta-adrenergic receptor-mediated PKA activation by substrate stiffness via microtubule dynamics in human MSCs. Biomaterials 2014, 35, 8348–8356. [Google Scholar] [CrossRef] [PubMed] [Green Version]

32. Zuppinger, C.; Gibbons, G.; Dutta-Passecker, P.; Segiser, A.; Most, H.; Suter, T.M. Characterization of cytoskeleton features and maturation status of cultured human iPSC-derived cardiomyocytes. Eur. J. Histochem. 2017, 61, 2763. [Google Scholar] [CrossRef] [PubMed] [Green Version]

33. Nguyen, N.; Nguyen, W.; Nguyenton, B.; Ratchada, P.; Page, G.; Miller, P.E.; Ghetti, A.; Abi-Gerges, N. Adult human primary cardiomyocyte-based model for the simultaneous prediction of drug-induced inotropic and pro-arrhythmia risk. Front. Physiol. 2017, 8, 1073. [Google Scholar] [CrossRef] [PubMed] [Green Version]

34. Nunes, S.S.; Miklas, J.W.; Liu, J.; Aschar-Sobbi, R.; Xiao, Y.; Zhang, B.; Jiang, J.; Masse, S.; Gagliardi, M.; Hsieh, A.; et al. Biowire: A platform for maturation of human pluripotent stem cell-derived cardiomyocytes. Nat. Methods 2013, 10, 781–787. [Google Scholar] [CrossRef] [Green Version]

35. Giacomelli, E.; Bellin, M.; Sala, L.; Van Meer, B.J.; Tertoolen, L.G.; Orlova, V.V.; Mummery, C.L. Three-dimensional cardiac microtissues composed of cardiomyocytes and endothelial cells co-differentiated from human pluripotent stem cells. Development 2017, 144, 1008–1017. [Google Scholar] [CrossRef] [Green Version]

36. Ronaldson-Bouchard, K.; Ma, S.P.; Yeager, K.; Chen, T.; Song, L.; Sirabella, D.; Morikawa, K.; Teles, D.; Yazawa, M.; Vunjak-Novakovic, G. Advanced maturation of human cardiac tissue grown from pluripotent stem cells. Nature 2018, 556, 239–243. [Google Scholar] [CrossRef]

03 3D-Neurospheres Derived from Human Induced Pluripotent Stem Cells are Appropriate for Screening Neurotoxicity

1. INTRODUCTION: AN OVERVIEW

Environmental stressors, such chemicals or pharmaceuticals, can be harmful to individuals at any point in their lives, including fetal development, youth, or adulthood. Predicting toxicology is challenging due to the combination of environmental chemicals' harmful effects and individuals' genetic predisposition. Conventional animal-based toxicity and safety tests have high costs, use large numbers of animals (mainly rats) and in many cases, they do not provide clearly translatable results for humans [**1,2,3**]. Consequently, in line with legislation, there is an increasing need to develop alternative testing methods which could handle thousands of drugs or chemicals with affordable time and cost and with human-relevant neurotoxicology (NT) outcome [**4,5,6,7**]. Development of new approach methods (NAM), would be important both for NT and developmental neurotoxicology (DNT) tests, providing data on the effect of chemicals and the potential adverse outcomes (AOs) [**6,8,9,10,11,12,13**].

More research are utilizing primary cell cultures and pluripotent stem cells (PSCs) to develop in vitro systems for neurotoxicity (NT) and developmental neurotoxicity (DNT) evaluations[**14,15,16,17**], 3D cell cultures are widely acknowledged to more accurately replicate the original tissue environment, including tissue-specific architecture, mechanical and biochemical features, cell-to-cell communication and signaling, and differentiation capability. In contrast, 2D cell culture systems are less complex and more artificial in this regard[**6,8,11**]. However, existing assays can still provide valuable insights into specific neurodevelopmental processes. A single in vitro assay is insufficient to capture the intricacies of in vivo development.

Therefore, a series of assays and applications tailored for specific purposes should be utilized to address the pertinent processes. Human induced pluripotent stem cell-derived neurospheres, cultivated on 3D scaffolds or self-forming, can create cell-to-cell connections and simulate specific neurodevelopmental processes[**10,18**]. This makes them a potential in vitro screening tool for neurotoxicity, developmental neurotoxicity, and drug development[**19,20,21**].

Neural stem cells (NSCs) are a multipotent and self-renewing group of cells found in the mammalian central nervous system (CNS). They appear in vivo during the development of embryonic neural tissue, coinciding with the formation of the neural tube. These cells have the capacity to differentiate into all neuronal cell types, as well as into glial cells, therefore they are able to emulate some fetal neurodevelopmental processes [**22,23**]. Moreover, NSCs can be differentiated in vitro from pluripotent stem cells (PSCs) thus providing an attractive and almost unlimited in vitro tool for toxicology studies including drug development [**24,25**]. Despite the developments mentioned above, still, a limited number of human iPSC derived 3D neuronal culture-based studies were published focusing on the development of NT or DNT models [**21,26,27,28,29,30,31**]. A limiting factor for the further development of such test methods is the lack of high-throughput screening (HTS) read-outs on 3D cell cultures [**16**], despite the developments using high-content image analysis (HCA) [**27**].Here, we present a reliable model system where hiPSC-derived NSCs are differentiated towards subtypes of neurons, astrocytes, and oligodendrocytes, forming free-floating 3D neurospheres in 96-well plate format. Over 6 weeks the various differentiation stages are characterized, and three selected stages are exposed with different compounds to investigate their cytotoxic effect. The neuronal spheroids created are utilized for neurotoxicity evaluations at several time points, representing different stages of differentiation. This makes them an ideal foundation for advancing the development of DNT test systems.

2. METHODS

2.1. Chemicals and Plasticware

The chemicals were bought from Sigma-Aldrich in St. Louis, MO, USA, and all cell culture supplies and plasticware were obtained from Thermo Fisher Scientific Inc. in Waltham, MA, USA, unless stated otherwise.

2.2. Human iPSC Culture

A human induced pluripotent stem cell (iPSC) line named Ctrl-2, obtained from peripheral blood mononuclear cells (PBMCs) of a healthy middle-aged Caucasian female donor, which was previously established and characterized, was utilized in this research(32,33) . Cells were cultured on BD Matrigel™ matrix (BD Biosciences,

Franklin Lakes, NJ, USA) with mTeSR™1 medium (Stem Cell Technologies, Vancouver, Canada), using Gentle Cell Dissociation Reagent for passages, according to the manufacturer's instruction. For mycoplasma screening, the Venor®GeM-Advance (Minerva Biolabs) Mycoplasma Detection Kit was used according to the manufacturer's protocol in every fifth passage during maintenance and before freezing. The cells were incubated at 37 °C in a humidified environment with 5% CO2. Cultures from passage 16 and 17 were utilized for differentiation in the study.

2.3. Neural Cell Differentiation and Sustenance

The Ctrl-2 hiPSC line was differentiated to neural stem cells (NSCs) by dual SMAD inhibition procedure [**34**], following the detailed protocol of Shi et al. [**35**]. Briefly, when hiPSC cultures reached 90% confluence, the culture was passaged onto poly-l-ornithine and laminin (POL/L; 0.002%/1 µg/cm^2) coated plates, using conventional iPSC passage (as detailed above). On the next day media was changed to neural induction medium (NIM; DMEM/F12: Neurobasal medium, supplemented with 1× N2, 2× B27, 2 mM glutamine, 1× non-essential amino acid (NEAA), 100 µM β-mercaptoethanol, 5 µg/mL insulin) supplemented with 10 µM SB431542, 500 ng/mL Noggin (R&D Systems, Inc., Minneapolis, MN, USA) and 5 ng/mL basic fibroblast growth factor (bFGF) to induce the neuroectodermal lineage. Neuronal induction media was applied until day 10 of the differentiation. The forming neural rosette-like structures were manually picked under a stereomicroscope (Olympus SZX2; Olympus Ltd. Tokyo, Japan) and re-plated onto POL/L (POL/L; 0.002%/1 µg/cm^2) plates. NSCs were expanded in neural maintenance medium (NMM; DMEM-F12: Neurobasal medium, supplemented with 1× N2, and 2× B27, 2 mM glutamine, 1× NEAA), supplemented with 10 ng/mL bFGF and 10 ng/mL Epidermal growth factor (EGF) and maintained in a monolayer on dishes coated with POL/L (0.002%/1 µg/cm^2). When reached 100% confluence, cells were passaged using Accutase (Sigma) and seeded as single cells (50,000 cells/cm^2) for further expansion on POL/L (0.002%/1 µg/cm^2) coated dishes. After 4 passages NSCs were frozen in 1 mL freezing medium (90% Fetal Bovine Serum, FBS; heat-inactivated, Thermo Fisher Sci.; Cat N.: 10500-064, LOT: 08F1180K; 10% DMSO; 2 million cells/vial), using Accutase passage. Before freezing the NSCs, a mycoplasma test was performed (see above), repeated every fifth passage during maintenance.

2.4. 3D Neurosphere Culture

After thawing, NSCs (generated as detailed above) were cultured on POL/L (0.002%/1 µg/cm^2) coated plates (50,000 cells/cm^2). When reached 100% confluence NSCs were propagated with Accutase treatment and single-cell suspension was plated onto a low-adherent 96-well plate with 10,000 cells/well in NMM medium. Neurospheres were formed within 48 h after plating and NMM half of the media was changed in every 3 days until analyzing the samples. Samples were collected at Day 0 (D0), Day 2 (D2), and weekly intervals from the end of the 1st week (D7) until the end of the 6th week (D14, D21, D28, D35, and D42).

2.5. Cryosectioning and Immunocytochemistry (ICC) Staining

3D neurospheres (untreated, vehicle or compound-treated) were fixed with 4% paraformaldehyde (PFA) in 0.1 mol/L phosphate buffer for 1 h at RT and washed 3 times with PBS. The fixed samples were cryoprotected in 30% sucrose in PBS containing 0.01% sodium azide at 4 °C until embedding in Shandon Cryomatrix gel (Thermo Fischer Scientific). The 16 μm parallel sections were made using cryostat (Leica CM 1850 Cryostat, Leica GmbH), mounted to Superfrost™ Ultra Plus Adhesion Slides (Thermo Fisher Scientific) and stored at −20 °C until use. After 10 min air-drying, the sections were blocked for 1 h at RT with blocking solution (3% BSA in PBS), supplemented with 0.2% TritonX-100. The sections were then incubated with primary antibodies overnight at 4 °C. Next day, sections were washed in PBS 3 times, and isotype-specific secondary antibodies were diluted in blocking buffer and applied for 1 h at RT. The sections were washed 3 times with PBS and covered using Vectashield® mounting medium containing DAPI (1.5 μg/mL; Vector Laboratories), that labelled the nuclei of the cells (at least 1 h at RT). Negative controls for the secondary antibodies were performed by omitting the primary antibodies. Immunoreactive sections were analyzed using a BX-41 epifluorescent microscope (objectives: 20× 0.50 NA; 40× 0.75 NA; Olympus) equipped with a DP-74 digital camera and its CellSens software (V1.18; Olympus). For confocal imaging, Olympus Fv10i-W compact confocal microscope system (objective: 60× 1.35 NA; Olympus) with Fv10i software (V2.1; Olympus) was applied. All images were further processed using the GNU Image Manipulation Program (GIMP 2.10.0) and NIH ImageJ analysis software (imagej.nih.gov/ij).

Quantification of the immunocytochemistry data was performed using ImageJ software according to Tieng et al. [**36**]. Briefly, images were taken by confocal microscopy at 120× magnification. The numbers of Ki-67-, NESTIN-, GFAP-, AQP4, TUBB3-, NF200kD-, MBP-, VAMP2-, and MAP2-immunoreactive pixels were measured in 5 neurosphere (highest diameter middle sections, 5 randomly selected fields/slide) at every time points. Data was normalized with DAPI positive nuclei number. Data were expressed as a percentage of marker/DAPI ratio ± SEM ($p < 0.05$).

2.6. Apoptosis Assay

Embedding and cryosectioning of 3D samples were conducted as previously described. The DeadEnd™ Colorimetric TUNEL System from Promega was utilized on the central cryosections with the largest diameter of the spheroids to identify apoptotic activity, in accordance with the manufacturer's recommendations. In brief, apoptosis was detected by immersing the slides in PBS for 5 min (at

RT), adding 20 μg/mL Proteinase K solution and incubating for 10–30 min (at RT). After 5–10 min treatment in Equilibration buffer, recombinant terminal deoxynucleotidyl transferase (rTdT) was added to the reaction mixture. Next, the sections were incubated for 60 min at 37 °C inside of a humidified chamber to allow the end-labelling reaction to occur. The reaction was terminated by immersing the slides in saline-sodium citrate for 15 min (RT). Endogenous peroxidases were blocked by immersing the slides in 0.3% hydrogen peroxide in PBS for 3–5 min (RT). Streptavidin-HRP was added to slides, incubated for 30 min (RT), stained with diaminobenzidine (DAB) solution for 5 min until a light brown background appeared. For hematoxylin–eosin (HE) staining Mayer's Hematoxylin solution was used for 3 min. Sections were rinsed with tap water and placed into distilled water for 30 s, then into 96% alcohol for 30 s. One percent Eosin solution in distilled water was used for 3 min. Stained sections were dehydrated through alcohols, clear in xylene and mount in DPX. Microphotographs were made with DP-74 digital camera (Olympus) using a light microscope (BX-41, objectives: 20× 0.50 NA; 40× 0.75 NA; Olympus) and CellSens software (V1.18; Olympus). NIH ImageJ analysis program was utilized to count the apoptotic and total number of cells stained with Hematoxylin. Five spheroids treated with Ctrl and five treated with ROT were randomly chosen for analysis. Middle sections were examined from each of the differentiation stages (D21, D28, and D42) in three separate experiments (n = 3).

2.7. Transmission Electron Microscopy (TEM)

Neurospheres (untreated, vehicle or compound-treated) were fixed at different differentiation stages in a fixative solution containing 3.2% PFA, 0.2% glutaraldehyde, 1% sucrose, 40 mM $CaCl_2$ in 0.1 M cacodylate buffer (pH 7.4) for 12 h at 4 °C. Samples for ultrastructural analysis were embedded in 1.5% agar (dissolved in dH_2O), post-fixed in 1% ferrocyanide-reduced osmium tetroxide [**37**], then dehydrated using graded series of ethanol, finally embedded in Spurr low viscosity epoxy resin medium. Thin slices were taken from the central area of the spheroids with the largest diameter, placed on copper slot grids covered with formwar (Agar Sci., Essex, UK), and then dyed with uranyl acetate and Reynolds's lead citrate. Sections were analyzed using a JEOL JEM 1011 transmission electron microscope from JEOL Ltd., Tokyo, Japan, which was fitted with a Morada 11-megapixel camera and operated with iTEM software from Olympus.

2.8. RT-qPCR Analysis

Each sample consisted of 12 spheroids, and 3 biological replicates were conducted (n = 3). RNA was extracted using the RNeasy Plus Mini Kit from Qiagen in Hilden, Germany. 600 ng of extracted RNA was utilized for reverse transcription using the Maxima First Strand cDNA Synthesis Kit for RT-qPCR with dsDNase from Thermo Fisher Scientific, following the manufacturer's instructions.Gene-specific primers were designed using the Primer3 software [**38**], specified with mFOLD software [**39**] and Primer-BLAST software [**40**]. Primers were optimized using two-fold serial dilution standard curves. As a reference, gene GAPDH was used. Each real-time PCR reaction contained 5 ng RNA-equivalent cDNA template, 400 nM of each primer and 50% SYBR Green JumpStart Taq ReadyMix (Sigma Aldrich) in a total volume of 15 μL. PCR reactions were set up using QIAgility liquid handling robot and performed on a Rotor-Gene Q cycler (Qiagen). The cycling parameters were as follows: 94 °C for 3 min initial denaturation followed by 40 cycles of 95 °C for 5 s, 60 °C for 15 s, and 72 °C for 30 s. Confirmation of primer specificity and absence of gDNA contamination was achieved using melting curve analysis and agarose gel electrophoresis. Three replicates of data were examined for each gene using the ddCT method [41].

2.9. XBP1-Assay of Endoplasmic Reticulum Stress

When unfolded proteins build up in the endoplasmic reticulum (ER), a 26-nucleotide fragment is spliced out from the X-box binding protein 1 mRNA (XBP1(U)) using a specific method. The truncated mRNA XBP1(S) is commonly employed as an indicator of endoplasmic reticulum stress. XBP1(S) expression was studied using both previously published primers [43] and new primers developed by the researchers [44] (Table S2). Cells were treated with 5 μM and 10 μM Tunicamycin as a positive control to generate ER-stress. RT-PCR experiments were conducted as previously described, utilizing Phusion Hot Start II High-Fidelity DNA Polymerase and 20 ng of the cDNA samples.

2.10. Toxicity Treatments and ATP Viability Assay

Concentration-response curves were generated by testing eleven renowned substances at seven different concentrations. The maximum dosage was established considering the compounds' solubility, ensuring that DMSO levels did not exceed 0.1% following dilution in the culture media. Each assay plate contained 4 technical replicates from each sample, and a total of 3 biological replicate assays were conducted (n = 3). The 3D cell cultures were treated with harmful substances for 72 hours as outlined. Vehicle control was utilized as a standard medium with the addition of 0.1% DMSO. The ATP viability assay was conducted using the CellTiter-Glo® 3D Cell Viability Assay following the manufacturer's instructions from Promega. Lysed neurospheres using 100 μL of CellTiter-Glo® 3D Reagent for 60 minutes at room temperature. The luminescence signal was measured using a Thermo VarioScan Flash plate reader from Thermo Fisher Scientific.

2.11. Determination of diametric and total protein in spheroids

Spheroids cultured in a 96-well plate were imaged using the 4x objective lens (0.1 numerical aperture) of an Olympus IX71 microscope equipped with a DP21 camera from Olympus. The photos were evaluated by measuring the diameters of the spheroids using the Olympus CellSens Dimension program (V1.11). Each number is the mean of 3 studies where 96 spheroids were measured in each. The 3D spheroids were individually lysed using RIPA Lysis and Extraction Buffer containing Halt™ Protease and Phosphatase Inhibitor Cocktail and Pierce™ Universal Nuclease for Cell Lysis. The lysates were sonicated, and the total protein concentration was measured using a Pierce BCA Protein Assay Kit following the manufacturer's guidelines. Because the D2, D7, and D14 samples had tiny spheroid sizes, three spheroids were combined, and the values were then calculated individually. Three tests were conducted, with 24 spheroids evaluated at each timepoint.

2.12. Neurite Outgrowth Assay

The approach developed by Harris et al. was adapted for measuring neurite outgrowth [**45**]. 3D spheroids were treated with different concentrations (vehicle, 0.1 μM, 0.5 μM, and 0.75 μM) of Rotenone (ROT) at D21 differentiation stage using the 72 h exposure scheme, similarly to the previous concentration-response experiments. After the treatment, the spheroids were plated on Matrigel-coated plates in NMM medium without compound, and 24 h later fixed with 4% PFA and immunostained against TUBB3, as described in detail under the immunostaining paragraph. First, the number of neurites was counted for each sample. Then, the "edge" of the spheroids was determined by drawing an "edge line" and every neurite length was measured from this "edge line" to the tip of each neurite. Total neurite length was calculated for each spheroid using the ImageJ software's Neurite Tracer plugin. In each experiment eight spheroids were treated in each experimental group (5 groups) and three independent experiments were performed (n = 3).

2.13. Statistical Analysis

The "n" value corresponds to the number of biological replicates for each tested concentration. Analysis of data is presented as the mean ± SEM. Significance of data was determined with paired T test for RT-qPCR (* $p < 0.01$) and with One-way ANOVA for concentration response (* $p < 0.05$; ** $p < 0.01$).

3. RESULTS

3.1. Three-Dimensional Spheroid Differentiation of iPSCs-Derived NSCs Revealed Complex Neuronal Cultures

We aimed to study the temporal differentiation of 3D neuronal spheroids derived from hiPSCs in suspension culture. We have previously thoroughly evaluated the ability of the initial neural stem cell (NSCs) population to differentiate into neurons using the dual-SMAD inhibition methodology [**32,33**]. These cells expressed the major NPC markers (NESTIN, SOX1 (SRY-Box 1), PAX6 (Paired Box 6) investigated on protein level with ICC. When the NPCs were terminally differentiated in a 2D culture system over 5 weeks, cortical neurons and glial cells were differentiated and formed a neuronal network, as we published recently [**32**]. In the present study differentiation in a 3D culture system was investigated in the course of 6 weeks (42 days).

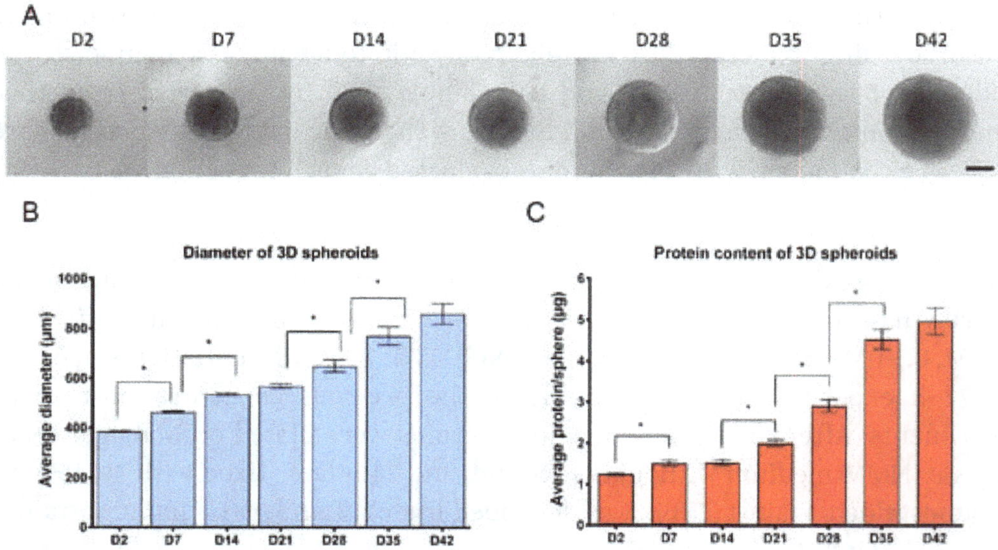

Figure 1. Growth properties of 3D neurospheres during the 6 weeks of differentiation (A) Representative microscopic view of 3D spheroids, investigated at weekly intervals (4×, scale bar: 200 µm). (B) The average diameter of 3D spheroids in µm measured by CellSens Dimension software (Olympus) (n = 3, in each experiment 96 spheroids were compared weekly trough 6-weeks). (C) Average total protein content of spheroids determined by Pierce BCA Protein Assay. Note that D2, D7 and D14 samples were measured by pooling three spheroids and individual values were calculated, while in all other timepoints spheroids were measured individually (n = 3, in each stage 24 spheroids were measured). ±SEM values are presented on graphs. (* $p < 0.05$).

In suspension culture upon withdrawing the two mitogens EGF and bFGF, NSCs formed compact 3D spheroids, the so-called neurospheres within 48 h. Growth properties of the structures were investigated by measuring the diameter of the individual spheres and their total protein content. Results showed a continuous growth of the spheres during the 6 weeks culture period, in terms of diametric growth and protein content (**Figure 1**). While the diameter increased linearly, the protein content increased more dynamically after week 4, resembling the cellular and structural changes during differentiation (**Figure 1**B,C).

This observation was in accordance with the expression of the cell proliferation marker Ki-67 (KI67), representing the proportion of dividing cells, monitored by ICC on protein level (**Figure** 2A,B) or by RT-qPCR on transcript level (**Figure 3**). The expression of Ki-67 and the number of Ki-67-positive cells were the highest in D2 and D7 samples, which showed a continuous decline over the differentiation period (**Figure** 2A,B or **Figure 3**). The forming 3D cell aggregates mainly expressed the early neuronal markers such as PAX6, NESTIN, and SOX1, which expressions decreased with maturation on a time-wise manner (RT-qPCR, **Figure 3**). Tubulin beta-3 chain (TUBB3) expression appeared very early in the samples, already at D2 as neuronal processes started to grow inside the spheres (ICC, **Figure** 2A,B). These changes were obvious when investigated at transcript level as well (RT-qPCR, TUBB3; **Figure 3**). It is important to note that no necrotic regions were detected in the center of the spheroids or in other regions, not even the highest diameter of spheroids reached 800 µm in average in D42 samples (**Figure 1**B or **Figure 2** first line). In semithin sections, cell density was found to be consistently high over the whole period under examination, confirming this fact. Distinct layers of fibers were visible on the surface starting from the 21st day.

A weekly investigation of the gene expression revealed a continuous progress in neuronal differentiation and increase in the level of maturation markers, such as the dendritic marker Microtubule-associated protein 2 (MAP2) or Microtubule-associated protein tau (MAPT), and RNA Binding Fox-1 Homolog 3 (RBFOX3, also known as NeuN) (**Figure 3**), which were in accordance with the protein data of immunofluorescent staining of the 3D spheroids, MAP2 and Neurofilament 200 kDa (NF200); (ICC, **Figure** 2A,B).

Terminal differentiation resulted in the formation of neuronal networks and synapses, from the stage of D28, post-synaptic marker PSD95 (now DLG4, Discs Large MAGUK Scaffold Protein 4) (**Figure 3** and **Figure 4**), and the major synaptic vesicle protein p38, Synaptophysin (SYNP) and Vesicle-associated membrane protein 2 (VAMP2) (**Figure 2** and **Figure 4**) expression appeared in maturing neurons. Synapse formation was assessed by transmission electron microscopy (TEM) revealing the presence of synaptic connections, presynaptic vesicles and postsynaptic density (Psd). Matured synapses were detected in D42 samples, where docked presynaptic vesicles were determined by identifiable contact point between the vesicle and the presynaptic membrane.

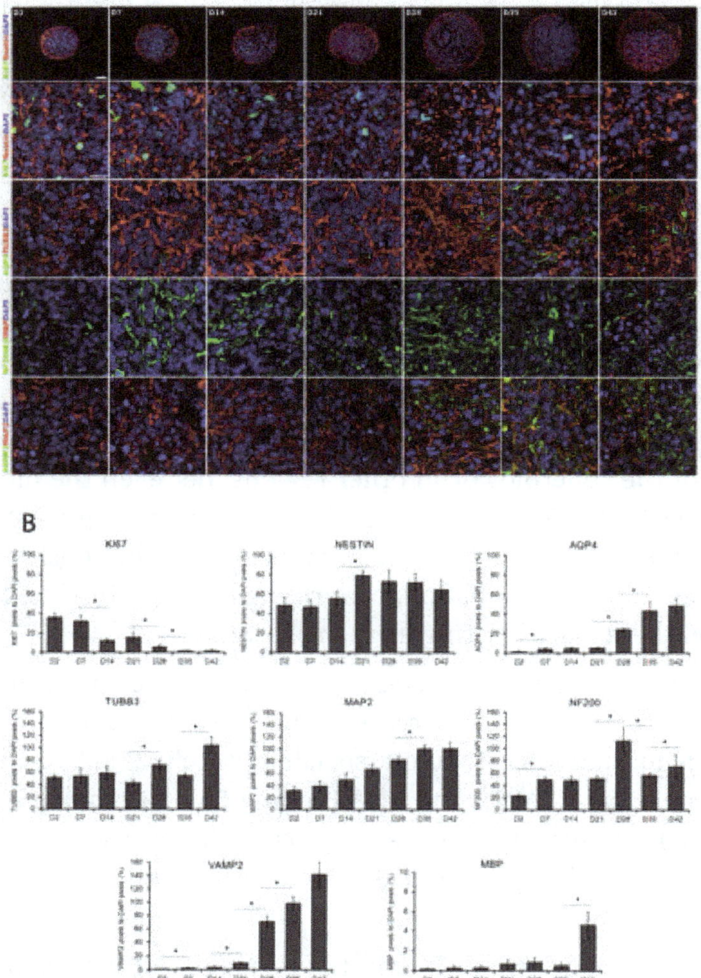

Figure 2. Immunocytochemical analysis of 3D spheroids. (A) Spheroids were fixed and cryosectioned then immunostained at weekly intervals from D2 until D42 stage. The first line represents the overview of the cryosectioned spheroids, while the rest of the panel shows higher magnifications. Relevant markers of proliferation (KI67), neural stem cells (NESTIN), neuronal differentiation (TUBB3 and MAP2), an intermediate filament of dendrites and axons (NF200), synaptic vesicles of neurons (VAMP2), astrocyte (AQP4), and oligodendrocyte (MBP) specific proteins were stained. Protein name IDs are indicated with colors, representing the color of the fluorophore used (e.g., green as Alexa 488; red as Alexa 594) Nuclei were counterstained with DAPI (in blue). Scale bar: 100 μm (first line only) and 25 μm. (B) Quantitative analysis of the immunostainings on confocal images. The numbers of Ki-67, NESTIN, AQP4, TUBB3, NF200kD, MBP, VAMP2, and MAP2 immunoreactive pixels were measured in 5 neurospheres (middle sections, 5 randomly selected fields/slide) at every time points. Data was normalized with DAPI positive nuclei number. Data were expressed as percentage of marker/DAPI ratio ± SEM (* $p < 0.05$).

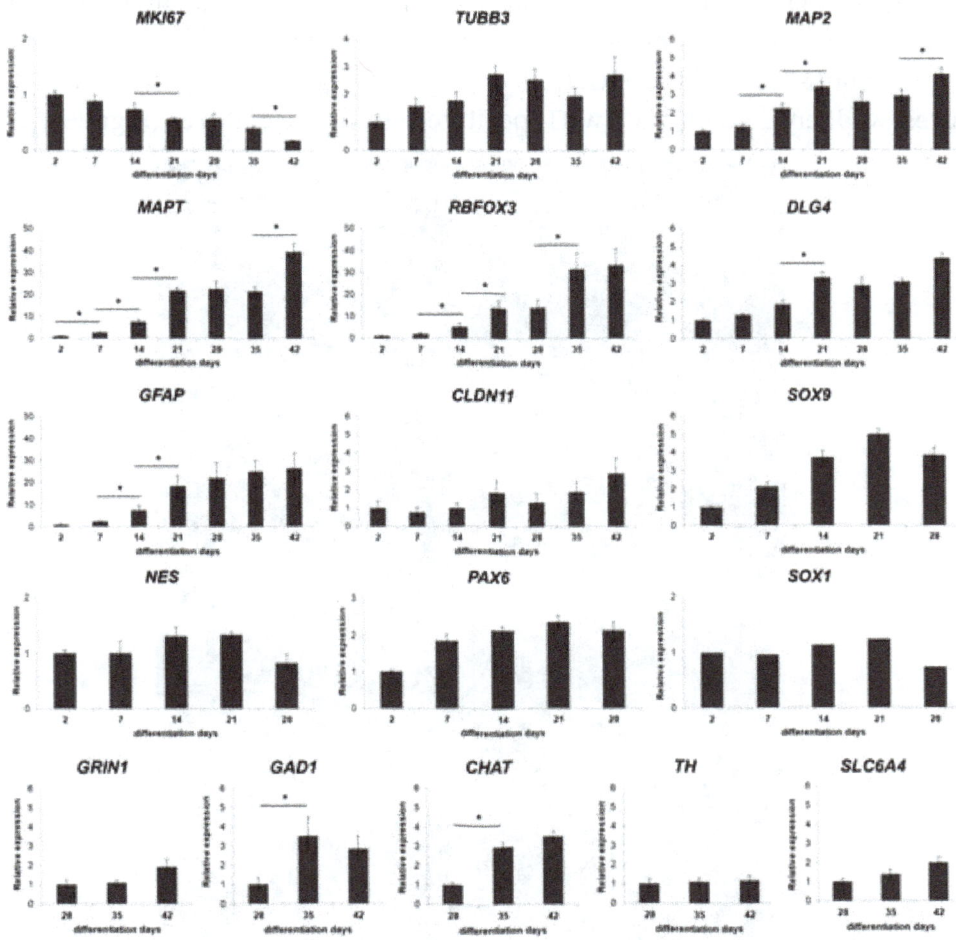

Figure 3. Real-time PCR measurements of relevant markers during the neuronal differentiation of the spheroids. Twelve 3D spheroids were pooled, lysed with RLT-buffer and used in RT-PCR analysis at each timepoints. Where the genes are already expressed in D2 samples, it is referred as 1. Day 2, 7, 14 and 21 values for GRIN1, CHAT, TH, GAD1, and SLC6A4 are not indicated as these genes were not expressed at those time points. Graphs represent normalized relative expression values, analyzed for each gene using the ddCT method [41]. Mean values and ± SEM of three biological replicates (n = 3) are presented on graphs, significance are determined by paired T test (*p < 0.01). Note that y axis's scales alter according to the different relative expression values.

Neuronal subtypes were investigated by the expression of glutamatergic (VGLUT1/2), GABAergic (GAD65/67), cholinergic (VAChT) and dopaminergic (TH) neurons with ICC and qRT-PCR (GRIN1: Glutamate Ionotropic Receptor NMDA Type Subunit 1; GAD1: Glutamate Decarboxylase 1; CHAT: Choline O-Acetyltransferase; TH: Tyrosine Hydroxylase; SLC6A4: Solute Carrier Family 6 Member 4) (**Figure 3** and **Figure 4**). The expression of these markers was detectable mainly from

D28 stage and gradually increased until the last investigated time point of the differentiation (D42), in line with the maturation process. It has to be remarked that the spontaneous differentiation of dopaminergic neurons was rare in the cultures, we identified only a few TH positive cells in the cultures (**Figure 4**).

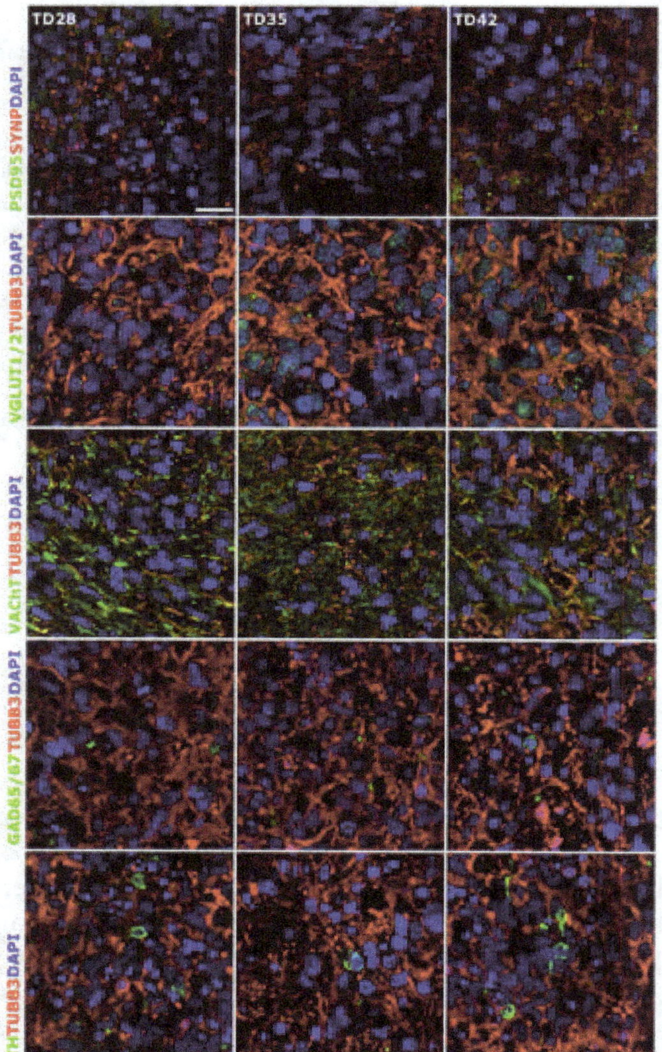

Figure 4. Immunocytochemical detection of neuronal subtypes in 3D neurospheres. Presence of synapses was determined with post-synaptic marker PSD95 and synaptic protein Synaptophysin (SYNP) double staining. Glutamatergic (VGLUT1/2), GABAergic (GAD65/67), cholinergic (VAChT) and dopaminergic (TH) neurons were detected in the developing 3D neurospheres from D28. All samples were stained with TUBB3 (in red) to label the neurites. Protein name IDs are indicated with colors, representing the color of the used fluorophore (e.g., green as Alexa 488; red as Alexa 594). Nuclei were counterstained with DAPI (in blue). Scale bar: 25 μm.

During the neuronal differentiation, astrocytes started to emerge after week 2, based on the Aquaporin-4 (AQP4) or the Glial fibrillary acidic protein (GFAP) expression both at mRNA and protein level (**Figure 2**, **Figure 3**). Oligodendrocyte differentiation followed a similar course, from D21 it was clearly detectable both at transcript (Claudin 11, CLDN11, formerly known as Oligodendrocyte marker 4; **Figure 3**) and protein level (Myelin basic protein, MBP; **Figure 2**A,B) which gradually increased from D35 with the maturation of the cells, however, still remained in a low expression level (**Figure 2**A,B or **Figure 3**). Our ICC results clearly show that the expression of mature neuronal and glial markers and neuron-neuron and neuron-glial interactions increased during the differentiation period, thus emulating the development of the human fetal neural tissue.

The transcript level results aligned with the proteins discovered by ICC, showing the successful differentiation of hiPSC-derived NSCs into brain cells. The 3D neurospheres exhibited a tissue-like differentiation resembling neuronal composition, including neurons, astrocytes, and oligodendrocytes, as confirmed by transcriptomic, proteomic, and ultrastructural analyses. The 3D spheroid technique offers a sophisticated neural cell culture that can be used as a model for early neuronal development.

3.2. Early 3D Neurospheres as a Neurotoxicity Model

We evaluated our 3D spheroid-based model in a cytotoxicity assay to monitor the vitality of cells within the neurospheres. Eleven compounds with well-known effects (drugs, pesticides, and chemicals) were selected and applied on the neurospheres in 7 different concentrations at D21 by acute (72 h) exposure. Concentration-response curves were generated and evaluated. The exposure scheme is presented in **Figure** 5A.

According to the results, Paraquat (PQ; EC50: 1.89 log µM), Rotenone (ROT; EC50: -0.61 log µM), Mercury(II) chloride ($HgCl_2$; EC50: 1.87 log µM) and Doxorubicin (DOX; EC50: 0.67 log µM) caused maximum cell death, Hexachlorophene (HE; EC50: 1.26 log µM) and Colchicine (COL; EC50: -0.49 log µM) had a strong effect on the viability, but did not kill all the cells in the investigated concentration range. Acrylamide (ACR; EC50: 3.5 log µM) and Rifampicin (RIF; EC50: > 2 log µM) also reduced the viability, while Valproic acid (VPA; EC50: > 2.6 log µM) and Paracetamol (PAR; EC50: > 2 log µM) had minimal effect on the viability of 3D neurospheres at D21 stage. Ibuprofen (IBU; EC50: > 2 log µM) as a non-neurotoxic agent was applied as negative control which indeed, did not decrease the viability of D21 3D neurospheres (**Figure** 5B,). Overall, the different compounds induced different levels of cytotoxicity in a concentration-dependent manner on the 3D neurosphere cultures.

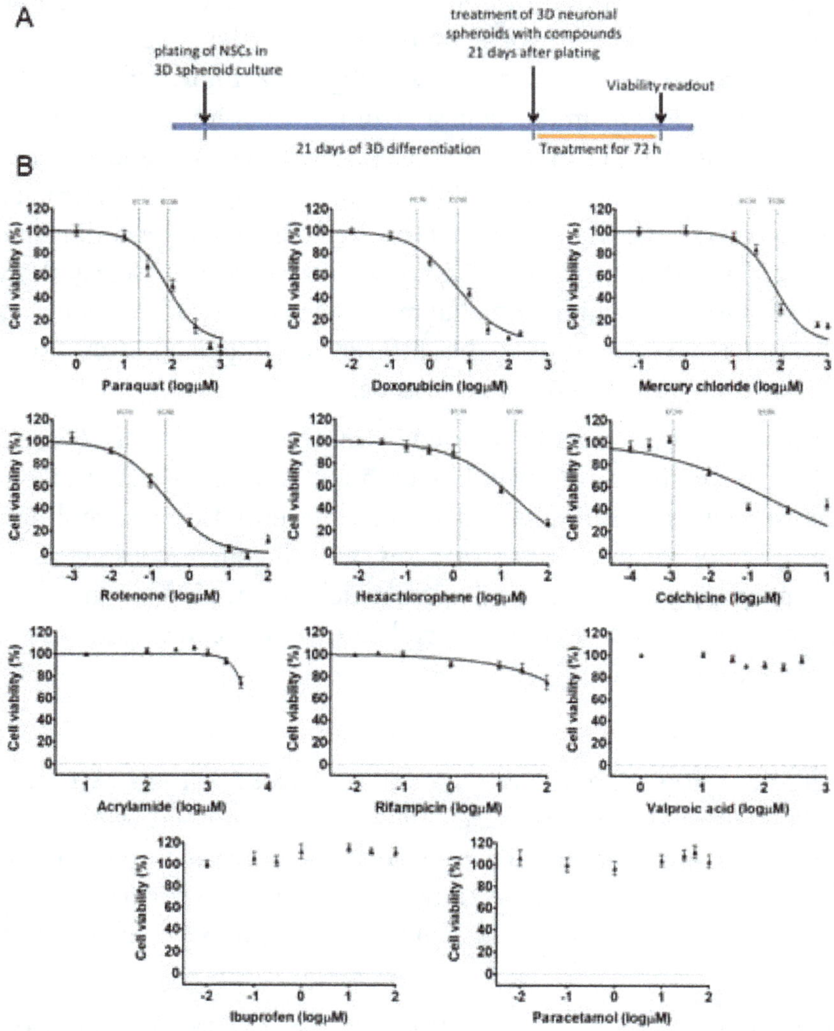

Figure 5. Cell viability measurement on D21 3D neurospheres after 72 h exposure. (**A**) Exposure scheme at D21 stage. (**B**) Concentration response curves of compounds, tested in 7 different concentrations, representing the cell viability (%) of treated D21 3D neurospheres (n = 3). Concentration values are presented in log μM ± SEM. EC10 and EC50 values are presented on graphs where applicable.

3.3. Various stages of differentiation in the cytotoxicity model are represented by neurospheres of different ages.

Next, we investigated the concentration-response of different differentiation stage-derived 3D neurospheres. D28 and D42 samples were analyzed in exposure schemes similar to that of the D21 samples for all the previously tested compounds. As detailed above, in D28 samples differentiated astrocytes expressing GFAP and AQP4 are present (**Figure 2**), axonal outgrowth is prevalent, and neuronal subtype-specific proteins start to appear (**Figure 2, Figure 3** and **Figure 4**). The D42 samples represent a more mature cell culture where synapsis of neurons was formed with established subtypes, mature astrocytes and a few oligodendrocytes are already present (**Figure 2, Figure 4**).

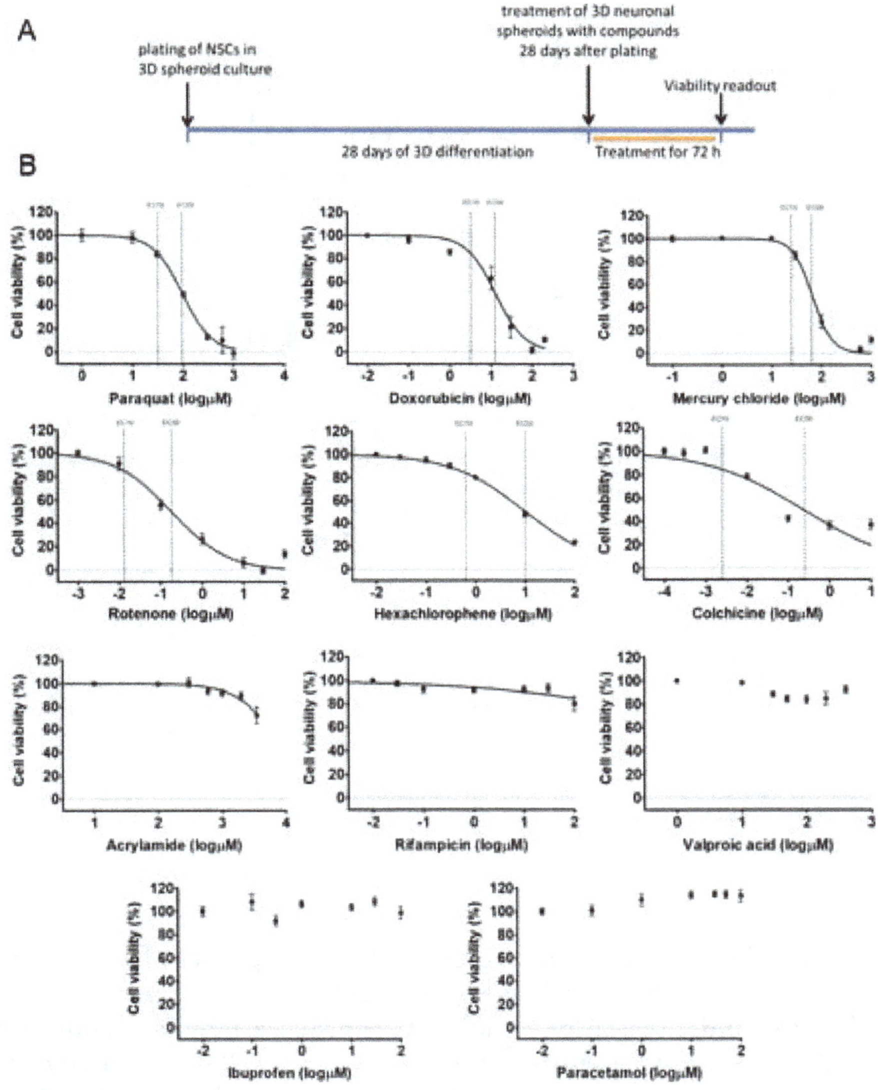

Figure 6. Cell viability measurement on D28 3D neurospheres after 72 h exposure with toxicants. (A) exposure scheme at D28 stage. (B) Concentration-response curves of compounds, tested in 7 different concentrations, representing the cell viability (%) of treated D28 3D neurospheres (n = 3). Concentration values are presented in log μM ± SEM. EC10 and EC50 values are presented on graphs where applicable.

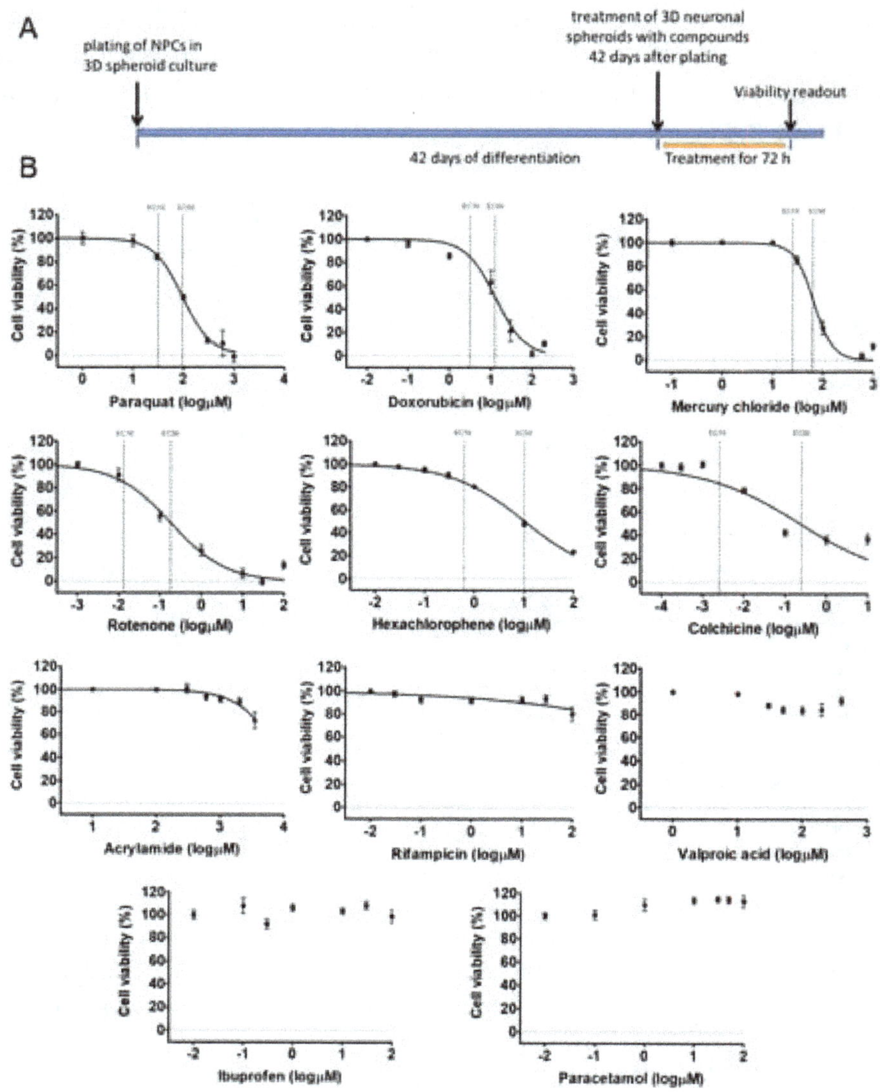

Figure 7. Cell viability measurement on D42 3D neurospheres after 72 h exposure with toxicants. (A) exposure scheme at D42 stage. (B) Concentration-response curves of compounds, tested in 7 different concentrations (see concentrations listed in Table S3), representing the cell viability (%) of treated D42 3D neurospheres (n = 3). Concentration values are presented in log μM ± SEM. EC10 and EC50 values are presented on graphs where applicable.

The results demonstrated that both the D28 and D42 stages are appropriate for conducting viability assays utilizing a 96-well plate format-based analysis without any alterations to the culture system. The EC50 and EC10 values were calculated for D28 and D42 samples for each drug, following the same method used for D21 samples. (**Figure** 6B or **Figure** 7B, **Table S4**). Some compounds (**Figure 5, Figure 6** and **Figure** 7) showed less toxic effect on more matured samples (e.g., ACR:

$EC50^{D21}$ = 4.1 μM vs. $EC50^{D42}$ = 3.6 μM) while it was the opposite action for other compounds (e.g., $HgCl_2$: $EC50^{D21}$ = 1.7 μM vs. $EC50^{D42}$ = 1.9 μM). Based on the data obtained, a concentration-related ranking of the toxicant could be generated for each differentiation stage (**Figure 8, Table S4**).

A

	Ranking of compounds based on EC50 values		
Rank	D21	D28	D42
1	Colchicine	Colchicine	Colchicine
2	Rotenone	Rotenone	Rotenone
3	Doxorubicin	Doxorubicin	Hexachlorophene
4	Hexachlorophene	Hexachlorophene	Doxorubicin
5	Paraquat	Mercury chloride	Paraquat
6	Mercury chloride	Paraquat	Mercury chloride
7	Paracetamol	Paracetamol	Paracetamol
8	Ibuprofen	Ibuprofen	Ibuprofen
9	Rifampicin	Rifampicin	Rifampicin
10	Valproic acid	Valproic acid	Valproic acid
11	Acrylamide	Acrylamide	Acrylamide

B

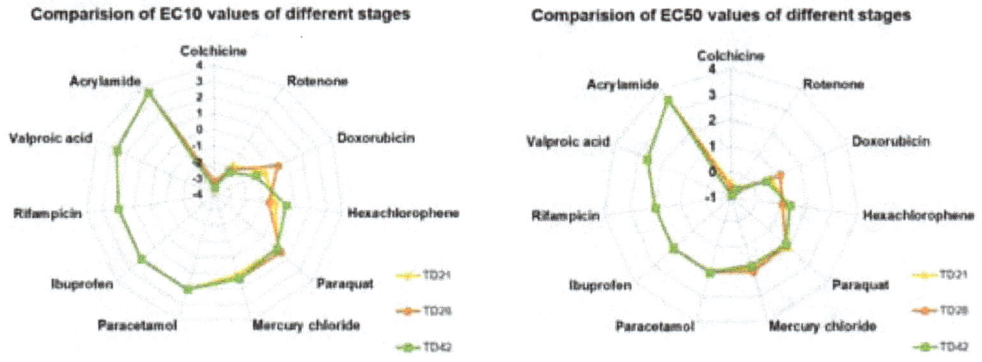

Figure 8. Comparison of the toxic effect of compounds. (A) Ranking of compounds at different differentiation stages based on EC50 values. Darker background color represents higher toxicity, while white color represents non-toxic compounds. (B) Radar chart showing the comparison of compounds based on the order of EC10 or EC50 values, at various differentiation stages (yellow line with rectangular: D21; orange line with circle: D28; green line with square: D42) . Concentration values are presented in log μM.

Ultimately, a concentration-response specific to the chemical was observed in all stages. An observed difference relevant to the differentiation stage indicates that the in vitro system can replicate the varied reactions of growing embryonic human neural tissue to diverse hazardous substances.

3.4. Specific Cellular Events can be Identified in the 3D Neurospheres

An ATP-based viability assay is capable of identifying cell death but is not appropriate for detecting other particular cellular occurrences. Because there are no approved tests for 3D tissues, we opted to study the impact of a harmful substance on a subcellular scale. We have chosen rotenone (ROT), a well-studied neurotoxic compound, known to interfere with the electron transport chain in mitochondria, to investigate the ultrastructure of the cells and especially mitochondria, followed by TEM. In parallel, a TUNEL assay was also applied to detect cell death. Based on the previously determined concentration-response curves and EC50 values, we treated the 3D neurospheres with 0.5 μM ROT for 72 h and analyzed the samples in the 3 differentiation stages.

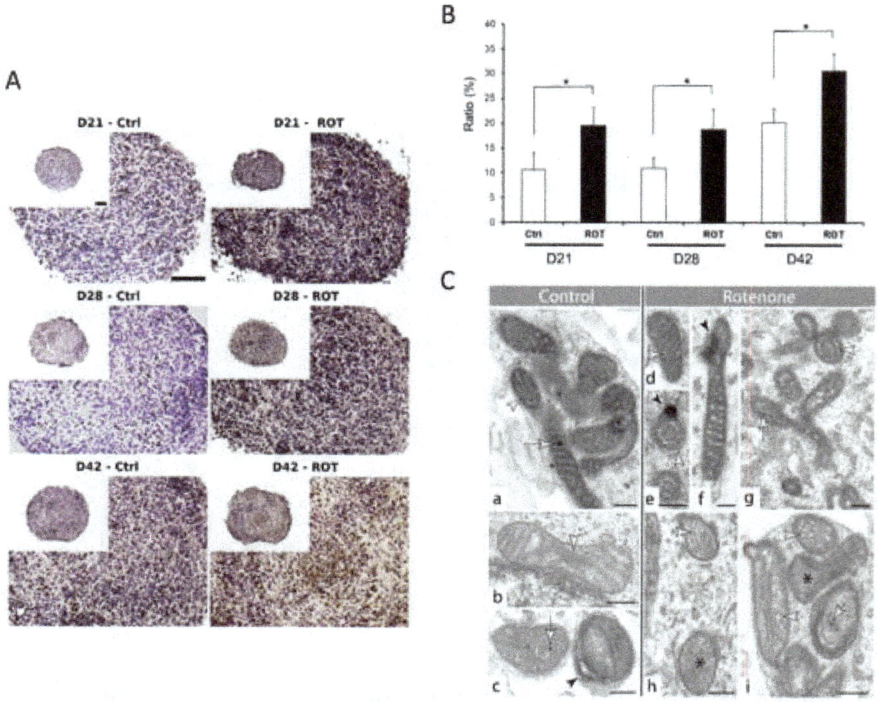

Figure 9. Effect of Rotenone (ROT) exposure on 3D neurospheres at three differentiation stages. (A) 3D neurospheres were treated with 0.5 μM ROT concentration for 72 h at three different maturation timepoints (D21, D28, and D42), fixed, sectioned and analyzed to detect the cellular effect of ROT by TUNEL assay (DeadEnd™ Colorimetric TUNEL System, Promega), compared to the vehicle (0.1% DMSO) treated control (scale bar: 100 μm). (B) ROT treatment revealed in average a 15% increase in the apoptotic cell number compared to the control in each stage (* $p < 0.05$). Average values are presented on graphs (n = 3). (C) Ultrastructure of mitochondria in control (panel a, b, c) and ROT treated (d–i) neurons in the 3D spheroids. See the alteration of the internal membrane (cristae) morphology (white arrowheads) in ROT treated cells (d, e, h, i). Black star: unidentifiable cristae morphology in lighter mitochondria (h, i); black arrowhead: membrane swirl in darker organelles (e, f); white arrows: matrix with and without matrix granules (control cells: a, c; treated cells: g, i) Note the density difference between these granules in control (c) and ROT treated mitochondria (panel i) (D21: a, d, f, h; D28: i; D42: b, c, g) (scale bar: 250 nm).

The data showed that ROT significantly increased the cell death in the spheroids (**Figure 9**A), compared to the vehicle-treated controls (**Figure 9**B), in accordance with the results of the ATP measurement (see **Figure 5**B or **Figure 6**B). Moreover, TEM revealed a change in the ultrastructure of the mitochondrial inner membrane, the cristae: Both shape and complexity were changed in the ROT treated samples, compared to the controls. Two types of mitochondria were detected, often in the same cell. Organelles with darker matrix were usually narrow and elongated, whereas lighter ones were more rounded. In control cells, cristae were straight, narrow, and long in both types. Matrix granules were observable more frequent in darker than in lighter mitochondria (**Figure 9**Ca–c). Effect of rotenone treatment was different on the two types of mitochondria. In darker organelles, cristae swelled and formed swirls. Several wide crista junctions became identifiable. In lighter mitochondria, cristae disintegrated and often became unrecognizable (**Figure 9**Cd–i). Matrix granules disappeared or showed decreased density (**Figure 9**Cc,i).

Finally, we used an ER-stress assay to detect if the observed change is compound-specific or an "overall" cell death event is detected with the ATP or TUNEL assay. The XBP1 assay was performed to identify ER-stress in the ROT treated samples, where ER stress was not expected. As a positive control, tunicamycin was used. The XBP1 assays demonstrated that ROT (using EC50 concentration) has no ER-stress inducing effect in the D21, D28 or D42 neurospheres (**Figure S6B**), while cell death was observed in the cryosectioned ROT-treated samples (**Figure 9**A), providing a strong evidence that compound-specific effects can be determined in 3D spheroids upon treatment. Immunocytochemical investigation reflected some disorganization of the treated group of spheroids compared to the controls, however other marked differences were not observed.

3.5. Neurite Outgrowth Assay Is Appropriate for Evaluating the Impact of Neurotrophic Compounds in the 3D Model.

Functional readouts that link the impact of a tested substance to a certain cell type are crucial for identifying their tissue-specific effect. 3D spheroids are a sophisticated cell culture containing neurons, astrocytes, and oligodendrocytes, which makes it difficult to assess subtle variations in neurite length caused by chemical exposure due to the constraints of existing detection methods. We examined whether neurite growth could be assessed using 3D neurospheres. We found that Matrigel-coated surface sufficiently supports the rapid and strong attachment of free-floating D21 3D neurospheres in order to generate a robust and reproducible procedure, where the effect of toxic compounds on neurite outgrowth can be investigated. The effect of different ROT concentrations were demonstrated comparing the total neurite outgrowth and the average number of neurites/spheroid ratio. ROT administration resulted significantly shorter and decreased number of neurites compared to the untreated and vehicle-treated control groups in all concentration levels in D21 spheroids (** $p < 0.01$) (**Figure 10**B).

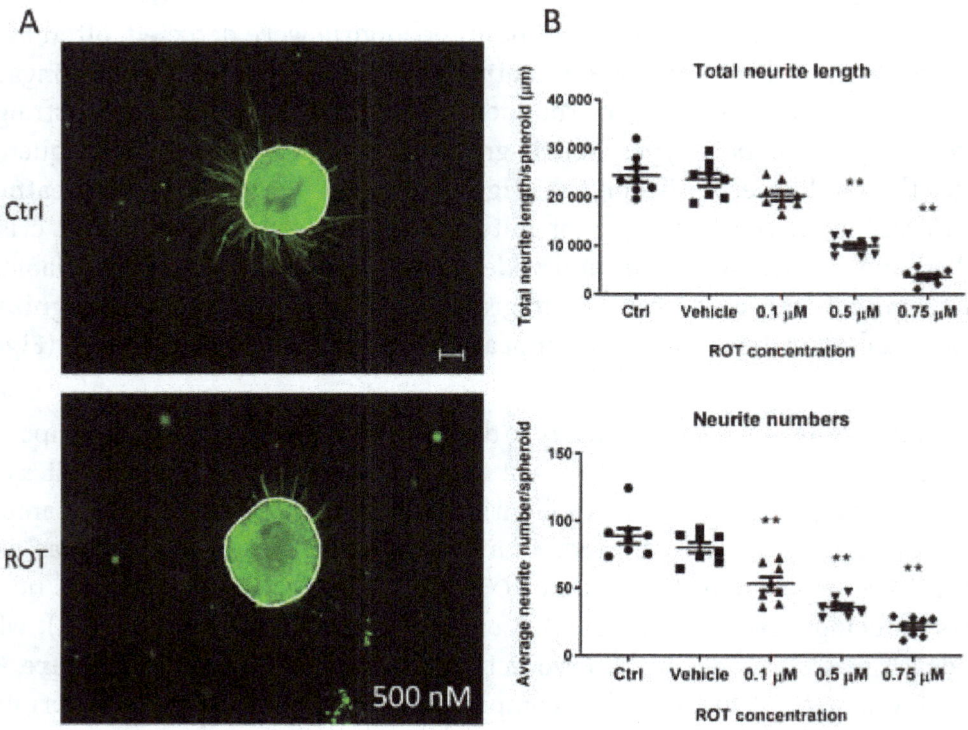

Figure 10. Neurite outgrowth measurement on D21 3D spheroids, exposed for 72 h with ROT. (A) Representative photograph of control (untreated) and ROT (0.5 µM) treated D21 spheroid immunolabeled with TUBB3 (in green). White lines represent the border of the spheroids where the neurite outgrowth was determined from, using ImageJ software (scale bar: 100 µm). (B) Total neurite length/spheroid (presented in µm ± SEM) and the average number of neurites/ spheroids were determined 24 h after plating the treated spheroids. Different symbols denote treatment groups. (n = 3, in each experiment 8 spheroids were treated in each group) ($p < 0.01$).**

4. DISCUSSION

The creation of in vitro platforms for neurotoxicology screenings is motivated by the pressing requirements of the chemical, food, cosmetic, and pharmaceutical sectors. Most neurotoxicity research are conducted in rats or primary cells produced from rodents, which leads to high expenses and less translational relevance of the findings because of interspecies variations. [3,46]. Major international initiatives have started to convert the traditional animal-based neurotoxicity tests to in vitro assays using both mammalian brain cells and human cells to detect and predict chemical hazards [**47,48**]. However, there is only a limited number of human neuronal cell lines (e.g., carcinoma cell lines such as SH-SY5Y; BE2-M17 or immortalized cell lines like LUHMES) are available and hard to obtain primary human CNS tissue suitable for NT studies. Overall, the highly complex structure of the human brain makes in vitro modeling very difficult. Human iPSCs could fill this niche and offer the advantage that other cells and tissue types (e.g., kidney, liver, cardiac, neuronal, intestinal) sharing the same individual genetic background can be created using specific differentiation protocols in a replicable manner. This may provide a very effective in vitro tool for toxicologist for capturing the individual variability in the human population [**49**]. For example, in 2D neurotoxicity screening, the usage of human iPSC derived neuronal cultures, especially the commercially available QC controlled neuron and astrocyte cultures, where the differentiation of iPSCs is not required for the "users", is dynamically increasing [**48**].Recently, several in vitro models have been developed to investigate the human central nervous system in a more natural way. However, the progress in the field of neurotoxicity (NT) and developmental neurotoxicity (DNT) utilizing 3D neuronal tissues has not advanced as quickly as illness or developmental modeling. The challenge is in balancing biological complexity and technical reproducibility, both essential for drug or toxicity screening. [**29**].

Human cell lines were crucial in developing the NT test. The LUHMES immortalized human fetal tissue-derived mesencephalic cell line can be effectively transformed into dopamine-like neurons by administering tetracycline [**50,51**] and provide a suitable system for neurotoxicology screenings [**52,53**] or Parkinson's disease-related drug testing [**54**] both in 2D or 3D cultures [**45,55,56,57**]. Despite the advantages in straightforward handling, they represent only one specific cell type of the CNS. New developments using stem cell-derived astrocytes or microglia in co-culture with LUHMES cells could reveal new potential both in NT and DNT tests [**58**], but also highlight that full-PSC derived systems could provide great advantages over the conventional cell lines. To develop an efficient, highly reproducible neurotoxicology test system, an improved 3D culture of microtissues differentiated from human PSCs would be beneficial. For example, in neuronal disease modeling, a major step that opened new perspectives, was the development of cortical layer-organized 3D brain microtissues, providing a complex system forming under in vitro conditions from human PSCs [**59,60**]. Yet, the limited capacity for high throughput in these intricate systems is a major obstacle for toxicological research currently.

Yet, the limited capacity for high throughput in these intricate systems is a major drawback for toxicological research. Li Huang and his colleagues showed that human brain organoids can be used as an in vitro model for central nervous system drug screening to assess structural, cellular, and molecular alterations. Currently experiencing a bottleneck.They used neurotoxic tranylcypromine in hiPSC-derived brain organoids leading to decreased proliferation activity and apoptosis induction [**61**]. HiPSC-derived cerebral organoids were treated with different concentrations of vincristine for 48 h, and the expansion of the treated organoids was measured, showing concentration-dependent neurotoxicity. Vincristine inhibited fibronectin, tubulin, and MMP10 expression in the cerebral organoids, which was specific for its well-known effect on microtubule dynamics [**62**]. Recently, iPSC-derived cortical neurons and astrocytes were co-cultured in 3D to detect calcium oscillations upon a chemical compound treatment, analyzing multiple parameters, highlighting the potential of such readouts in neurotoxicity assessment [**31**]. Another study has presented a novel 3D heterotypic glioblastoma-brain sphere (gBS) model applied for screening new anti-glioblastoma agents [**63**]. This new application highlighted the flexibility of iPSC-derived platforms to be used in disease modeling, drug testing, and toxicology. In this study, we have analyzed the complexity of our hiPSC-derived 3D neurosphere system demonstrating intensive glial-neuron interaction with the astrocytes and oligodendrocytes present in the neurospheres. Complex characterization was performed with gene expression, protein level analysis in line with immunocytochemical investigations, including morphological evidence of neurocrine communication at the end of the examined period. Morphologically, synapses are composed of precisely opposed pre- and postsynaptic membranes decorated with electron-dense thickening, synaptic cleft filled with a fine meshwork of electron-dense material, and presynaptic vesicles [**64**]. One of the two populations of presynaptic vesicles belong to the active zone matrix, is the docked vesicles [**65**]. The membrane of them is in contact with the presynaptic membrane, therefore they form the readily releasable pool (RRP) of synaptic vesicles. [**66**].

The system displayed resemblances in structure and development characteristics to a prior work involving the creation and analysis of 3D organoids during an 8-week period. [**29**]. In our system, there was no need to use BDNF, GDNF, or a special electrophysiology media; a basal medium was sufficient to promote the differentiation of complex spheroids within 6 weeks of culture. Although the spheroids showed a continuous growth and development/maturation, the homogeneity of the plates was not compromised, both the diameter and total protein content of the spheroids within the 96-well plate showed very low variation at a given time point, represented by the low SEM values (**Figure 1**). Low variability of samples and high homogeneity is crucial when the aim is the development of a reliable HTS for DNT studies. Here, we performed a medium-throughput 96-well plate assay on 3D neurospheres to detect the cytotoxic effect of the selected compounds, based on ATP-release measurements. We tested drugs, pesticides and well-known chemicals with or without neurotoxic effect in different stages of the neuronal differentiation. Our results highlighted a compound-specific and differentiation stage-related effect of the tested chemicals, providing the possibility to determine EC50 and EC10 values for the compounds. For example, colchicine has a strong toxic effect on neurospheres with very similar EC50 values in all differentiation stages. Its effect can be detrimental, it blocks basic cellular (protein assembly, endocytosis, exocytosis, cellular motility, etc.) and neuronal functions at the same time (assembly of tubulin filaments in the microtubules of neurites), which we supposed to happen in all differentiation stages in our neurospheres. A comparable neurotoxic effect was described on iPSC derived 2D cultures of NSCs, neurons, and astrocytes [**67**], and LUHMES cells [**57**]. Comparing EC10 or EC50 values, doxorubicin, for instance, showed that D42 samples were the most sensitive to treatment. Intensive protein synthesis could occur in both neurons and glial cells, affecting processes like neurotransmitter synthesis, axonal growth, and oligodendrocyte maturation. Blocking the transcription machinery could significantly impact cell viability. (see **Table 1** for a summary).

Table 1. Known effects of the used compounds.

Compound Name (CAS Number)	Known Effects of the Compound
Acrylamide 79-06-1	• Water-soluble crystalline amide that polymerizes rapidly; • Widely used in chemical industry (e.g., water treatment industry, paper industry, textile treatment industry) and cosmetics; • Occurs in food upon heat treatment—both during home cooking or industrial processing of food—[**68**];neurotoxic: occupational exposures [**69,70**]; • Could cross the placental barrier and appears in breast milk [**71**]; and • Probable oral lethal human dose is between 50–500 mg/kg.
Colchicine 64-86-8	• Can bind to tubulin and inhibit tubulin polymerization leading to inhibition in mitosis; • Interacts with the P-glycoprotein transporter (MDR1/ABCB1) and the CYP3A4 enzyme (both involved in toxin metabolism) [**72,73**]; • Medication used to treat gout and Behçet's disease; • Probable oral lethal dose in humans is less than 5 mg/kg; and • In vitro cytotoxicity limit: 0.02 μM.

Compound Name (CAS Number)	Known Effects of the Compound
Doxorubicin 25316-40-9	• Intercalating chemotherapy drug; • Inhibiting the movement of topoisomerase II, which leads to the blocking of both replication and transcription; and • LD50: 21.8 mg/kg (rat, subcutaneous).
Hexachlorophene 70-30-4	• Disinfectant; • Blocks the electron transport chain through acting on membrane-anchoring subunit of succinate dehydrogenase (SDHD) and Glutamate dehydrogenase 1, mitochondrial (GLUD1); • Probable oral lethal dose in humans is not determined; LD50: 66 mg/kg (rat, oral); and • In vitro cytotoxicity limit: 1.86 μM.
Ibuprofen 15687-27-1	• Drug (pain killer); • Effectively reduces fever, as a non-steroid anti-inflammatory drug (NSAID), acts on inhibiting cyclooxygenase (COX) enzymes (COX-1 and 2); and • Overdose symptoms appear in individuals consumed more than 99 mg/kg; LD50: 636 mg/kg (rat, oral).
Mercury(II) chloride 7487-94-7	• Component of pesticides; • Corrosive, toxic; • could accumulate in the kidney; • Probable oral lethal dose is 5–50 mg/kg; and • In vitro cytotoxicity limit: 1.37 μM.
Paracetamol 103-90-2	• Drug (pain killer); • Ioverdosing could cause liver toxicity; and • Hepatic toxicity in humans occurred with acute overdoses more than 10 g; LD50: 2400 mg/kg (rat, oral).
Paraquat 75365-73-0	• Herbicide; • Neurotoxic: occupational exposures leading to Parkinson's disease [**74**]; • Widely investigated neurotoxic mechanism [**75,76**]; and • Probable oral lethal dose in humans is 35 mg/kg.
Rifampicin 13292-46-1	• Antibiotic; • Stops RNA synthesis in bacteria; • Could cause liver toxicity; • Robable lethal oral dose in humans is 14–60 gLD50: 1570 mg/kg (rat); and • In vitro cytotoxicity limit: 4.37 μM.

Compound Name (CAS Number)	Known Effects of the Compound
Rotenone 83-79-4	• Pesticide; • Inhibits mitochondrial Complex I of the electron transport chain; • In rats Parkinson's disease- like symptoms were developed, →considered as an environmental risk factor for PD [77]; • Probable lethal dose in human 0.3–0.5 g/kg; and • In vitro cytotoxicity limit: 0.22 μM.
Valproic acid 1069-66-5	• Drug used in epilepsy, bipolar disorders, and for the prevention of seizures; • Known to block voltage-gated sodium channels and increase brain levels of gamma-aminobutyric acid (GABA); • Well-known teratogen induces different congenital malformations and neural tube defects (NTDs); and • LD50: 670 mg/kg (rat, oral).
Note: probable lethal dose data is provided upon PubChem database (**https://pubchem.ncbi.nlm.nih.gov/**), in vitro multicellular cytotoxicity "comptox" data were collected from EPA's Chemical dashboard (**https://comptox.epa.gov/dashboard**).	

Hexachlorophene disrupts the electron transport chain by targeting GLUD1, leading to alterations in the metabolism of the excitatory neurotransmitter glutamate. This phenomenon may account for the varying sensitivity of neurospheres at different stages of differentiation when exposed to a short-term treatment.. Likewise, less cytotoxic effect was reported on iPSC derived 2D cultures of NSCs, early neurons (14 days old) and astrocytes when 10 or 100 μM HE was exposed for 24 h [**67**], while more pronounced cytotoxicity and neurite outgrowth inhibition of LUHMES cells were reported [**57**].

Valproate is classified as a chemical that is positive for developmental neurotoxicity. However, the compound did not have any noticeable effect on cell viability in the tested concentration range. This could be due to the fact that the cells being treated are not in the early stages of neurodevelopment (neural tube stage), but are instead growing neurons and astrocytes. When LUHMES cells were exposed the EC50 value of VPA was determined as >100 μM, and significant inhibition of neurite outgrowth was detected. While the EC50 value was in a similar range with our 3D neurosphere-driven data, we did not investigate its effect on neurite outgrowth. Here, we also have to clarify that cytotoxicity read-out alone is not suitable to predict DNT, although it is suitable to predict the neurotoxic effect of compounds or detect necrosis in differentiating cultures, more relevant end-points (e.g., proliferation, migration, apoptosis, network formation, synaptogenesis, and growth of neurites) must be investigated for evaluating the DNT effect of a compound [**18**]. In the case of pesticide rotenone, which inhibits mitochondrial Complex I of the electron transport chain, strong cell death was detected. The effect of ROT exposure was investigated extensively. In iPSC-derived neuron-astroglia 2D cell cultures the activation of the Nrf2/ARE pathway was documented upon ROT-induced oxidative stress, which led to the activation of astrocytes and cell death of neurons [**67,78,79**]. Using LUHMES cells this robust cytotoxic effect was not obvious while a prominent neurite growth inhibition was reported [**57**]. Using "BrainSpheres" system [**30**], where ICC-based morphology analysis, ROS measurements and viability were compared in different developmental times and exposure schemes, dopaminergic-neuron selective toxicity and general cytotoxic concentration were determined [**30**]. Importantly, increased cell death and mitochondrial dysfunction were detected in our ROT exposed 3D neurospheres, similar to others' results [**30**]. Ibuprofen did not impact neuronal cell viability within the tested concentration range, aligning with previous in vitro and in vivo findings.

Neurite outgrowth assays are well established in conventional 2D neuronal cultures, derived from cell lines, primary tissues, or iPSCs [**57,80,81**], however, the adaptation to 3D cultures is less tested. Determining the radial migration and neuronal density distribution within the migration area of NPCs grown as spheroids is rather described [**27**]. Here we adapted a simple system which provides a tissue-specific functional readout for neurospheres upon exposure, which can be automated using high content imaging (HCI) systems [**45**]. Based on our results, it is sensitive enough to distinguish different concentration of toxic compounds, does not require complicated read-out systems which was proved by testing the effect of ROT, previously confirmed to inhibit neurite growth of LUHMES cells [**57**]. Although these results agree with the reported neurite outgrowth inhibition effect, we cannot exclude the influence of cytotoxicity on the reduction of the overall neurite length we observed. Combining with LDH or lactate sampling, metabolite measurements from the media or terminal transcriptomic or proteomic assays, a complex dataset can be collected, and the effect of a given compound can be investigated systematically on the molecular level, as well to identify adverse effects. Similar to the RT-qPCR and ICC investigation that we used to characterize our 3D neurospheres these methods can be used when the effect of a given compound is investigated. Although we performed immunocytochemistry on treated spheroids using rotenone only, others successfully used such investigations to gain DNT readouts, for example detecting cell migration, neurite outgrowth, Ca^{2+} reabsorption, synaptogenesis, and PPAR pathway disruption [**29,30,57,82,83**].

When assessing our concentration-response findings, we encountered a challenge due to the absence of relevant in vitro human data for comparison. This shows that the absence of EC values and distinct readouts often makes it challenging to compare the different test systems accurately. Table 1 summarizes that human in vitro neurotoxicity values are not available for every chemical due to incomplete databases. Despite several programs and efforts to gather and standardize test methods and assess the data generated, there is still significant work needed in the development of in vitro neurotoxicity test methodologies. [**1**,**16**].

6. AT A GLANCE

We introduce a hiPSC-based 3D in vitro system designed for assessing neurotoxicity (NT). Human induced pluripotent stem cells (iPSCs) were used to create 3D neurospheres in a 96-well plate and monitored over a 6-week period. Alterations in complexity and uniformity were examined using immunocytochemistry and transmission electron microscopy. The transcriptional activity of key developmental, structural, and cell-type-specific indicators was examined weekly to demonstrate the differentiation process of neurons, astrocytes, and oligodendrocytes. Neurospheres were treated with several hazardous substances such as paraquat, acrylamide, and ibuprofen, some of which have neurotoxic effects. The neurospheres were then analyzed at different stages of differentiation using an ATP-based cell viability assay specifically designed for 3D tissues. Concentration responses were studied following a short-term (72-hour) exposure. The particular impact of rotenone was studied using various methods including ER-stress assay, TUNEL assay, immunocytochemistry, electron microscopy, and a 3D-spheroid based neurite outgrowth assay. Exposure to various toxic substances showed different vulnerability patterns based on the stage of development, suggesting that hiPSC-based 3D neurosphere models could be valuable for assessing neurotoxicity and potentially replacing animal models in research and pharmaceutical settings.

REFERENCES

1. Krewski, D.; Acosta, D., Jr.; Andersen, M.; Anderson, H.; Bailar, J.C., 3rd; Boekelheide, K.; Brent, R.; Charnley, G.; Cheung, V.G.; Green, S., Jr.; et al. Toxicity testing in the 21st century: A vision and a strategy. J. Toxicol. Environ. Health Part B Crit. Rev. 2010, 13, 51–138. [Google Scholar] [CrossRef]

2. Tsuji, R.; Crofton, K.M. Developmental neurotoxicity guideline study: Issues with methodology, evaluation and regulation. Congenit. Anom. (Kyoto) 2012, 52, 122–128. [Google Scholar] [CrossRef]

3. Hartung, T. Thoughts on limitations of animal models. Parkinsonism Relat. Disord. 2008, 14, S81–S83. [Google Scholar] [CrossRef] [PubMed]

4. Crofton, K.M.; Mundy, W.R.; Shafer, T.J. Developmental neurotoxicity testing: A path forward. Congenit. Anom. (Kyoto) 2012, 52, 140–146. [Google Scholar] [CrossRef] [PubMed]

5. Bal-Price, A.; Crofton, K.M.; Leist, M.; Allen, S.; Arand, M.; Buetler, T.; Delrue, N.; FitzGerald, R.E.; Hartung, T.; Heinonen, T.; et al. International STakeholder NETwork (ISTNET): Creating a developmental neurotoxicity (DNT) testing road map for regulatory purposes. Arch. Toxicol. 2015, 89, 269–287. [Google Scholar] [CrossRef] [PubMed] [Green Version]

6. Bal-Price, A.; Hogberg, H.T.; Crofton, K.M.; Daneshian, M.; FitzGerald, R.E.; Fritsche, E.; Heinonen, T.; Hougaard Bennekou, S.; Klima, S.; Piersma, A.H.; et al. Recommendation on test readiness criteria for new approach methods in toxicology: Exemplified for developmental neurotoxicity. ALTEX 2018, 35, 306–352. [Google Scholar] [CrossRef]

7. Westerink, R.H. Do we really want to REACH out to in vitro? Neurotoxicology 2013, 39, 169–172. [Google Scholar] [CrossRef]

8. Bal-Price, A.K.; Hogberg, H.T.; Buzanska, L.; Lenas, P.; van Vliet, E.; Hartung, T. In vitro developmental neurotoxicity (DNT) testing: Relevant models and endpoints. Neurotoxicology 2010, 31, 545–554. [Google Scholar] [CrossRef]

9. Sachana, M.; Rolaki, A.; Bal-Price, A. Development of the Adverse Outcome Pathway (AOP): Chronic binding of antagonist to N-methyl-d-aspartate receptors (NMDARs) during brain development induces impairment of learning and memory abilities of children. Toxicol. Appl. Pharmacol. 2018, 354, 153–175. [Google Scholar] [CrossRef]

10. Fritsche, E.; Grandjean, P.; Crofton, K.M.; Aschner, M.; Goldberg, A.; Heinonen, T.; Hessel, E.V.S.; Hogberg, H.T.; Bennekou, S.H.; Lein, P.J.; et al. Consensus statement on the need for innovation, transition and implementation of developmental neurotoxicity (DNT) testing for regulatory purposes. Toxicol. Appl. Pharmacol. 2018, 354, 3–6. [Google Scholar] [CrossRef]

11. Harrill, J.A.; Freudenrich, T.; Wallace, K.; Ball, K.; Shafer, T.J.; Mundy, W.R. Testing for developmental neurotoxicity using a battery of in vitro assays for key cellular events in neurodevelopment. Toxicol. Appl. Pharmacol. 2018, 354, 24–39. [Google Scholar] [CrossRef] [PubMed]

12. Alepee, N.; Bahinski, A.; Daneshian, M.; De Wever, B.; Fritsche, E.; Goldberg, A.; Hansmann, J.; Hartung, T.; Haycock, J.; Hogberg, H.; et al. State-of-the-art of 3D cultures (organs-on-a-chip) in safety testing and pathophysiology. ALTEX 2014, 31, 441–477. [Google Scholar] [CrossRef] [PubMed]

13. Bal-Price, A.K.; Sunol, C.; Weiss, D.G.; van Vliet, E.; Westerink, R.H.; Costa, L.G. Application of in vitro neurotoxicity testing for regulatory purposes: Symposium III summary and research needs. Neurotoxicology 2008, 29, 520–531. [Google Scholar] [CrossRef] [PubMed]

14. Pampaloni, F.; Reynaud, E.G.; Stelzer, E.H. The third dimension bridges the gap between cell culture and live tissue. Nat. Rev. Mol. Cell Biol. 2007, 8, 839–845. [Google Scholar] [CrossRef]

15. F-W Greiner, J.; Kaltschmidt, B.; Kaltschmidt, C.; Widera, D. Going 3D-Cell Culture Approaches for Stem Cell Research and Therapy. Curr. Tissue Eng. 2013, 2, 8–19. [Google Scholar] [CrossRef]

16. Pamies, D.; Hartung, T. 21st Century Cell Culture for 21st Century Toxicology. Chem. Res. Toxicol. 2017, 30, 43–52. [Google Scholar] [CrossRef] [Green Version]

17. Edmondson, R.; Broglie, J.J.; Adcock, A.F.; Yang, L. Three-dimensional cell culture systems and their applications in drug discovery and cell-based biosensors. Assay Drug Dev. Technol. 2014, 12, 207–218. [Google Scholar] [CrossRef] [Green Version]

18. Bal-Price, A.; Pistollato, F.; Sachana, M.; Bopp, S.K.; Munn, S.; Worth, A. Strategies to improve the regulatory assessment of developmental neurotoxicity (DNT) using in vitro methods. Toxicol. Appl. Pharmacol. 2018, 354, 7–18. [Google Scholar] [CrossRef]

19. Smirnova, L.; Hogberg, H.T.; Leist, M.; Hartung, T. Developmental neurotoxicity—Challenges in the 21st century and in vitro opportunities. ALTEX 2014, 31, 129–156. [Google Scholar] [CrossRef] [Green Version]

20. Schmidt, B.Z.; Lehmann, M.; Gutbier, S.; Nembo, E.; Noel, S.; Smirnova, L.; Forsby, A.; Hescheler, J.; Avci, H.X.; Hartung, T.; et al. In vitro acute and developmental neurotoxicity screening: An overview of cellular platforms and high-throughput technical possibilities. Arch. Toxicol. 2017, 91, 1–33. [Google Scholar] [CrossRef] [Green Version]

21. Hofrichter, M.; Nimtz, L.; Tigges, J.; Kabiri, Y.; Schroter, F.; Royer-Pokora, B.; Hildebrandt, B.; Schmuck, M.; Epanchintsev, A.; Theiss, S.; et al. Comparative performance analysis of human iPSC-derived and primary neural progenitor cells (NPC) grown as neurospheres in vitro. Stem Cell Res. 2017, 25, 72–82. [Google Scholar] [CrossRef] [PubMed]

22. Gage, F.H. Mammalian neural stem cells. Science 2000, 287, 1433–1438. [Google Scholar] [CrossRef] [PubMed]

23. Breunig, J.J.; Haydar, T.F.; Rakic, P. Neural stem cells: Historical perspective and future prospects. Neuron 2011, 70, 614–625. [Google Scholar] [CrossRef] [PubMed] [Green Version]

24. Thomson, J.A.; Itskovitz-Eldor, J.; Shapiro, S.S.; Waknitz, M.A.; Swiergiel, J.J.; Marshall, V.S.; Jones, J.M. Embryonic stem cell lines derived from human blastocysts. Science 1998, 282, 1145–1147. [Google Scholar] [CrossRef] [Green Version]

25. Takahashi, K.; Tanabe, K.; Ohnuki, M.; Narita, M.; Ichisaka, T.; Tomoda, K.; Yamanaka, S. Induction of pluripotent stem cells from adult human fibroblasts by defined factors. Cell 2007, 131, 861–872. [Google Scholar] [CrossRef] [Green Version]

26. Qian, X.; Nguyen, H.N.; Song, M.M.; Hadiono, C.; Ogden, S.C.; Hammack, C.; Yao, B.; Hamersky, G.R.; Jacob, F.; Zhong, C.; et al. Brain-Region-Specific Organoids Using Mini-bioreactors for Modeling ZIKV Exposure. Cell 2016, 165, 1238–1254. [Google Scholar] [CrossRef] [Green Version]

27. Schmuck, M.R.; Temme, T.; Dach, K.; de Boer, D.; Barenys, M.; Bendt, F.; Mosig, A.; Fritsche, E. Omnisphero: A high-content image analysis (HCA) approach for phenotypic developmental neurotoxicity (DNT) screenings of organoid neurosphere cultures in vitro. Arch. Toxicol. 2017, 91, 2017–2028. [Google Scholar] [CrossRef]

28. Hogberg, H.T.; Bressler, J.; Christian, K.M.; Harris, G.; Makri, G.; O'Driscoll, C.; Pamies, D.; Smirnova, L.; Wen, Z.; Hartung, T. Toward a 3D model of human brain development for studying gene/environment interactions. Stem Cell Res. Ther. 2013, 4, S4. [Google Scholar] [CrossRef] [Green Version]

29. Pamies, D.; Barreras, P.; Block, K.; Makri, G.; Kumar, A.; Wiersma, D.; Smirnova, L.; Zang, C.; Bressler, J.; Christian, K.M.; et al. A human brain microphysiological system derived from induced pluripotent stem cells to study neurological diseases and toxicity. ALTEX 2017, 34, 362–376. [Google Scholar] [CrossRef] [Green Version]

30. Pamies, D.; Block, K.; Lau, P.; Gribaldo, L.; Pardo, C.A.; Barreras, P.; Smirnova, L.; Wiersma, D.; Zhao, L.; Harris, G.; et al. Rotenone exerts developmental neurotoxicity in a human brain spheroid model. Toxicol. Appl. Pharmacol. 2018, 354, 101–114. [Google Scholar] [CrossRef]

31. Sirenko, O.; Parham, F.; Dea, S.; Sodhi, N.; Biesmans, S.; Mora-Castilla, S.; Ryan, K.; Behl, M.; Chandy, G.; Crittenden, C.; et al. Functional and Mechanistic Neurotoxicity Profiling Using Human iPSC-Derived Neural 3D Cultures. Toxicol. Sci. Off. J. Soc. Toxicol. 2019, 167, 58–76. [Google Scholar] [CrossRef] [PubMed]

32. Chandrasekaran, A.; Avci, H.X.; Ochalek, A.; Rosingh, L.N.; Molnar, K.; Laszlo, L.; Bellak, T.; Teglasi, A.; Pesti, K.; Mike, A.; et al. Comparison of 2D and 3D neural induction methods for the generation of neural progenitor cells from human induced pluripotent stem cells. Stem Cell Res. 2017, 25, 139–151. [Google Scholar] [CrossRef] [PubMed]

33. Zhou, S.; Szczesna, K.; Ochalek, A.; Kobolak, J.; Varga, E.; Nemes, C.; Chandrasekaran, A.; Rasmussen, M.; Cirera, S.; Hyttel, P.; et al. Neurosphere Based Differentiation of Human iPSC Improves Astrocyte Differentiation. Stem Cells Int. 2016, 2016, 4937689. [Google Scholar] [CrossRef] [PubMed] [Green Version]

34. Chambers, S.M.; Fasano, C.A.; Papapetrou, E.P.; Tomishima, M.; Sadelain, M.; Studer, L. Highly efficient neural conversion of human ES and iPS cells by dual inhibition of SMAD signaling. Nat. Biotechnol. 2009, 27, 275–280. [Google Scholar] [CrossRef] [PubMed] [Green Version]

35. Shi, Y.; Kirwan, P.; Livesey, F.J. Directed differentiation of human pluripotent stem cells to cerebral cortex neurons and neural networks. Nat. Protoc. 2012, 7, 1836–1846. [Google Scholar] [CrossRef] [PubMed]

36. Tieng, V.; Stoppini, L.; Villy, S.; Fathi, M.; Dubois-Dauphin, M.; Krause, K.H. Engineering of midbrain organoids containing long-lived dopaminergic neurons. Stem Cells Dev. 2014, 23, 1535–1547. [Google Scholar] [CrossRef]

37. White, D.L.; Mazurkiewicz, J.E.; Barrnett, R.J. A chemical mechanism for tissue staining by osmium tetroxide-ferrocyanide mixtures. J. Histochem. Cytochem. Off. J. Histochem. Soc. 1979, 27, 1084–1091. [Google Scholar] [CrossRef] [Green Version]

38. Rozen, S.; Skaletsky, H. Primer3 on the WWW for general users and for biologist programmers. Bioinform. Methods Protoc. 1999, 132, 365–386. [Google Scholar] [CrossRef] [Green Version]

39. Zuker, M. Mfold web server for nucleic acid folding and hybridization prediction. Nucleic Acids Res. 2003, 31, 3406–3415. [Google Scholar] [CrossRef]

40. Ye, J.; Coulouris, G.; Zaretskaya, I.; Cutcutache, I.; Rozen, S.; Madden, T.L. Primer-BLAST: A tool to design target-specific primers for polymerase chain reaction. BMC Bioinform. 2012, 13, 134. [Google Scholar] [CrossRef] [Green Version]

41. Livak, K.J.; Schmittgen, T.D. Analysis of relative gene expression data using real-time quantitative PCR and the 2(-Delta Delta C(T)) Method. Methods 2001, 25, 402–408. [Google Scholar] [CrossRef] [PubMed]

42. Yoshida, H.; Haze, K.; Yanagi, H.; Yura, T.; Mori, K. Identification of the cis-acting endoplasmic reticulum stress response element responsible for transcriptional induction of mammalian glucose-regulated proteins. Involvement of basic leucine zipper transcription factors. J. Biol. Chem. 1998, 273, 33741–33749. [Google Scholar] [CrossRef] [PubMed] [Green Version]
43. Van Schadewijk, A.; van't Wout, E.F.; Stolk, J.; Hiemstra, P.S. A quantitative method for detection of spliced X-box binding protein-1 (XBP1) mRNA as a measure of endoplasmic reticulum (ER) stress. Cell Stress Chaperones 2012, 17, 275–279. [Google Scholar] [CrossRef] [PubMed] [Green Version]
44. Kobolak, J.; Molnar, K.; Varga, E.; Bock, I.; Jezso, B.; Teglasi, A.; Zhou, S.; Lo Giudice, M.; Hoogeveen-Westerveld, M.; Pijnappel, W.P.; et al. Modelling the neuropathology of lysosomal storage disorders through disease-specific human induced pluripotent stem cells. Exp. Cell Res. 2019, 380, 216–233. [Google Scholar] [CrossRef] [PubMed]
45. Harris, G.; Eschment, M.; Orozco, S.P.; McCaffery, J.M.; Maclennan, R.; Severin, D.; Leist, M.; Kleensang, A.; Pamies, D.; Maertens, A.; et al. Toxicity, recovery, and resilience in a 3D dopaminergic neuronal in vitro model exposed to rotenone. Arch. Toxicol. 2018, 92, 2587–2606. [Google Scholar] [CrossRef] [PubMed] [Green Version]
46. Baumann, J.; Gassmann, K.; Masjosthusmann, S.; DeBoer, D.; Bendt, F.; Giersiefer, S.; Fritsche, E. Comparative human and rat neurospheres reveal species differences in chemical effects on neurodevelopmental key events. Arch. Toxicol. 2016, 90, 1415–1427. [Google Scholar] [CrossRef] [PubMed]
47. Tukker, A.M.; de Groot, M.W.; Wijnolts, F.M.; Kasteel, E.E.; Hondebrink, L.; Westerink, R.H. Is the time right for in vitro neurotoxicity testing using human iPSC-derived neurons? ALTEX 2016, 33, 261–271. [Google Scholar] [CrossRef] [Green Version]
48. Tukker, A.M.; Wijnolts, F.M.J.; de Groot, A.; Westerink, R.H.S. Human iPSC-derived neuronal models for in vitro neurotoxicity assessment. Neurotoxicology 2018, 67, 215–225. [Google Scholar] [CrossRef]
49. Fritsche, E.; Barenys, M.; Klose, J.; Masjosthusmann, S.; Nimtz, L.; Schmuck, M.; Wuttke, S.; Tigges, J. Current Availability of Stem Cell-Based In Vitro Methods for Developmental Neurotoxicity (DNT) Testing. Toxicol. Sci. Off. J. Soc. Toxicol. 2018, 165, 21–30. [Google Scholar] [CrossRef] [Green Version]
50. Lotharius, J.; Falsig, J.; van Beek, J.; Payne, S.; Dringen, R.; Brundin, P.; Leist, M. Progressive degeneration of human mesencephalic neuron-derived cells triggered by dopamine-dependent oxidative stress is dependent on the mixed-lineage kinase pathway. J. Neurosci. Off. J. Soc. Neurosci. 2005, 25, 6329–6342. [Google Scholar] [CrossRef] [Green Version]

51. Scholz, D.; Poltl, D.; Genewsky, A.; Weng, M.; Waldmann, T.; Schildknecht, S.; Leist, M. Rapid, complete and large-scale generation of post-mitotic neurons from the human LUHMES cell line. J. Neurochem. 2011, 119, 957–971. [Google Scholar] [CrossRef] [PubMed]
52. Zuberek, M.; Stepkowski, T.M.; Kruszewski, M.; Grzelak, A. Exposure of human neurons to silver nanoparticles induces similar pattern of ABC transporters gene expression as differentiation: Study on proliferating and post-mitotic LUHMES cells. Mech. Ageing Dev. 2018, 171, 7–14. [Google Scholar] [CrossRef] [PubMed]
53. Hollerhage, M.; Moebius, C.; Melms, J.; Chiu, W.H.; Goebel, J.N.; Chakroun, T.; Koeglsperger, T.; Oertel, W.H.; Rosler, T.W.; Bickle, M.; et al. Protective efficacy of phosphodiesterase-1 inhibition against alpha-synuclein toxicity revealed by compound screening in LUHMES cells. Sci. Rep. 2017, 7, 11469. [Google Scholar] [CrossRef] [PubMed]
54. Zhang, X.M.; Yin, M.; Zhang, M.H. Cell-based assays for Parkinson's disease using differentiated human LUHMES cells. Acta Pharmacol. Sin. 2014, 35, 945–956. [Google Scholar] [CrossRef] [Green Version]
55. Smirnova, L.; Harris, G.; Delp, J.; Valadares, M.; Pamies, D.; Hogberg, H.T.; Waldmann, T.; Leist, M.; Hartung, T. A LUHMES 3D dopaminergic neuronal model for neurotoxicity testing allowing long-term exposure and cellular resilience analysis. Arch. Toxicol. 2016, 90, 2725–2743. [Google Scholar] [CrossRef] [Green Version]
56. Tong, Z.B.; Hogberg, H.; Kuo, D.; Sakamuru, S.; Xia, M.; Smirnova, L.; Hartung, T.; Gerhold, D. Characterization of three human cell line models for high-throughput neuronal cytotoxicity screening. J. Appl. Toxicol. JAT 2017, 37, 167–180. [Google Scholar] [CrossRef] [Green Version]
57. Delp, J.; Gutbier, S.; Klima, S.; Hoelting, L.; Pinto-Gil, K.; Hsieh, J.H.; Aichem, M.; Klein, K.; Schreiber, F.; Tice, R.R.; et al. A high-throughput approach to identify specific neurotoxicants/developmental toxicants in human neuronal cell function assays. ALTEX 2018, 35, 235–253. [Google Scholar] [CrossRef] [Green Version]
58. Brull, M.; Spreng, A.S.; Gutbier, S.; Loser, D.; Krebs, A.; Reich, M.; Kraushaar, U.; Britschgi, M.; Patsch, C.; Leist, M. Incorporation of stem cell-derived astrocytes into neuronal organoids to allow neuro-glial interactions in toxicological studies. ALTEX 2020. [Google Scholar] [CrossRef] [Green Version]
59. Lancaster, M.A.; Renner, M.; Martin, C.A.; Wenzel, D.; Bicknell, L.S.; Hurles, M.E.; Homfray, T.; Penninger, J.M.; Jackson, A.P.; Knoblich, J.A. Cerebral organoids model human brain development and microcephaly. Nature 2013, 501, 373–379. [Google Scholar] [CrossRef]

60. Kadoshima, T.; Sakaguchi, H.; Nakano, T.; Soen, M.; Ando, S.; Eiraku, M.; Sasai, Y. Self-organization of axial polarity, inside-out layer pattern, and species-specific progenitor dynamics in human ES cell-derived neocortex. Proc. Natl. Acad. Sci. USA 2013, 110, 20284–20289. [Google Scholar] [CrossRef] [Green Version]

61. Huang, J.; Liu, F.; Tang, H.; Wu, H.; Li, L.; Wu, R.; Zhao, J.; Wu, Y.; Liu, Z.; Chen, J. Tranylcypromine Causes Neurotoxicity and Represses BHC110/LSD1 in Human-Induced Pluripotent Stem Cell-Derived Cerebral Organoids Model. Front. Neurol. 2017, 8, 626. [Google Scholar] [CrossRef] [PubMed] [Green Version]

62. Liu, F.; Huang, J.; Liu, Z. Vincristine Impairs Microtubules and Causes Neurotoxicity in Cerebral Organoids. Neuroscience 2019, 404, 530–540. [Google Scholar] [CrossRef] [PubMed]

63. Plummer, S.; Wallace, S.; Ball, G.; Lloyd, R.; Schiapparelli, P.; Quinones-Hinojosa, A.; Hartung, T.; Pamies, D. A Human iPSC-derived 3D platform using primary brain cancer cells to study drug development and personalized medicine. Sci. Rep. 2019, 9, 1407. [Google Scholar] [CrossRef]

64. Sudhof, T.C. The presynaptic active zone. Neuron 2012, 75, 11–25. [Google Scholar] [CrossRef] [Green Version]

65. Bell, M.E.; Bourne, J.N.; Chirillo, M.A.; Mendenhall, J.M.; Kuwajima, M.; Harris, K.M. Dynamics of nascent and active zone ultrastructure as synapses enlarge during long-term potentiation in mature hippocampus. J. Comp. Neurol. 2014, 522, 3861–3884. [Google Scholar] [CrossRef] [PubMed] [Green Version]

66. Wang, S.S.H.; Held, R.G.; Wong, M.Y.; Liu, C.; Karakhanyan, A.; Kaeser, P.S. Fusion Competent Synaptic Vesicles Persist upon Active Zone Disruption and Loss of Vesicle Docking. Neuron 2016, 91, 777–791. [Google Scholar] [CrossRef] [PubMed] [Green Version]

67. Pei, Y.; Peng, J.; Behl, M.; Sipes, N.S.; Shockley, K.R.; Rao, M.S.; Tice, R.R.; Zeng, X. Comparative neurotoxicity screening in human iPSC-derived neural stem cells, neurons and astrocytes. Brain Res. 2016, 1638, 57–73. [Google Scholar] [CrossRef] [Green Version]

68. Mottram, D.S.; Wedzicha, B.L.; Dodson, A.T. Acrylamide is formed in the Maillard reaction. Nature 2002, 419, 448–449. [Google Scholar] [CrossRef]

69. Dearfield, K.L.; Abernathy, C.O.; Ottley, M.S.; Brantner, J.H.; Hayes, P.F. Acrylamide: Its metabolism, developmental and reproductive effects, genotoxicity, and carcinogenicity. Mutat. Res. 1988, 195, 45–77. [Google Scholar] [CrossRef]

70. Kjuus, H.; Goffeng, L.O.; Heier, M.S.; Sjöholm, H.; Øvrebø, S.; Skaug, V.; Paulsson, B.; Törnqvist, M.; Brudal, S. Effects on the peripheral nervous system of tunnel workers exposed to acrylamide and N-methylolacrylamide. Scand. J. Work Environ. Health 2004, 21–29. [Google Scholar] [CrossRef] [Green Version]

71. Sorgel, F.; Weissenbacher, R.; Kinzig-Schippers, M.; Hofmann, A.; Illauer, M.; Skott, A.; Landersdorfer, C. Acrylamide: Increased concentrations in homemade food and first evidence of its variable absorption from food, variable metabolism and placental and breast milk transfer in humans. Chemotherapy 2002, 48, 267–274. [Google Scholar] [CrossRef] [PubMed] [Green Version]

72. Mundy, W.R.; Tilson, H.A. Neurotoxic effects of colchicine. Neurotoxicology 1990, 11, 539–547. [Google Scholar] [PubMed]

73. Goldschmidt, R.B.; Steward, O. Comparison of the neurotoxic effects of colchicine, the vinca alkaloids, and other microtubule poisons. Brain Res. 1989, 486, 133–140. [Google Scholar] [CrossRef]

74. Tanner, C.M.; Kamel, F.; Ross, G.W.; Hoppin, J.A.; Goldman, S.M.; Korell, M.; Marras, C.; Bhudhikanok, G.S.; Kasten, M.; Chade, A.R.; et al. Rotenone, paraquat, and Parkinson's disease. Environ. Health Perspect. 2011, 119, 866–872. [Google Scholar] [CrossRef] [PubMed] [Green Version]

75. Rappold, P.M.; Cui, M.; Chesser, A.S.; Tibbett, J.; Grima, J.C.; Duan, L.; Sen, N.; Javitch, J.A.; Tieu, K. Paraquat neurotoxicity is mediated by the dopamine transporter and organic cation transporter-3. Proc. Natl. Acad. Sci. USA 2011, 108, 20766–20771. [Google Scholar] [CrossRef] [PubMed] [Green Version]

76. Kanthasamy, A.; Jin, H.; Charli, A.; Vellareddy, A.; Kanthasamy, A. Environmental neurotoxicant-induced dopaminergic neurodegeneration: A potential link to impaired neuroinflammatory mechanisms. Pharmacol. Ther. 2019, 197, 61–82. [Google Scholar] [CrossRef]

77. Betarbet, R.; Sherer, T.B.; MacKenzie, G.; Garcia-Osuna, M.; Panov, A.V.; Greenamyre, J.T. Chronic systemic pesticide exposure reproduces features of Parkinson's disease. Nat. Neurosci. 2000, 3, 1301–1306. [Google Scholar] [CrossRef]

78. Pistollato, F.; Canovas-Jorda, D.; Zagoura, D.; Bal-Price, A. Nrf2 pathway activation upon rotenone treatment in human iPSC-derived neural stem cells undergoing differentiation towards neurons and astrocytes. Neurochem. Int. 2017, 108, 457–471. [Google Scholar] [CrossRef]

79. Zagoura, D.; Canovas-Jorda, D.; Pistollato, F.; Bremer-Hoffmann, S.; Bal-Price, A. Evaluation of the rotenone-induced activation of the Nrf2 pathway in a neuronal model derived from human induced pluripotent stem cells. Neurochem. Int. 2017, 106, 62–73. [Google Scholar] [CrossRef]

80. Radio, N.M.; Mundy, W.R. Developmental neurotoxicity testing in vitro: Models for assessing chemical effects on neurite outgrowth. Neurotoxicology 2008, 29, 361–376. [Google Scholar] [CrossRef] [Green Version]

81. Ryan, K.R.; Sirenko, O.; Parham, F.; Hsieh, J.H.; Cromwell, E.F.; Tice, R.R.; Behl, M. Neurite outgrowth in human induced pluripotent stem cell-derived neurons as a high-throughput screen for developmental neurotoxicity or neurotoxicity. Neurotoxicology 2016, 53, 271–281. [Google Scholar] [CrossRef] [PubMed]

82. Hellwig, C.; Barenys, M.; Baumann, J.; Gassmann, K.; Casanellas, L.; Kauer, G.; Fritsche, E. Culture of human neurospheres in 3D scaffolds for developmental neurotoxicity testing. Toxicol. Int. J. Publ. Assoc. BIBRA 2018, 52, 106–115. [Google Scholar] [CrossRef] [PubMed]

83. Pamies, D.; Bal-Price, A.; Chesne, C.; Coecke, S.; Dinnyes, A.; Eskes, C.; Grillari, R.; Gstraunthaler, G.; Hartung, T.; Jennings, P.; et al. Advanced Good Cell Culture Practice for human primary, stem cell-derived and organoid models as well as microphysiological systems. ALTEX 2018, 35, 353–378. [Google Scholar] [CrossRef] [PubMed]

04 VERTICAL FUNCTIONALIZED SILICON MICROPILLARS FOR THREE-DIMENSIONAL CULTIVATION OF HUMAN PLURIPOTENT STEM CELL-DERIVED CORTICAL PROGENITORS

1. INTRODUCTION

In biology, developing tissues' microarchitecture is fundamental to allow correct cell differentiation and organization into appropriate structures that relate to specific physiological functions [**1,2**]. Standard in vitro cell culture models are mainly set in reductionist monolayer settings, conditions that intrinsically lack any structural architecture. This condition often represents a poor proxy to extrapolate cell growth in vivo, thus substantially affecting cell performance and biological assays outcomes [**3,4**]. Indeed, with respect to whole tissues, monolayer cultured cells are usually more responsive to toxic or therapeutic agents [**5,6**]. Additionally, cell culture on rigid surfaces can enhance cell proliferation, but might impact cell differentiation due to the partial cell interactions [7].

In this view, more appropriate three-dimensional (3D) cell culture environments can allow more physiological cell-to-cell contact, assisting cell growth and allowing better modelling of developmental processes [**8,9,10**]. A 3D environment also facilitates cells to organize into tissue-like structures that better mimic the in vivo function of cells, thus enhancing physiological relevance and predictive accuracy [**11,12,13,14**]. In the last few years, there has been a gradual development and adoption of technologies that enable tissue-like 3D cultures. Both scaffold-free organoid-based technologies and natural or synthetic scaffold-based culture systems have been developed [7]. In particular, since different tissue types show definite assemblies associated with their functional organization, scaffold-based methods allow assisted mimicking of complex tissue geometrical topographies, such as cerebral cortex, thus facilitating effective biofabrication of in vitro 3D tissue-like models [**15**,**16**,**17**]. With this purpose, silicon-based micro-fabricated culture substrates with well-defined continuous and discontinuous topographies, including the development of surfaces patterned with grooves, nanopillars or nanowires for the study of neural guidance and polarity, have been extensively developed in order to create scaffolds for a variety of applications [**18**,**19**,**20**,**21**,**22**,**23**,**24**].

In the present study, we exploited vertically-aligned silicon micropillar arrays to reproduce the developing cerebral cortex 3D architecture, where effective control over neural columns width, resembling the mammalian neocortex, is required for a large spectrum of applications. In the developing cerebral cortex, cortical progenitors are oriented from the ventricular to the pial surface with an apical-basal polarity. They divide to form radial glia and neuroblasts, the latter can migrate using the apico-basal oriented radial glia fascicles of the subventricular zone (SVZ) as a scaffold, thus forming the different cortical layers [**25**,**26**]. Here we focused on mimicking the radially-oriented cortical radial glia fibers, as they are the key players in controlling the expansion, radial migration and differentiation of cortical progenitors, thus allowing for the establishment of the correct multilayered cerebral cortex structure. We show that the scaffold material and structures are compatible with human cortical progenitors' maintenance. Immunofluorescence imaging analysis and RT-PCR results reveal that silicon vertical micropillar arrays efficiently promote the expansion and stemness preservation of human cortical progenitors, when compared to monolayer growth conditions. Furthermore, the precise orientation of the micropillars allows the radial migration, movement that is distinctive of cortical progenitors in vivo. These results indicate that vertically-aligned silicon micropillar arrays can offer an optimal system for human cortical progenitor growth and migration, and a potentially interesting platform for cortical tissue engineering.

2. MATERIALS AND METHODS

2.1. Vertically-Aligned Silicon Micropillar Array Fabrication

Silicon slides containing vertically-aligned micropillar arrays have been realized on silicon surface through a CMOS like process at the Micro-Nano Facility of Fondazione Bruno Kessler (FBK). The silicon slides are composed of a central zone containing a matrix of vertically-aligned micropillars (height: 250–600 μm). Slides with different micropillar diameters have been obtained, with a diameter of 10 or 15 μm that leads to an aspect ratio that varies from 1:25 to 1:17. These significant proportions are particularly hard to achieve for pillar-like structures. The classical MEMS devices usually have aspect ratio of 1:12, for this reason the Bosch process used to realize the surfaces has been tuned in order to be able to reach higher aspect ratio.

The slide surface used for cellular seeding and culturing is 14 mm long and 5 mm wide these sizes were specifically designed to allow each slide to be accommodated in a well of a 12-well cell culture plate. The design foresees a range of distances between the micropillars, from 20 to 50 μm to evaluate the advantages of smaller and larger spaces between the micropillars for cellular deposition and growth. To realize the structures, the silicon wafer was first oxidized, patterned through soft lithography, then the silicon dioxide (SiO_2) was patterned through dry etching, and finally a deep reactive ion etching (DRIE) process was used to realize the micropillar-like structures. The DRIE process consists of a two-step process: first an isotropic plasma etch, second the deposition of a passivation layer that protects the lateral part of the structure. This two-step process is called Bosch process and it is repeated several times to realize nearly vertical wall. The time lapse of each of the two steps defines the roughness of the vertical wall as the process feed rate while the maximal depth that can be reached is defined by the power of the radio frequency bias that accelerates the ions toward the surface.

Since the fabrication process does not damage the mask, the same stamp can be employed for many subsequent cycles in a very reproducible manner.

During slides production, the micropillars on the open edge of the structures are systematically damaged during the DRIE process. This effect is connected with the presence of a blank space between slides, this void space increments the effective power of the ions impacting on the surfaces and then destroy or modify the shape of the first micropillars row. These defects have been eliminated in the cutting step. The cutting diamond disk was placed over the border, in order to cut away the defected micropillars and leaving a sharp edge.

2.2. Cell Cultures

Human cortical progenitors used in this study were differentiated from a commercial control hiPSC line (Gibco, Thermo Fisher Scientific, Monza, Italy) as previously described [**27,28**]. Briefly, hiPSCs commitment to a neural lineage and subsequently to the dorsal telencephalic lineage was performed by using N2B27 supplemented with human recombinant Noggin (500 ng/mL, Peprotech, London, UK), SB431542 (20 mM, Santa Cruz Biotechnologies, Heidelberg, Germany) and Fibroblast Growth Factor-2 (4 ng/mL, Peprotech). Cells were then detached and seeded on poly-ornithine and laminin-coated plastic dishes (Sigma-Aldrich, Milan, Italy) in medium supplemented with 10 μM Rock inhibitor Y27632 (Sigma-Aldrich).

At day 10, neural rosettes containing cortical progenitor cells were manually collected and plated on poly-ornithine/laminin-treated culture dishes in N2B27 medium containing epidermal growth factor (10 ng/mL), fibroblast growth factor-2 (10 ng/mL) and brain-derived neurothrophic factor (20 ng/mL). Confluent cultures were passed as small multicellular clumps at a ratio of 1:3 using trypsin and amplified until passages 8–10. Cryopreserved stocks of human cortical progenitors were prepared from confluent cultures by trypsinization and resuspension in freezing medium (10% DMSO and 90% foetal calf serum).

Neuronal differentiation of hCPs was induced as previously described. Briefly, hCPs were plated at high density (10^5 cells per cm^2) on laminin-treated silicon vertical micropillar arrays. Cells were allowed to grow for four days and then switched in N2B27 medium without growth factors and cultured for 35 days. The medium was changed every four days.

To visualize the cells for fluorescent imaging analyses and time-lapse experiments, hiPSC-derived cortical progenitors were transduced with a lentiviral vector carrying eGFP cDNA under Cytomegalovirus (CMV) promoter and containing a puromycin selection cassette [**29**].

Procedure for generation and expansion of mouse NS cells (i.e., radial glia-like neural progenitors) were previously described [**30,31,32**]. In this study we used the LC1 NS cell line grown in standard conditions in expansion medium composed of Euromed-N medium (Euroclone) supplemented with 1% N2 (Thermo Fisher Scientific) and 20 ng/mL human recombinant epidermal growth factor (20 ng/mL) and fibroblast growth factor-2 (20 ng/mL).

Human cortical progenitors and mouse NS cells were seeded on silicon slides pre-coated with mouse laminin (Thermo Fisher Scientific).

2.3. Scanning Electron Microscopy (SEM)

Cultures were fixed for 30 min at 4 °C in 25% Glutaraldehyde and 0.1 M cacodylic acid in distilled water (pH 7.2). Then, samples were washed three times with 0.1 M cacodylic acid and dehydrated by the exposure to 50%, 70%, 90% and (2×) 100% v/v ethanol concentration, 10 min each. After being air-dried under an air flow, samples were gold coated by evaporation of a thin gold layer on top of the sample surface (thickness 6 nm, 1.5 nm Cr adhesion layer). Silicon micropillar-based devices deprived of cells did not require any treatment prior to SEM image acquisition. SEM micrographs were acquired by using a TESCAN VEGA III scanning electron microscope (Tescan Analytics, Fuveau, France) (operating voltage 4 kV, working distance 18 mm, stage tilting angle 45°).

2.4. Cell Growth/Viability Assay

Analysis of cell growth/viability of all cell types employed in this work (hCPs and mouse NS cells) was performed by MTT assay (Sigma-Aldrich). Briefly, MTT powder was dissolved into culture medium at a final concentration of 1.5 mg/mL. For culture incubation with MTT solution, cell medium was removed, cultures rinsed twice with PBS (Thermo Fisher Scientific) and incubated with MTT solution for 1h at 37 °C. Following incubation, MTT solution was removed, cells were air-dried and violet MTT precipitates dissolved with isopropanol. The absorbance was read at 570 nm wavelength with a microplate reader (Tecan Infinite M200PRO, Tecan Italia, Milan, Italy).

2.5. Immunocytochemistry

To process samples for immunofluorescence analyses, cultures were fixed in 4% paraformaldehyde for 30 min at room temperature (RT), permeabilized in PBS containing 0.5% Triton X-100 for 15 min at RT and then blocked in blocking solution (PBS containing 0.3% Triton X-100 and 5% FCS) for 1 h at RT. Samples were next incubated overnight at 4 °C with primary antibody diluted in antibody solution (PBS containing 0.2% Triton X-100 and 2% FCS), then washed three times with PBS and incubated for 2 h at RT with secondary antibodies. Samples were then counterstained with 1 µg/mL Hoechst 33,258 (Thermo Fisher Scientific) and further rinsed with PBS before proceeding with visualization. Fluorescent signals and Z-Stack of eGFP^{+ve} human cortical progenitors (12 slices of 7.7 µm each, shown at 7 fps) were detected using a Leica DMi8 microscope equipped with an Andor Zyla 4.2 PLUS, monochromatic, sCMOS sensor, 4.2 megapixel camera. Acquired images were processed with the open-source Fiji software (v2.0.0, open source under the GNU General Public License, Madison, WI, USA) [**33**].

Antibodies used in this study: primary mouse monoclonal anti-NESTIN antibody (R&D Systems, Minneapolis, MN, USA, 1:300), primary mouse monoclonal β3-TUBULIN antibody (Promega, Milan, Italy, 1:1000), primary rabbit polyclonal anti-SOX2 antibody (Millipore, Milan, Italy, 1:200), primary rabbit polyclonal anti-MAP2 antibody (Santa Cruz, Heidelberg, Germany, 1:200), primary mouse monoclonal anti-TBR2 antibody (ABCAM, Cambridge, UK, 1:500), primary mouse monoclonal anti CUX1 (ABCAM, 1:200), AlexaFluor-488 or -568 conjugated secondary antibodies (Thermo Fisher Scientific, 1:500).

2.6. Time Lapse Analysis

Time-lapse movies of live GFP-expressing cells migrating along micropillars were acquired with a Zeiss Axio Observer Z1 inverted microscope equipped with the Apotome 2 module for structured illumination and a 2.83 Megapixel AxioCam 503 mono D (all from Zeiss Italia, Castiglione Olona, Italy). Time-lapses were acquired as z-stacks (10 µm z-step) using a plan-apochromatic 10×/0.3 objective, with a frame interval of 30 min for 12.5 h. The movies shown are maximum intensity projections. Optimal focus selection was performed by manual extraction of each focus z-slices from original z-stack time-lapses to select the best focused z position for each time point, then adjusted for brightness and contrast and saved as 7 fps AVI files using Fiji software [**33**].

2.7. RNA Isolation and Quantitative RT-PCR (qRT-PCR)

Total RNA was isolated by using TRIzol Reagent (Thermo Fisher Scientific) following the manufacturer's protocol, then retro-transcribed with iScript cDNA Synthesis Kit (BioRad, Segrate, Italy). cDNA was used to verify the expression of specific target genes by qRT-PCR (quantitative RT PCR), using the SsoAdvanced Universal SYBR Green Supermix Kit. Specific primers sets were used (RT-qPCR data were analyzed according to the comparative ΔΔCt method and normalized by using β-Actin housekeeping gene. Sequence of primers used in this study:

Nestin forward 5′-GGAGAAGGACCAAGAACTG-3′, reverse 5′-ACCTCCTCTGTGGCATTC-3′; β3-tubulin forward 5′-TCAGCGTCTACTACAACGAGGC-3′, reverse 5′-GCCTGAAGAGATGTCCAAAGGC-3′; β-Actin forward 5′-GACAGGATGCAGAAGGAGATTACTG-3′, reverse 5′-CTCAGGAGGAGCAATGATCTTGAT-3′.

2.8. Statistical Analysis

Analyses were performed using either a two-sided unpaired Student's t-test or a one-way analysis of variance with a Dunnett's post hoc test. Experiments were repeated three times in triplicate and values were considered statistically significant for $p < 0.05$ (*), $p < 0.01$ (**), $p < 0.001$ (***), $p < 0.0001$ (****).

3. RESULTS AND DISCUSSION

3.1. Generation of Vertically-Aligned Silicon Micropillar Array Structures

Biomimetic cortical-like 3D platforms have been created based on different approaches, such as cell spheroids, organoids and engineered constructs based on hydrogels [**34,35,36**]. These structures present advantages based on cell self-assembly or enabling spatial self-organization. Nonetheless fine control over the 3D micro-architecture, phenotype and reproducibility have been reported to be challenging [**37**]. To overcome these limitations, we sought to develop a novel scaffold-based approach mimicking the structural organization of the developing cerebral cortex by ideally controlling network topography.

Mammalian cerebral cortex is a complex layered structure organized in columns generated during developmental stages by means of cortical progenitors (CPs) and neuroblasts that move radially along radial glia fibers serving as scaffolds for directed columnar migration [**25,26**]. Our aim here is to fabricate a 3D culture platform that mimics in vitro these cerebral radial structures, being able to optimally support the outer growth (from the bottom to the top) of CPs such as that occurring in vivo during cortical neurogenesis. With this aim we designed micropatterned structures containing topographically ordered micropillar arrays. Micropatterned substrates with different geometries have been reported in the form of discontinuous micro-grooved configurations and discontinuous geometries like nanopillar arrays made from a several materials comprising polymers, such as PS, PLGA and PDMS together with hard materials, such as silicon and quartz [**18,38,39,40,41**]. In particular, in the neural field pillars and cone geometries at micron scale have been shown to control the outgrowth of neuronal processes, guiding neurite outgrowth alignment and cell growth [**20,38,42,43**].

Here, we produced a novel 3D neural cell culture platform based on silicon substrates displaying arrays of micropillars fabricated by lithographic patterning (see Methods) of crystalline silicon (Si) wafers. Such technique enables the fabrication of discontinuous micropillars exhibiting at the same time anisotropic geometry. The silicon structures consist of a rectangular seeding surface of 0.7 cm^2 containing vertically arranged micropillars (**Figure 1**A,B).

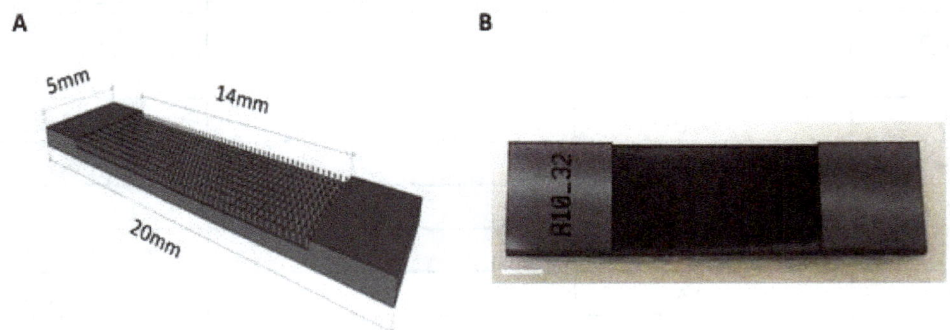

Figure 1. Design, size and morphology of 3D silicon micropillar array slides. (A) Schematic structure of a silicon slide containing vertically-aligned micropillars (micropillars are not in scale). (B) The image shows a 3D silicon slide. Scale bar: 1 mm.

Silicon-based nanostructures exhibit conceivable applications in several fields. As examples, plasmonic nanostructures based on array of silicon nanopillars could be used for surface enhanced Raman spectroscopy (SERS) or to control the wettability of a silicon surface [**44,45,46,47**]. Silicon micropillar arrays can be assembled by lithographic techniques allowing tight control over the size and density of the micropillars, differently from randomly generated rough surfaces as those presented in several other works [**17,43,48,49**]. Accordingly, they allow greatest control over the topographic structure of the system, thus warranting high reproducibility and robustness of the experiments. Additionally, differently from other materials, silicon surfaces hold particular technological impacts and potential.

The size of the slide was specifically designated to easily accommodate in a well of a tissue culture 12-multiwell plate. By varying the reaction conditions of growth, we can produce pillars that have 10–15 µm diameter and height that can be regulated in the range of 200–600 µm. For this study we used silicon slides with 250 µm tall micropillars. Different micropillars topographies were successfully fabricated by using different masks. We produced 12 distinctive layouts of silicon micropillar arrays, coded as A1 to S6, with variable micropillar density and topographies (square grid-aligned and hexa grid-staggered micropillar arrays and with variable distances between the micropillars; see **Table 1**).

Table 1. List of different silicon slide arrays fabricated and tested in this work.

Slide Code	Pillar Diameter (µm)	Distance Among Pillars (µm)	Topography
A1	10	20	Alligned
A2	10	30	Alligned
A3	10	40	Alligned
A4	15	20	Alligned
A5	15	30	Alligned
A6	15	40	Alligned
S1	10	20	Staggered
S2	10	30	Staggered
S3	10	40	Staggered
S4	15	20	Staggered
S5	15	30	Staggered
S6	15	40	Staggered

Additionally, to set up the best conditions for cell growth, we fabricated both oxidized silicon (SiO_2) and silicon nitride (Si_3N_4) vertically-aligned silicon micropillar arrays.

The fabrication accuracy and morphology of the structures at the nanoscale were evaluated by measuring the distance between the micropillars and their diameter by scanning electron microscopy (SEM). Cross-sectional SEM images were produced to derive the internal structure of the samples (**Figure** 2A,B) and top-view SEM images to derive the density of the silicon micropillar arrays.

We found that while the distance between micropillars was quite accurate, the diameter of the micropillars varied depending on the height of the structure. Indeed, the diameters at the bottom of the micropillars were reduced of about 40% (~5–7 µm) with respect to the top of the same micropillar.

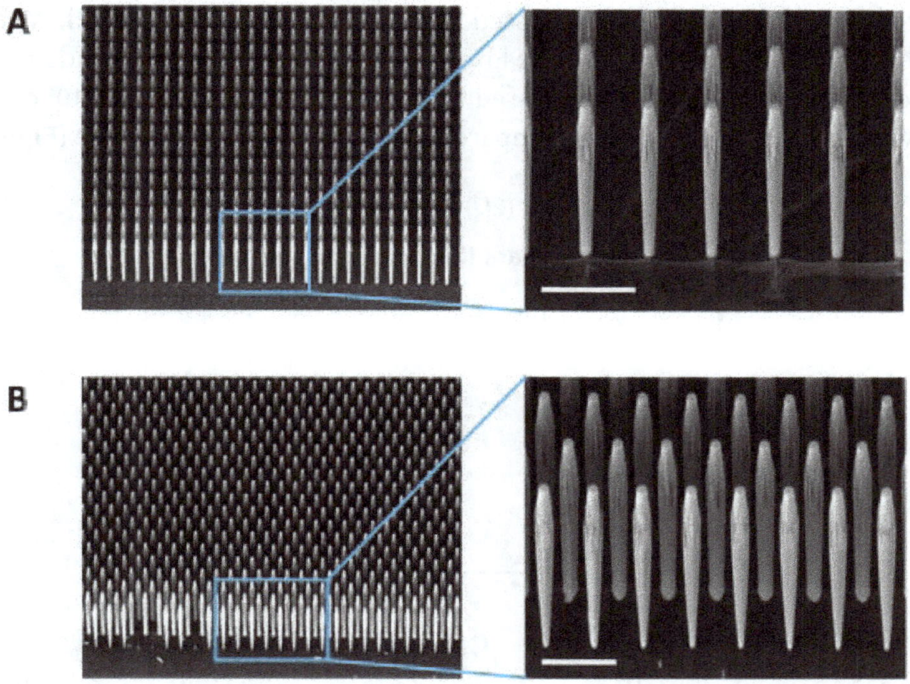

Figure 2. Silicon micropillars can be arranged with different topographies. Silicon micropillar arrays are perfectly vertically-aligned with a height that can be tuned in a 200–600 μm range. Specific spacing, density and morphology of the silicon pillars can be arranged by changing the mask of lithographic process. Low and high magnification of cross-sectional SEM images of aligned (A) and staggered (B) micropillar arrays. Scale bar: 50 μm.

This effect is particularly noticeable on the first row of micropillars, and we assumed that this is mainly due to the fact that the chemical-physical processes on which the Bosch process is based depending on the area exposed to the engraving process. Therefore, the etching rate is different in the areas between the micropillars than in the areas between the slides. Therefore, we assume that the first row of micropillars is etched much faster than the others and that this is the cause of the reduction of the diameter of the micropillar. Up to now, we were able to reach structures with a diameter of 15 μm and a height of 600 μm, nevertheless further tests to improve this aspect ratio are ongoing.

3.2. Culturing Human Cortical Progenitors on Vertically-Aligned Silicon Micropillar Arrays

To establish which human cortical progenitors (hCPs) density was the most comparable to the standard 2D monolayer method used as control and to detect potential toxic effects of silicon material, we first performed a cell viability assay. hCPs were seeded on laminin-coated samples A6–S6 with cell density ranging from 2×10^4 to 8×10^4 cells per 3D device (i.e., 2.8×10^4 and 1.1×10^5 cells per cm^2) and cultured for 48 h before being processed in an MTT assay (see **Section 2**). We found that cell viability was reduced for the lowest cell density (2×10^4 cells) and increased for the highest (8×10^4 cells), compared to the 2D culture. Indeed, 4×10^4 cells per 3D device showed no differences compared to the 2D monolayer culture (**Figure 3**).

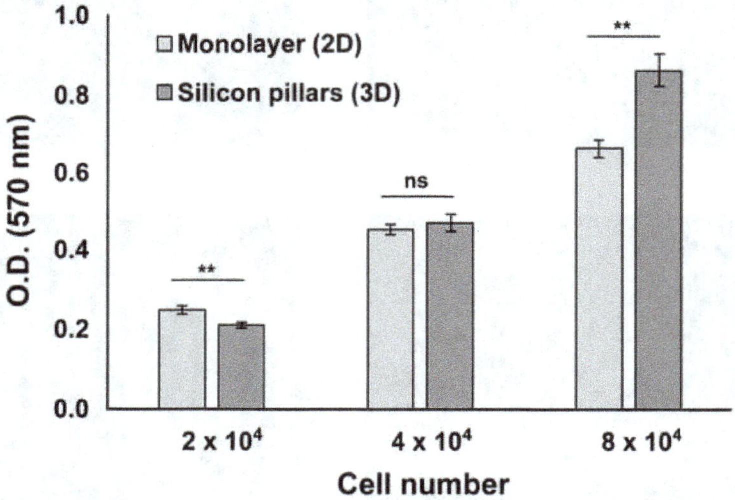

Figure 3. hCPs seeded on silicon micropillar arrays maintain their viability. MTT assay performed on hCPs plated on 3D silicon slide and in standard 2D monolayer shows that hCPs efficiently maintain their viability. Different cell densities were assessed 48 h after seeding. $p < 0.01$ (**), not significant (ns).

We found no significant difference between oxidized silicon or silicon nitride material (not shown), thus indicating that these 3D structures are fully compatible with living cells without affecting cell growth. Moreover, our silicon micropillar arrays might also allow for increased hCPs proliferation activity in long-term cultures by offering a 3D environment in which the cells can also exploit the third (vertical) dimension for growth. Additionally, we did not detect any significant difference between different topographic layouts and silicon types (oxidized silicon or silicon nitride) tested in terms of cell adhesion, viability and growth (not shown).

As further confirmation of these results, an analogous MTT analysis was performed on mouse radial glia-like NS cells plated at the same aforesaid cell densities. NS cell analysis gave similar results to the hCPs, indicating that 4×10^4 cells per 3D device represents the preferred cell density. This was then selected as standard seeding density in the subsequent experiments in this work. The compatibility of oxidized silicon or silicon nitride for in vitro functional studies on neurons has been already reported, nevertheless, this is the first study to report compatibility with hCPs [**50**]. Furthermore, contrary to other studies employing silicon uncoated surfaces, we used surface topographies coated with laminin to optimize cell adhesion as also been reported by others [**51,52,53**]. In addition, these results demonstrate that our silicon micropillar arrays can be functionalized according to the cells' needs. We then performed SEM analysis in order to monitor the behaviour of the hCPs seeded on the arrays in terms of interaction with the vertical silicon micropillars. We found that cells at high density interact with each other and with the micropillars establishing a uniform network (**Figure** 4A).

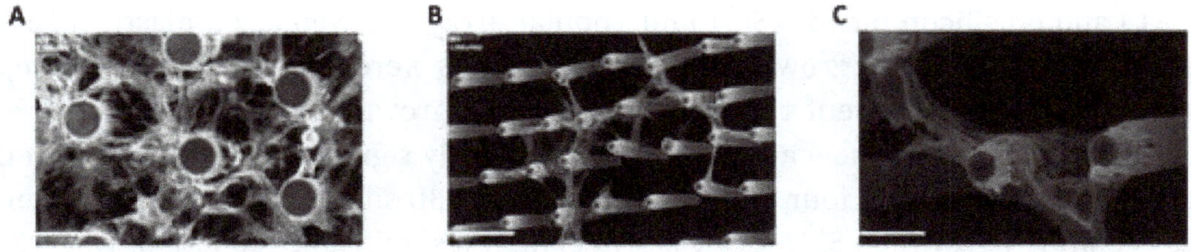

Figure 4. hCPs seeded on silicon slide establish close interactions with micropillars. (A) Top-view SEM image showing hCPs seeded at standard density on silicon micropillars. (B,C) Cross-sectional SEM images showing hCPs seeded at low density on silicon structures to visualize single cells-micropillars interactions. Scale bar: 20 µm (A,B) and 10 µm (C).

Interestingly, hCPs plated at low density show an increased propensity to adhere to the micropillars rather than to the bottom flat surface of the device, with cells that can be found at different heights of the micropillars (**Figure** 4B,C). Cells formed 3D neural networks and suspended bridges throughout the micropillar height and along and between the micropillar walls. A similar formation of suspended neural process bridges has also been reported with microtowers, microfibres and 2PP-DLW fabricated microstructures [**54,55,56,57**]. In order to visualize the cells seeded on the silicon micropillar arrays with an inverted microscope, the device has to be set upside down, facing the microscope objectives. To facilitate this operation, we fabricated, by 3D-printing technique, a slide holder support to be placed on a glass bottom dish that allows to visualize the slide with a tilt of 45 degrees, so as to have a 3D visual prospect of the cells. Also, a glass bottom dish was used to place the holder. To visualize live cultures, we generated eGFP^{+ve} hCPs by infection with lentiviral particles allowing constitutive expression of eGFP cDNA (see Methods). eGFP^{+ve} hCPs were used to live monitor the interactions of hCPs with the device and the single silicon micropillars by time-lapse analysis, and to capture the dynamics of cells movements among the micropillars. We found that hCPs move within the chip and interact with each other and with micropillars. In particular, hCPs can move along the whole micropillar from the bottom to the top (Movie S1) in a manner that resembles the in vivo migration along the radial glia during cortical neurogenesis, and extend processes embracing the micropillars (Movie S2). We also noticed the progressive neurite extension surrounding micropillars at the same height, which might represent the way for the cells to preferentially form a layered architecture.

3.3. hCPs Seeded on Silicon Micropillar Arrays Proliferate and form 3D Layered Structures

We next assessed the proliferation of hCPs seeded on different silicon 3D devices in order to find the silicon type better supporting hCPs stable long-term growth. To this aim, hCPs were plated and maintained for several days on silicon oxide (SiO_2) and on silicon nitride (Si_3N_4) micropillar arrays, as well as on plastic dishes as standard monolayer growth conditions. Cultures were analysed by MTT-based growth assays at different time points. Resulting growth curves from the three experimental groups show a modest, yet statistically significant, reduction in cell growth within the first four days for both types of 3D silicon devices. After seven days cultures grown on Si_3N_4 devices still exhibit a significant reduction, whereas cultures on SiO_2 device show no difference with respect to the standard monolayer conditions. At the later time point considered, 14 days, a statistically significant difference was detected for the cells seeded on SiO_2 3D silicon device, which resulted in increased growth when compared to the other experimental groups (**Figure 5**).

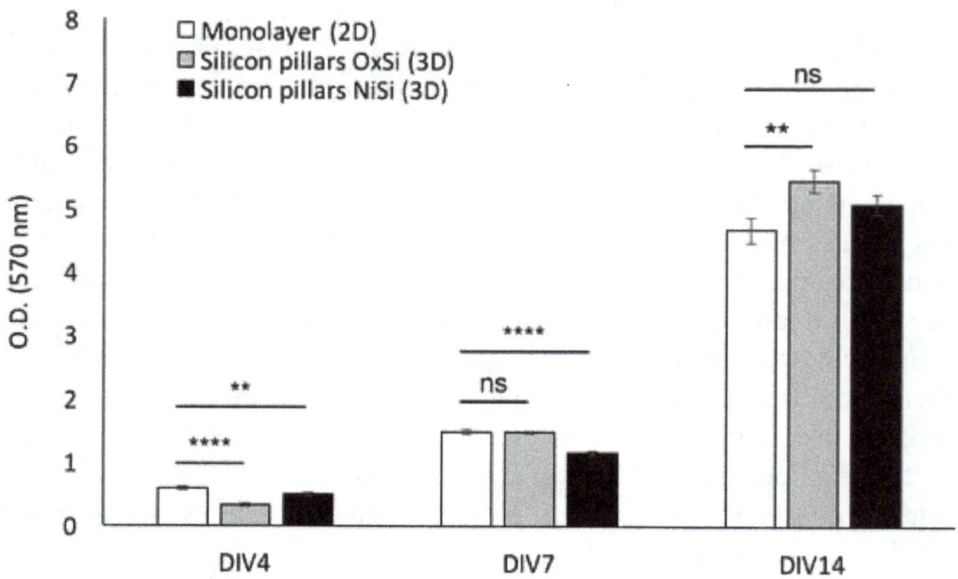

Figure 5. hCPs seeded on silicon slides maintain their proliferation capability. Cell growth analysis (MTT assays) performed on hCPs seeded on oxidized silicon (OxSi) or nitride silicon (NiSi) micropillar arrays. Standard 2D monolayer cultures were used as control. Cultures were assessed at different days in vitro (DIV) after seeding. $p < 0.01$ (**), $p < 0.0001$ (****), not significant (ns).

These results indicate that growth on silicon 3D silicon devices improves hCPs long-term maintenance. Additionally, since oxide silicon 3D arrays resulted to be more compatible and efficient in sustaining hCPs long-term survival and growth with respect with the nitride silicon devices, for the next experiments we employed the former type. Immunofluorescence imaging analysis of hCPs grown on silicon

3D micropillar arrays for two weeks show that cells are well distributed inside the device, filling the whole space among the micropillars (**Figure** 6A).

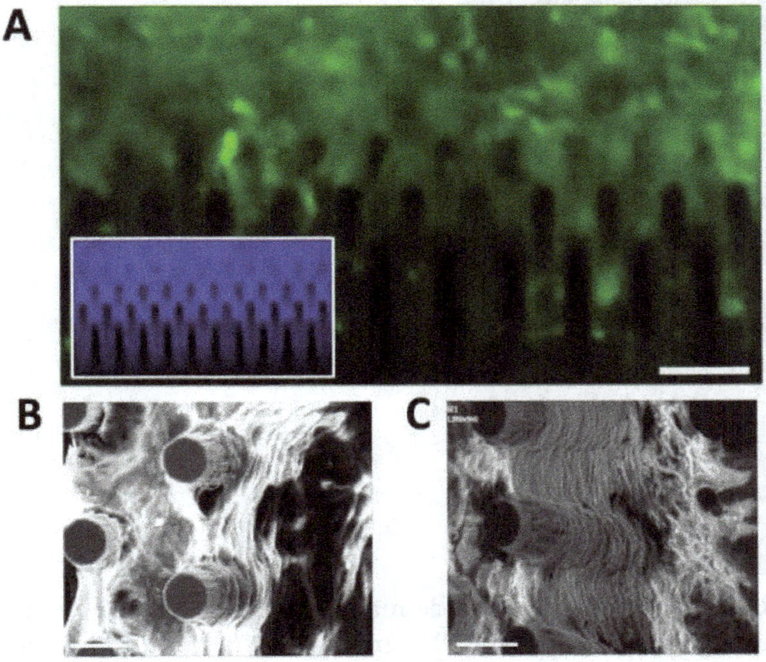

Figure 6. hCPs cultured on silicon micropillar arrays establish layered structures. (A) Picture of eGFP^{+ve} hCPs cultured for 14 days on silicon slides showing the establishment of a high-density 3D culture. Inset shows the same culture stained with Hoechst. (B,C) SEM images of hCPs maintained on silicon pillars device for 14 days. Cultures exhibit the generation of multiple cell layers. Scale bar: 50 µm (A) and 20 µm (B,C).

Additionally, SEM imaging shows that the cells form a complex three-dimensional multilayered-like structure by growing among the micropillars and interacting with each other, finally establishing regular horizontal layers (**Figure** 6B,C).

3.4. Human Chondroprogenitor Cells Cultivated on Silicon Micropillar Arrays Maintain Their Ability to differentiate into many cell types and preserve their specific location-based characteristics

We then assessed if growth on silicon 3D arrays might interfere with hCPs (i) multipotency and (ii) preservation of their cortical regional identity. To assess these issues, we first performed an immunostaining analysis for SOX2 and NESTIN, two key neural multipotent markers, on hCP cultures expanded for 14 days on silicon 3D arrays or in standard monolayer conditions. To this respect, we found that silicon 3D cultures show the great majority of cells to co-express SOX2 and NESTIN, comparably to the cultures maintained in standard monolayer conditions previously characterized to efficiently preserve hCPs multipotency (**Figure 7**A,B).

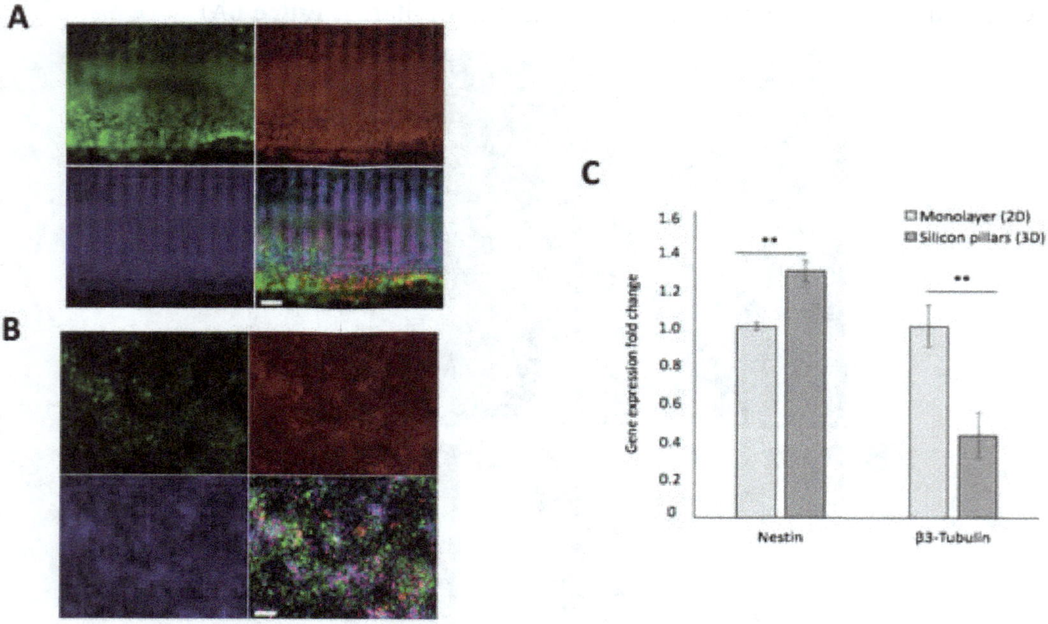

Figure 7. hCPs seeded on silicon slide maintain their neural immature identity. Immunostaining of hCPs for NESTIN (green), SOX2 (red) and nuclear staining with Hoechst (blue) in 3D culture (A) and 2D culture (B) cultured for 14 days. (C) Quantitative RT-PCR assay showing the expression levels of Nestin and β3-Tubulin transcripts in hCPs grown in 2D or 3D cultures. Scale bar: 100 μm (A) and 50 μm (B). $p < 0.01$ (**), not significant (ns).

To extend this result, we measured the transcript levels of Nestin and of the neuronal marker β3-Tubulin by quantitative RT-PCR (**Figure 7**C). This assay showed a 30% increase and a 60% decrease on the expression levels of Nestin and β3-Tubulin, respectively, in cultures maintained on silicon 3D arrays with respect to standard monolayer conditions (**Figure 7**C). These results further confirmed that growth on our silicon 3D devices does not alter hCP's multipotency. Furthermore, growth on silicon 3D arrays further lowers the occurrence of spontaneous neuronal differentiation in the cultures.

We then investigated the capability of hCPs cultured in silicon 3D arrays to retain their original cortical identity. To assess this issue, we first performed an immunostaining analysis for TBR2, a key maker of cortical progenitors, on hCP cultures expanded for 14 days on silicon 3D arrays or in standard monolayer conditions. We found that TBR2 immunoreactivity was maintained in nearly all of the cells in the silicon 3D cultures (**Figure 8**A). Finally, we tested the ability of hCPs plated in silicon 3D arrays to undergo neuronal maturation giving rise cortical glutamatergic neurons. To this end, hCPs were cultured for 5 days on 3D silicon devices and then exposed for 35 days to differentiative conditions and processed for immunofluorescent analysis for β3-TUBULIN, the mature neuronal marker MAP2 and the cortical neuronal marker CUX1. We found that differentiated cultures exhibited the presence of β3-TUBULIN^{+ve} neuronal cells (**Figure 8**B, left panel) and the appearance of neurons co-expressing MAP2 and CUX1 (**Figure 8**B).

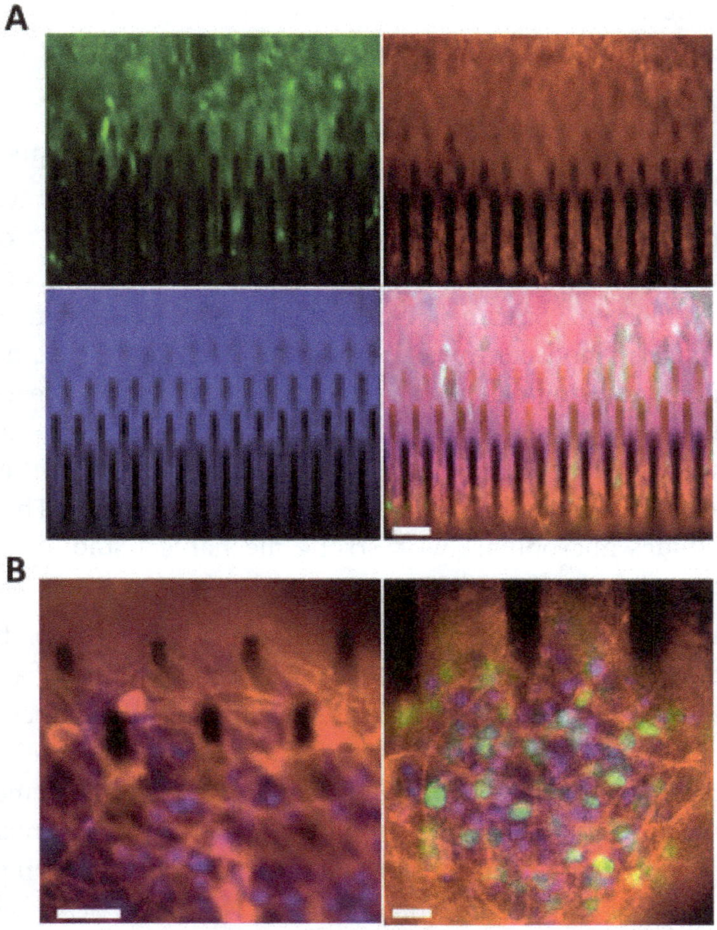

Figure 8. hCPs seeded on silicon micropillar arrays preserve their cortical regional identity and upon exposure to differentiative conditions, generate cortical glutamatergic neurons. (A) eGFP^{+ve} hCPs cultured for 14 days on 3D silicon devices preserve the expression of the cortical progenitor marker TBR2 (red). Nuclei are stained with Hoechst (blue). Scale bar: 50 μm. (B) hCPs cultured for 5 days on 3D silicon devices and then exposed for 35 days to differentiative conditions maturate into cortical glutamatergic neurons. Left: cultures stained for the pan-neuronal neuronal marker β3-TUBULIN (red). Nuclei are stained with Hoechst (blue). Scale bar: 10 μm. Right: cultures stained for the mature neuronal marker MAP2 (red) and for the cortical neuronal marker CUX1 (green). Nuclei are stained with Hoechst (blue). Scale bar: 10 μm.

The results show that human cortical progenitor cells (hCPs) maintained their ability to develop into many cell types and maintain their cortical characteristics when cultivated on silicon micropillar arrays. Additionally, they were able to produce glutamatergic cortical neurons. Additional research are needed to determine if the cortical neurons grown in the 3D environment can arrange themselves into distinct upper and deeper cortical layers.

4. CONCISE SUMMARY

We have detailed a new culture platform for human cardiac progenitor cells (hCPs) development utilizing 3D vertically-aligned silicon micropillar arrays. This design imitates the radially-oriented cortical radial glia fibers that play a crucial role in regulating the expansion, radial migration, and differentiation of hCPs during embryonic development. Silicon micropillar arrays can be organized in various topographic patterns and can measure micropillar heights that have not been previously examined using neural progenitors. The structures created effectively blend the benefits of small-scale surface patterns, without requiring intricate manufacturing methods. Our fabrication technology enables the creation of biocompatible 3D devices with great versatility and consistency. The micrometre-sized base provides micropillars with strong mechanical stability and creates a close connection with the living hCPs.

Other scaffold-based methods have been reported for the biofabrication of in vitro 3D tissue-like models [**15,16,17**]. In particular, some of these systems, especially the ones based on 3D polymeric materials, i.e., microfibres and hydrogel scaffolds, offer a highly useful and strong method for creating large-scale 3D tissue cultures. Additionally, these systems have been shown to be extremely flexible in terms of production, biocompatibility, biodegradability, mechanical properties and functionalization with chemicals or oligopeptides in order to implement their adhesion and/or ECM mimicking properties [**16**]. The 3D vertically-aligned silicon micropillar arrays here described exhibited a lower flexibility with respect to these microfibers and hydrogel scaffolds, nevertheless they represent highly reproducible scaffolds in which both the height and the topography of the pillars can be finely regulated. Similar pillar-like structures have been previously reported by Limongi and colleagues and characterized for their ability to allow culturing of functional neuronal and glial cells in a 3D manner, allowing the formation of viable and functional neuronal networks [**17**]. In particular, the pillars there reported were different from ours since they were designed to reach limited height (cylindrical pillars of 10 μm in height and 10 μm in diameter) and to include a patterning in the nanoscale on their sidewall, leading to a spatial modulation in the z direction. Similarly, culturing platform containing arrays of microchannels arranged into ordered 2D arrays (with maximum height of ~3 μm and amplitudes ranging from

~10 to ~1.5 μm) have been reported [**15**]. These structures were shown to host neuronal cells strongly guiding their axons' growth direction and with additional advantage to enable coupling to devices for active sensing and stimulation at the local scale.

We need to further investigate the true capabilities of our 3D vertically-aligned silicon micropillar arrays in promoting hCPs neuronal maturation to create cortical-like tissue similar to self-assembled brain organoid technology, but with the added benefit of enhanced reproducibility inherent in the scaffold-assisted method. In the future, we plan to enhance the capabilities of our 3D vertically-aligned silicon micropillar arrays by integrating them with a compartmentalized microfluidic device. This integration will allow us to have complete control over the culture environment and minimize medium volumes and associated costs. The knowledge obtained will facilitate the creation of useful tools for studying cortex development in humans and for cortical tissue engineering.

5. AT A GLANCE

Silicon is a favorable material for tissue engineering due to its ability to create micropatterned scaffolding structures that mimic biological tissues. By employing precise fabrication techniques, aligned 3D network architectures can be constructed. In this study, we used vertically-aligned silicon micropillar arrays as culture systems for human induced pluripotent stem cell-derived cortical progenitors. Our goal was to replicate the radial cortical radial glia fibers that are crucial in regulating the growth, migration, and specialization of cortical progenitor cells during embryonic development, which are essential for forming the proper multilayered structure of the cerebral cortex. Our study demonstrates that silicon vertical micropillar arrays effectively enhance the proliferation and maintenance of stemness in human cortical progenitor cells compared to traditional monolayer growth settings. Moreover, the vertically aligned micropillars facilitate the radial migration characteristic of cortical progenitors in their natural environment. The results suggest that vertical silicon micropillar arrays are an ideal method for the development and migration of human cortical progenitors. Moreover, comparable formations offer an appealing foundation for cortical tissue engineering.

REFERENCES

1. Davenport, R.J. What controls organ regeneration? Science 2005, 309, 84. [Google Scholar] [CrossRef] [PubMed] [Green Version]

2. Griffith, L.G.; Swartz, M.A. Capturing complex 3D tissue physiology in vitro. Nat. Rev. Mol. Cell Biol. 2006, 7, 211–224. [Google Scholar] [CrossRef] [PubMed]

3. Vergani, L.; Grattarola, M.; Nicolini, C. Modifications of chromatin structure and gene expression following induced alterations of cellular shape. Int. J. Biochem. Cell Biol. 2004, 36, 1447–1461. [Google Scholar] [CrossRef] [PubMed]
4. Thomas, C.H.; Collier, J.H.; Sfeir, C.S.; Healy, K.E. Engineering gene expression and protein synthesis by modulation of nuclear shape. Proc. Natl. Acad. Sci. USA 2002, 99, 1972–1977. [Google Scholar] [CrossRef] [PubMed] [Green Version]
5. Bhadriraju, K.; Chen, C.S. Engineering cellular microenvironments to cell-based drug testing improve cell-based drug testing. Drug Discov. Today 2002, 7, 612–620. [Google Scholar] [CrossRef]
6. Sun, T.; Jackson, S.; Haycock, J.W.; MacNeil, S. Culture of skin cells in 3D rather than 2D improves their ability to survive exposure to cytotoxic agents. J. Biotechnol. 2006, 122, 372–381. [Google Scholar] [CrossRef]
7. Knight, E.; Przyborski, S. Advances in 3D cell culture technologies enabling tissue-like structures to be created in vitro. J. Anat. 2015, 227, 746–756. [Google Scholar] [CrossRef] [Green Version]
8. Abbott, R.D.; Kaplan, D.L. Strategies for improving the physiological relevance of human engineered tissues. Trends Biotechnol. 2015, 33, 401–407. [Google Scholar] [CrossRef] [Green Version]
9. LaPlaca, M.C.; Vernekar, V.N.; Shoemaker, J.T.; Cullen, D.K. Three-dimensional neuronal cultures. In 3D Tissue Engineering; Berthiaume, F., Morgan, J.R., Eds.; Artech House: Boston, MA, USA, 2010; Chapter 11; pp. 187–204. [Google Scholar]
10. Bercu, M.M.; Arien-Zakay, H.; Stoler, D.; Lecht, S.; Lelkes, P.I.; Samuel, S.; Or, R.; Nagler, A.; Lazarovici, P.; Elchalal, U. Enhanced survival and neurite network formation of human umbilical cord blood neuronal progenitors in three-dimensional collagen constructs. J. Mol. Neurosci. 2013, 51, 249–261. [Google Scholar] [CrossRef]
11. Cukierman, E.; Pankov, R.; Yamada, K.M. Cell interactions with three-dimensional matrices. Curr. Opin. Cell Biol. 2002, 14, 633–639. [Google Scholar] [CrossRef]
12. Mazzoleni, G.; Di Lorenzo, D.; Steimberg, N. Modelling tissues in 3D: The next future of pharmacotoxicology and food research. Genes Nutr. 2009, 4, 13–22. [Google Scholar] [CrossRef] [Green Version]
13. Vinci, M.; Gowan, S.; Boxall, B.; Patterson, L.; Zimmermann, M.; Court, W.; Lomas, C.; Mendiola, M.; Hardisson, D.; Eccles, S.A. Advances in establishment and analysis of three-dimensional tumor spheroid-based functional assays for target validation and drug evaluation. BMC Biol. 2012, 10, 29. [Google Scholar] [CrossRef] [Green Version]

14. Lai, Y.; Cheng, K.; Kisaalita, W. Three-dimensional neuronal cell cultures more accurately model Voltage Gated Calcium Channel functionality in freshly dissected nerve tissue. PLoS ONE 2012, 7, 45074. [Google Scholar] [CrossRef]

15. Cavallo, F.; Huang, Y.; Dent, E.W.; Williams, J.C.; Lagally, M.G. Neurite guidance and three-dimensional confinement via compliant semiconductor scaffolds. ACS Nano 2014, 8, 12219–12227. [Google Scholar] [CrossRef]

16. McNamara, M.C.; Sharifi, F.; Wrede, A.H.; Kimlinger, D.F.; Thomas, D.G.; Vander Wiel, J.B.; Chen, Y.; Montazami, R.; Hashemi, N.N. Microfibers as physiologically relevant platforms for creation of 3D cell cultures. Macromol. Biosci. 2017, 17, 1700279. [Google Scholar] [CrossRef] [Green Version]

17. Limongi, T.; Cesca, F.; Gentile, F.; Marotta, R.; Ruffilli, R.; Barberis, A.; Dal Maschio, M.; Petrini, E.M.; Santoriello, S.; Benfenati, F.; et al. Nanostructured superhydrophobic substrates trigger the development of 3D neuronal networks. Small 2013, 9, 402–412. [Google Scholar] [CrossRef]

18. Johansson, F.; Carlberg, P.; Danielsen, N.; Montelius, L.; Kanje, M. Axonal outgrowth on nano-imprinted patterns. Biomaterials 2006, 27, 1251–1258. [Google Scholar] [CrossRef]

19. Bucaro, M.A.; Vasquez, Y.; Hatton, B.D.; Aizenberg, J. Fine-tuning the degree of stem cell polarization and alignment on ordered arrays of high-aspect-ratio nanopillars. ACS Nano 2012, 6, 6222–6230. [Google Scholar] [CrossRef]

20. Dowell-Mesfin, N.M.; Abdul-Karim, M.A.; Turner, A.M.; Schanz, S.; Craighead, H.G.; Roysam, B.; Turner, J.N.; Shain, W. Topographically modified surfaces affect orientation and growth of hippocampal neurons. J. Neural Eng. 2004, 1, 78–90. [Google Scholar] [CrossRef]

21. Kwiat, M.; Elnathan, R.; Pevzner, A.; Peretz, A.; Barak, B.; Peretz, H.; Ducobni, T.; Stein, D.; Mittleman, M.; Ashery, U.; et al. Highly ordered large-scale neuronal networks of individual cells—Toward single cell to 3D nanowire intracellular interfaces. ACS Appl. Mater. Interfaces 2012, 4, 3542–3549. [Google Scholar] [CrossRef]

22. Yu, M.; Huang, Y.; Ballweg, J.; Shin, H.; Huang, M.; Savage, D.E.; Lagally, M.G.; Dent, E.W.; Blick, R.H.; Williams, J.C. Semiconductor Nanomembrane Tubes: Three-Dimensional Confinement for Controlled Neurite Outgrowth. ACS Nano 2011, 26, 2447–2457. [Google Scholar] [CrossRef] [PubMed] [Green Version]

23. Paul, F.; Huang, Y.; Cangellaris, O.V.; Huang, W.; Dent, E.W.; Gillette, M.U.; Williams, J.C. Toward intelligent synthetic neural circuits: Directing and accelerating neuron cell growth by self-rolled-up silicon nitride microtube array. ACS Nano 2014, 25, 11108–11117. [Google Scholar]

24. Mazzini, G.; Carpignano, F.; Surdo, S.; Aredia, F.; Panini, N.; Torchio, M.; Erba, E.; Danova, M.; Scovassi, A.I.; Barillaro, G. 3D Silicon Microstructures: A new tool for evaluating biological aggressiveness of tumor cells. IEEE Trans. Nanobiosci. 2015, 14, 797–805. [Google Scholar] [CrossRef] [PubMed]

25. McConnell, S.K. Constructing the cerebral cortex: Neurogenesis and fate determination. Neuron 1995, 15, 761–768. [Google Scholar] [CrossRef] [Green Version]

26. Solozobova, V.; Wyvekens, N.; Pruszak, J. Lessons from the embryonic neural stem cell niche for neural lineage differentiation of pluripotent stem cells. Stem Cell. Rev. Rep. 2012, 8, 813–829. [Google Scholar] [CrossRef] [Green Version]

27. Boissart, C.; Poulet, A.; Georges, P.; Darville, H.; Julita, E.; Delorme, R.; Bourgeron, T.; Peschanski, M.; Benchoua, A. Differentiation from human pluripotent stem cells of cortical neurons of the superficial layers amenable to psychiatric disease modeling and high-throughput drug screening. Transl. Psychiatry 2013, 3, 294. [Google Scholar] [CrossRef]

28. Corti, S.; Faravelli, I.; Cardano, M.; Conti, L. Human pluripotent stem cells as tools for neurodegenerative and neurodevelopmental disease modeling and drug discovery. Expert Opin. Drug Discov. 2015, 10, 615–629. [Google Scholar] [CrossRef]

29. Brilli, E.; Reitano, E.; Conti, L.; Conforti, P.; Gulino, R.; Consalez, G.G.; Cesana, E.; Smith, A.; Rossi, F.; Cattaneo, E. Neural stem cells engrafted in the adult brain fuse with endogenous neurons. Stem Cells Dev. 2013, 22, 538–547. [Google Scholar] [CrossRef] [Green Version]

30. Conti, L.; Pollard, S.M.; Gorba, T.; Reitano, E.; Toselli, M.; Biella, G.; Sun, Y.; Sanzone, S.; Ying, Q.L.; Cattaneo, E.; et al. Niche-independent symmetrical self-renewal of a mammalian tissue stem cell. PLoS Biol. 2005, 3, 283. [Google Scholar] [CrossRef] [Green Version]

31. Pollard, S.; Conti, L.; Smith, A. Exploitation of adherent neural stem cells in basic and applied neurobiology. Regen. Med. 2006, 1, 111–118. [Google Scholar] [CrossRef]

32. Pollard, S.M.; Conti, L. Investigating radial glia in vitro. Prog. Neurobiol. 2007, 83, 53–67. [Google Scholar] [CrossRef] [PubMed]

33. Schindelin, J.; Arganda-Carreras, I.; Frise, E.; Kaynig, V.; Longair, M.; Pietzsch, T.; Preibisch, S.; Rueden, C.; Saalfeld, S.; Schmid, B.; et al. Fiji: An open-source platform for biological-image analysis. Nat. Methods 2012, 9, 676–682. [Google Scholar] [CrossRef] [PubMed] [Green Version]

34. Gjorevski, N.; Ranga, N.; Lutolf, M.P. Bioengineering approaches to guide stem cell-based organogenesis. Development 2014, 141, 1794–1804. [Google Scholar] [CrossRef] [PubMed] [Green Version]

35. Kratochvil, M.J.; Seymour, A.J.; Li, T.L.; Sergiu, P.P.; Kuo, C.J.; Heilshorn, S.C. Engineered materials for organoid systems. Nat. Rev. Mater. 2019, 4, 606–622. [Google Scholar] [CrossRef]

36. Seliktar, D. Designing cell-compatible hydrogels for biomedical applications. Science 2012, 336, 1124–1128. [Google Scholar] [CrossRef]

37. Fang, Y.; Eglen, R.M. Three-dimensional cell cultures in drug discovery and development. Slas Discov. 2017, 22, 456–472. [Google Scholar]

38. Simitzi, C.; Efstathopoulos, P.; Kourgiantaki, A.; Ranella, A.; Charalampopoulos, I.; Fotakis, C.; Athanassakis, I.; Stratakis, E.; Gravanis, A. Laser fabricated discontinuous anisotropic microconical substrates as a new model scaffold to control the directionality of neuronal network outgrowth. Biomaterials 2015, 67, 115–128. [Google Scholar] [CrossRef]

39. Yao, L.; Wang, S.; Cui, W.; Sherlock, R.; O'Connell, C.; Damodaran, G.; Gorman, A.; Windebank, A.; Pandit, A. Effect of functionalized micropatterned PLGA on guided neurite growth. Acta Biomater. 2009, 5, 580–588. [Google Scholar] [CrossRef]

40. Rajnicek, A.; Britland, S.; McCaig, C. Contact guidance of CNS neurites on grooved quartz: Influence of groove dimensions, neuronal age and cell type. J. Cell Sci. 1997, 110, 2905–2913. [Google Scholar]

41. Cecchini, M.; Bumma, G.; Serresi, M.; Beltrami, F. PC12 differentiation on biopolymer nanostructures. Nanotechnology 2007, 18, 505103. [Google Scholar] [CrossRef]

42. Hanson, J.N.; Motala, M.J.; Heien, M.L.; Gillette, M.; Sweedler, J.; Nuzzo, R.G. Textural guidance cues for controlling process outgrowth of mammalian neurons. Lab Chip 2009, 9, 122–131. [Google Scholar] [CrossRef] [PubMed] [Green Version]

43. Mattotti, M.; Micholt, L.; Braeken, D.; Kovacic, D. Characterization of spiral ganglion neurons cultured on silicon micro-pillar substrates for new auditory neuro-electronic interfaces. J. Neural Eng. 2015, 12, 026001. [Google Scholar] [CrossRef] [PubMed] [Green Version]

44. Schmidt, M.S.; Hubner, J.; Boisen, A. Large Area Fabrication of Leaning Silicon Nanopillars for Surface Enhanced Raman Spectroscopy. Adv. Mater. 2012, 24, 11–18. [Google Scholar] [CrossRef] [PubMed]

45. Magno, G.; Belier, B.; Barbillon, G. Al/Si Nanopillars as Very Sensitive SERS Substrates. Materials 2018, 11, 1534. [Google Scholar] [CrossRef]

46. Vereecke, G.; Xu, X.M.; Tsai, W.K.; Yang, H.; Armini, S.; Delande, T.; Doumen, G.; Kentie, F.; Shi, X.; Simms, I.; et al. Partial Wetting of aqueous solutions on high aspect ratio nanopillars with hydrophilic surface finish. ECS J. Solid State Sci. Technol. 2014, 3, 3095–3100. [Google Scholar] [CrossRef]

47. Liu, C.; Sun, J.; Li, J.; Xiang, C.; Che, L.; Wang, Z.; Zhou, X. Long-range spontaneous droplet self-propulsion on wettability gradient surfaces. Sci. Rep. 2017, 7, 7552. [Google Scholar] [CrossRef]

48. Park, Y.S.; Yoon, S.Y.; Park, J.S.; Lee, J.S. Deflection induced cellular focal adhesion and anisotropic growth on vertically aligned silicon nanowires with differing elasticity. NPG Asia Mater. 2016, 8, 249. [Google Scholar] [CrossRef] [Green Version]

49. Tullii, G.; Giona, F.; Lodola, F.; Bonfadini, S.; Bossio, C.; Varo, S.; Desii, A.; Criante, L.; Sala, C.; Pasini, M.; et al. High-aspect-ratio semiconducting polymer pillars for 3D cell cultures. ACS Appl. Mater. Interfaces 2019, 11, 28125–28137. [Google Scholar] [CrossRef] [Green Version]

50. Medina Benavente, J.J.; Mogami, H.; Sakurai, T.; Sawada, K. Evaluation of silicon nitride as a substrate for culture of PC12 cells: An interfacial model for functional studies in neurons. PLoS ONE 2014, 9, 90189. [Google Scholar] [CrossRef]

51. Liliom, H.; Lajer, P.; Berces, Z.; Csernyus, B.; Szabò, A.; Pinke, D.; Low, P.; Fekete, Z.; Pongracz, A.; Schlett, K. Comparing the effects of uncoated nanostructured surfaces on primary neurons and astrocytes. J. Biomed. Mater. Res. A 2019, 107, 2350–2359. [Google Scholar] [CrossRef]

52. Fan, Y.W.; Cui, F.Z.; Hou, S.P.; Xu, Q.Y.; Chen, L.N.; Lee, I.S. Culture of neural cells on silicon wafers with nano-scale surface topograph. J. Neurosci. Methods 2002, 120, 17–23. [Google Scholar] [CrossRef]

53. Chen, W.S.; Guo, L.Y.; Tang, C.C.; Tsai, C.K.; Huang, H.H.; Chin, T.Y.; Yang, M.L.; Chen-Yang, Y.W. The effect of laminin surface modification of electrospun silica nanofiber substrate on neuronal tissue engineering. Nanomaterials 2018, 8, 165. [Google Scholar] [CrossRef] [PubMed] [Green Version]

54. Turunen, S.; Joki, T.; Hiltunen, M.L.; Ihalainen, T.O.; Narkilahti, S.; Kellomaki, M. Direct laser writing of tubular microtowers for 3D culture of human pluripotent stem cell-derived neuronal cells. ACS Appl. Mater. Interfaces 2017, 9, 25717–25730. [Google Scholar] [CrossRef] [PubMed]

55. Sharifi, F.; Patel, B.B.; Dzuilko, A.K.; Montazami, R.; Sakaguchi, D.S.; Hashemi, N. Polycaprolactone microfibrous scaffols to navigate neural stem cells. Biomacromolecules 2016, 17, 3287–3297. [Google Scholar] [CrossRef] [PubMed] [Green Version]

56. Timashev, P.S.; Vedunova, M.V.; Guseva, D.; Ponimaskin, E.; Deiwick, A.; Mishchenko, T.A.; Mitroshina, E.V.; Koroleva, A.V.; Pimashkin, A.S.; Mukhina, I.V.; et al. 3D in vitro platform produced by two-photon polymerization for the analysis of neural network formation and function. Biomed. Phys. Eng. Exp. 2016, 2, 035001. [Google Scholar] [CrossRef] [Green Version]

57. Koroleva, A.; Gill, A.A.; Ortega, I.; Haycock, J.W.; Schilie, S.; Gittard, S.D.; Chichkov, B.N.; Claeyssens, F. Two-photon polymerization-generated and micromolding-replicated 3D scaffolds for peripheral neural tissue engineering applications. Biofabrication 2012, 4, 025005. [Google Scholar] [CrossRef]

05 HUMAN BONE MARROW MESENCHYMAL STEM CELLS EXPRESS TENDON AND CYTOKINE MARKERS IN A HYALURONATE/POLY-LACTIC-CO-GLYCOLIC ACID (PLGA)/FIBRIN THREE-DIMENSIONAL (3D) SCAFFOLD.

1. INTRODUCTION: AN OVERVIEW

Tissue engineering approaches for tendon healing and regeneration aim to enhance current treatments or offer novel therapeutic options. 3D bioengineered systems can enhance our comprehension of tendinopathy physiopathology and the involvement of stem cells in tendon regeneration. 3D scaffold design and construction, combined with specialized bioreactor setups, could create advanced 3D in vitro culture and differentiation systems to study how cells respond to specific external biochemical and mechanical cues. [**1**]. The 3D scaffold provides a model of fidelity via its provision of a microenvironment with defined stiffness and elastic modulus as well as the necessary surfaces for cell attachment [**2,3,4**].Detailed understanding of cell behavior when incorporated into specific biomaterials allows to develop designs with specific functionalization. These functionalization may, for instance, stimulate local stem cells, attract specific circulating nucleated blood cells, such as macrophages, and induce their polarization into M2 phenotype to accelerate tissue regeneration and healing following the biomaterials in vivo implantation [**5**]. For example, human Mesenchymal Stem Cells (hMSCs) are largely used in tissue engineering strategies, and their immune-modulatory activity in the development of tendon pathologies have been explored, but the precise mechanisms involved remain undetermined [**6,7,8,9,10**]. Neutrophils and macrophages enter damaged tendons, possibly interacting with MSCs and triggering cytokine release to aid in repair. They help break down the extracellular matrix, cause inflammation, and cell death. In the later stages of tendon healing, they release anti-inflammatory cytokines to reduce inflammation and support tendon restructuring. [**11,12,13**].

Among the biomaterials described for tendon tissue engineering [**14**], a promising emerging strategy is the use of a complex biomimetic matrix with a hydrogel component and extracellular matrix mimicking properties [**15,16**]. Tenocyte precursors can be harvested from different sources, including periosteum [**17,18**], bone marrow [**19,20,21**], tendon [**21,22**], and adipose tissue [**21,23**]. To overcome the intrinsic poor mechanical properties of the hydrogel, they can be merged with more force resistant biopolymers. Cells and biomaterials alone are not sufficient to achieve optimal levels of differentiation and matrix organization. Mechanical stimulation has a key role in tenogenic differentiation induction [**19**]. Scaffolds are therefore required to display an appropriate elastic behavior to deliver strain [**24**] or compression [**25**] inputs. Strain is a tenogenic differentiation signal [**26,27,28,29**], and several bioreactors have been used to impart tenogenic mechanical stimuli to cells in culture [**19,30,31,32,33,34,35**]. For example, Rinoldi et al. designed and fabricated 3D multilayered composite scaffolds, where an electrospun nanofibrous substrate was coated with a thin layer of GelMA-alginate composite hydrogel carrying MSCs. MSCs were subsequently differentiated by the addition of bone morphogenetic protein 12 (BMP-12) and, to mimic the natural function of tendons, the scaffolds were mechanically stimulated using a custom-built bioreactor [**34**]. Grier et al. described an aligned collagen-glycosaminoglycan scaffold able to enhance tenogenic differentiation of MSCs via cyclic tensile strain within a bioreactor, in the absence of growth factor supplementation [**36**]. Another protocol, proposed by Youngstrom et al., promoted tenogenic differentiation of MSCs cultivated on decellularized tendon scaffolds with the application of 3% cyclic strain for one hour per day for 11 days [**31**]. Additionally, several growth factors and other small molecules can stimulate transcriptional activation of genes involved in tenogenic differentiation [**15,37,38**]. Growth Differentiation Factor 5 (GDF-5), for instance, induces the expression of genes linked to the neo-tendon phenotype [**39,40,41**].

Tendinopathies associated with physical activity and age-related degeneration are a major medical issue [**23**], and recent healing and regeneration studies include the use of human Bone Marrow Mesenchymal Stem Cells (hBM-MSCs) [**42,43,44**]. hBM-MSCs are a multipotent population present in bone marrow that can be readily differentiated in vitro [**45,46**] into cells of three mesodermal lineages, namely adipocytes, chondrocytes and osteoblasts under appropriate conditions [**47,48,49,50**]. MSCs-based therapies include direct transplantation of MSCs populations, growth factor-loaded scaffolds for local MSCs recruitment or implantation of scaffolds containing in vitro culture-expanded MSCs populations

[51,52]. We previously described an engineered multiphase three-dimensional (3D) scaffold as an in vitro model for tendon regeneration studies. The multiphase 3D construct was totally absorbable and consisted of a braided hyaluronate elastic band merged with a fibrin hydrogel containing hBM-MSCs and poly-lactic-co-glycolic acid nano-carriers (PLGA-NCs) themselves loaded with human Growth Differentiation Factor 5 (hGDF-5) [**53**]. In that work, the PLGA nano-carriers were transient scaffold components to ensure sustained and controlled delivery of hGDF-5 with benefits beyond those associated with standard culture medium supplementation [**53,54**]. The study found that human bone marrowderived mesenchymal stem cells showed an early commitment to becoming tendons following three days of culture in dynamic settings..

This work explores the impact of a scaffold called HY-FIB on hBM-MSCs in a 3D environment for 11 days, with or without mechanical stimulation, and without any specific biochemical differentiation signal.. HY-FIB was assembled with hBM-MSCs as previously described [**53**] including PLGA-NCs stratified within the 3D fibrin structure. Importantly, the PLGA-NCs carried an inactive form of human Growth Differentiation Factor 5 (ihGDF-5) enabling the overall 3D scaffold structure to be safely evaluated with or without mechanical input. Gene expression of type 1 Collagen, decorin, scleraxis, and tenomodulin were considered; type 3 collagen was also monitored, as negative control. Histology and quantitative immunofluorescence were used to monitor cell behavior and their interaction with the synthetic extracellular matrix. Moreover, to understand whether HY-FIB microenvironment configuration would stimulate any cell inflammation responses, the cells expression of cytokine markers was also monitored, including pro-inflammatory cytokines and anti-inflammatory ones. The results provide strong evidence that HY-FIB environment plus mechanical signaling, promoted tenogenic markers expression, collagen production and better pro-repair cytokine balance by hBM-MSCs.

2. MATERIALS AND METHODS

2.1. hBM-MSCs Isolation and Harvesting

Human bone marrow mesenchymal stem cells (hBM-MSCs) were obtained from the bone marrow of three independent healthy donors (age 36, 38, 44 years). The donors gave written informed consent in accordance with the Declaration of Helsinki to the use of their filter residual bone marrow aspirate for research purposes, with approval from the University Hospital of San Giovanni di Dio e Ruggi d'Aragona (Salerno, IT). Review Board authorization number: (24988 achieved on April 9, 2015).

Briefly, total bone marrow aspirate was directly seeded at a concentration of 50,000 total nucleated cells/cm^2 in T75 plastic flask in Minimum Essential Medium Alpha (α-MEM) supplemented with 1% Glutagro™, 10% Fetal Bovine Serum (FBS), and 1% Pen/Strep and incubated at 37 °C in 5% CO_2 atmosphere and 95% relative humidity [55]. After 72h, non-adherent cells were removed by medium change, and the adherent cells were further fed twice a week with new medium. On day 14, colonies of adherent hBM-MSCs were detached and re-seeded at 4000 cells/cm^2 in the same culture conditions. Once the cell cultures reached 70–80% confluence, cells were detached using 0.05% trypsin-0.53mM EDTA and washed with PBS 1× (Corning Cellgro, Manassas, VA, USA), counted using Trypan Blue (Sigma-Aldrich, Milan, IT) and subcultured at a concentration of 4 × 10^3 cells/cm^2. Flow Cytometry analysis was performed on hBM-MSCs obtained at Passage 1 examining levels of CD90, CD105, CD73 CD14, CD34, CD45, and HLA-DR expression (Miltenyi Biotec, DE).

2.2. ihGDF-5 Effect on hBM-MSCs

These sets of experiments were performed to assure the absence of any effect of inactivated human GDF-5 (ihGDF-5, Cloud-Clone Corp., USA) on both tenogenic markers stimulation and cytokines expression by hBM-MSCs. Cells were seeded on coverslips in 12 well plates at a concentration of 4 × 10^3 cells/cm^2. Once the cultures reached 60% confluence, cells were treated with either 1.6 ng/mL or 100 ng/mL of ihGDF-5. Cells were fed twice a week with new medium and fresh ihGDF-5 supplementation for up to 16 days. Untreated cells for matched time-points studied were used for control purposes. Passage 3 cells were seeded in the 3D environment (~8 × 10^5 cells/mL) and were fed twice a week with new medium, without any growth factor added.

PLGA carriers were not tested because they cannot be supplemented to the cells planar monolayer culture, indeed, in static conditions their sedimentation on cells reduced oxygen exchange and prevented cells survival (data not shown).

2.3. Immunofluorescence and immunohistochemical assays

Cells were fixed with 3.7% formaldehyde for 30 min at room temperature (RT) followed by permeabilization with 0.1% Triton X-100 for 5 min and blocking with 1% Bovine Serum Albumine (BSA) for 1h. For type 1 and type 3 Collagen staining, cells were incubated overnight at 4 °C with a mouse monoclonal anti-type 1 Collagen antibody (1:100, Sigma-Aldrich) and a rabbit polyclonal anti-type 3 Collagen antibody (1:100, Santa Cruz Biotechnology). Following incubation with the primary antibody, cells were incubated for 1h at RT with the DyLight 649 anti-mouse IgG (1:500, BioLegend, CA) and the Alexa FluorTM 488 goat anti-rabbit IgG (1:500; Thermo Fisher Scientific, USA). Cell nuclei were stained with DAPI solution (1:1000) for 5 min. Images acquisition was at 20× magnification on a fluorescent microscope (Eclipse Ti-E Inverted Microscope; NIKON Instruments Inc., USA).

For 3D scaffold immunohistochemical analysis, slices were permeabilized with 0.1% Triton X-100 for 5 min, and non-specific staining blocked with 1% BSA for 1h at RT. For type 1 Collagen staining, slices were incubated overnight at 4 °C with a rabbit polyclonal anti-type 1 Collagen antibody (1:200, AbCam). Following incubation with the primary antibody, slices were incubated for 1h at RT with Alexa Fluor™ 488 goat anti-rabbit IgG (1:400, Thermo Fisher Scientific, USA) antibody. Subsequently, cell nuclei were stained with DAPI solution (1:1000) and incubated for 5 min. Images were acquired as described above. Image quantification was performed using image analysis software (ImageJ, National Institutes of Health, USA) [56,57] by measuring the red and green areas where type 1 and type 3 collagen, respectively, are expressed. A minimum of 10 image fields was used for the image analysis at each time point. Signal intensity at each time point was normalized by the cell number (e.g., by amount of cell nuclei revealed by DAPI staining).

Sirius red staining was performed using the Picrosirius Red Stain Kit (Polysciences, Inc., USA). Sections of 15 μm of thickness were stained in hematoxylin for 8 min, then washed in water for 2 min. The sections were dipped into phosphomolybdic acid for 2 min, then washed in water for 2 m. Then they were dipped into Picrosirius Red F3BA Stain for 60 min and dipped into HCl 0.1M solution for 2 min. The sections were dehydrated in increasing ethanol gradient solutions (70–75–95–100%) and finally dipped into xylene for 5 min. Eukitt medium was used to mount the samples.

2.4. RNA Isolation and Gene Expression Profile by Quantitative Reverse Transcription PCR (RT-qPCR)

Total RNA was extracted from hBM-MSCs seeded into the 3D construct of each experimental group using QIAzol® Lysis Reagent (Qiagen, DE), chloroform (Sigma-Aldrich, Milan, IT) and the RNeasy Mini Kit (Qiagen, DE). For each sample, 300 ng of total RNA was reverse-transcribed using the iScriptTM cDNA synthesis kit (Bio-Rad, Milan, IT). Relative gene expression analysis was performed in a LightCycler® 480 Instrument (Roche, IT), using the SsoAdvancedTM Universal SYBR® Green Supermix (Bio-Rad) with the validated primers for COL1A1, COL3A1, DCN, IL-1β, IL-6, IL-10, IL-12A, SCX-A, TGF-β1, TNF, and TNMD (Bio-Rad), and following MIQE guidelines [58]. Amplification was performed in a 10 μL final volume, including 2 ng of complementary DNA (cDNA) as template. Specificity of the formed products was addressed via melting curve analysis. Triplicate experiments were performed for each condition explored, and data were normalized to glyceraldehyde-3-phosphate dehydrogenase (GAPDH) expression (reference gene), applying the geNorm method [59] to calculate reference gene stability between the different conditions (calculated with CFX Manager software; M <0.5). Fold changes in gene expression were determined by the $2^{-\Delta\Delta Cp}$ method, and are presented as relative levels versus hBM-MSCs just loaded within the HY-FIB system.

2.5. PLGA-NCs Fabrication, Size, Morphology, and ihGDF-5 Release Profile

PLGA nano-carriers were produced using Supercritical Emulsion Extraction (SEE) technique, which allows for fast manufacture of polymer nano-carriers by extracting the oily phase organic solvent with dense gas in a countercurrent packed tower operating continuously. [**60**]. In detail, ihGDF-5 (Cloud-Clone Corp., USA) was dissolved into 1% (w/v) human serum albumin (hSA; Sigma-Aldrich, Milan, IT) containing 0.06% polyvinyl alcohol (PVA). Human serum albumin (hSA) was included as an ihGDF-5 stabilizer. This solution was added to the oily phase formed in an Ethyl Acetate (EA, purity 99.9%) and PLGA (RG 504H, 38,000–54,000 kDa, Evonik, DE) at 5% (w/w) solution. All emulsions were processed immediately after their preparation.

SEE technology operative pressure and temperature conditions in the high-pressure column were set at 8 MPa and 38 °C, respectively, with a dense gas flow of Carbon Dioxide (CO_2) set at 1.4 kg/h with Liquid/Gas ratio of 0.1 (w/w) [**61**]. Carrier suspensions were collected at the bottom of the extraction column, washed, and lyophilized. Each run allowed the recovery of 98% of the loaded biopolymer. Empty and loaded NCs were produced using the same process conditions.

Carrier particle size distributions (PSDs) were measured using a laser granulometer (mod. Mastersizer S; Malvern Instruments Ltd., Worcestershire, UK), based on dynamic light scattering (DLS). Sizes are expressed as volume mean size (MS) with standard deviation (SD) in nanometers (nm). The shape and morphology of the PLGA-NCs were investigated by field emission-scanning electron microscopy (FE-SEM; mod. LEO 1525; Carl Zeiss, Oberkochen, D). Samples were placed on a double-sided adhesive carbon tape previously glued to an aluminum stub and coated with a gold film (250 A thickness) using a sputter coater (mod.108 A; Agar Scientific, Stansted, UK). ihGDF-5 release profile was monitored in vitro from 20(±0.3) mg of carriers suspended in 1mL of α-MEM, placed in an incubator at 37 °C, and stirred continuously at 1× g. Every 24 h, samples were centrifuged at 160× g for 10 min and the supernatant completely removed and replaced with fresh media to maintain sink conditions. Released ihGDF-5 concentrations from collected samples were then measured with an Enzyme Linked Immunosorbent Assay (ELISA, Cloud-Clone Corp., USA). Release experiments were performed in triplicate (n = 3), and the curve describing the mean profile calculated as ng/g (protein released/PLGA-NCs) versus time.

2.6. HY-FIB Preparation and Characterization

For each sample, a mixture of 50 mg/mL fibrinogen from human plasma (Sigma-Aldrich, Milan, IT), 15,600 U/mL aprotinin (Sigma-Aldrich, Milan, IT), and α-MEM (Corning, NY, USA) supplemented with 10% FBS (referred to as growing media,

GM) was added at a 1:1:1 ratio to 100 mg of PLGA-NCs (ihGDF-5 loading: 350 ng/g) and, then, to an average of 8 × 10^5 cells. A homogeneous cells/PLGA-NCs/fibrinogen suspension was then embedded into a mold (30 × 20 × 4.5 mm) where the braided band had been previously positioned. Free ends were left to enable HY-FIB fixing into the bioreactor. Upon addition of 100 U/mL thrombin (Sigma-Aldrich, Milan, IT), the mold was placed in a 37 °C humidified incubator for 30 min to allow fibrin polymerization. When the hydrogel was formed, the band was entrapped inside a uniformly distributed hydrogel. The construct was then transferred from the mold to either a standard polystyrene culture plate or to the bioreactor culture chamber, each containing 30 mL of the culture media, and placed in an incubator at 37 °C in a 5% CO_2 atmosphere and 95% relative humidity.

HY-FIB morphology was observed by field emission-scanning electron microscopy (FE-SEM; mod. LEO 1525; Carl Zeiss, Oberkochen, Germany). Samples were fixed in 4% PFA (4 °C, overnight) and then dehydrated by multiple passages across ethanol:water solutions (10 min each) with increasing concentrations of ethanol (10%, 20%, 30%, 50%, 70%, 90%), ending in a 100% dehydrating liquid (3 changes, 10 min each).

Samples were then lyophilized in a Critical Point Dryer (mod. K850 Emitech, Assing, Rome IT), placed on a double-sided adhesive carbon tape previously glued to an aluminum stub and coated with a gold film (250 A thickness) using a sputter coater (mod.108 A; Agar Scientific, Stansted, United Kingdom) before observation.

HY-FIB mechanical characterization was performed according to the ASTM 1708 by a dynamometer (CMT 6000 SANS, Shenzen, China) equipped with a 1 kN load cell. The sample was conditioned in Dulbecco's Modified Essential Medium (DMEM) for 1 h, and then shaped to obtain a specimen with gauge length (Lo) of 22 mm and width (W) of 5 mm. Sample thickness (S) was measured with a thickness gauge brand at three different averaged points. Monoaxial deformation was applied to the sample at a speed of 10 mm/min, and force (F) and elongation (L) during traction were recorded. The elastic modulus and ultimate tensile strength (both expressed in MPa) were calculated from the stress/strain plot. For the immuno-histochemical analysis, at different time points, a portion of HY-FIB was fixed in 4% PFA (4 °C, overnight), cryo-protected in 30% sucrose overnight, mounted in OCT embedding compound, frozen at -20°C and then cut in slices of 10 μm of thickness using a cryostat. The remaining portion of HY-FIB was placed in QIAzol® Lysis Reagent for total RNA extraction.

2.7. Dynamic Culture

HY-FIB was clamped at both free ends, one motionless and one sliding (operated by a linear motor actuator) arm, into the bioreactor system culture chamber, described in detail elsewhere [**23**]. A maximal load, set by pre-tensioning, was relaxed to a minimum value cycling at a pre-determined frequency. In addition, continuous feedback signals provided by strain gauges located onto the fixed arm, allowed the maintenance of a defined load on the scaffold in response to physical system modifications, by automatic adjustment of the pre-tensioning position.

2.8. Finite Element Modeling

Finite Element Modeling (FEM) was implemented by using COMSOL Multiphysics Software (rel. 5.3a®) to assess the stress distribution into 3D constructs when a 10% mechanical cyclic strain stimulus is applied. All components were obtained using primitive geometries and Boolean operations. Linear elasticity equations were set as boundary conditions for the scaffold. A sensitivity study of the mesh obtained the most computationally efficient solution. The specific parameters used in the model are listed in **Table 1**. The simulation considered only the stress within the fibrin 3D environment neglecting any further contribution of the band, cells and PLGA-NCs.

Table 1. Finite Element Modeling (FEM) parameters used.

Parameters	Value	Unit
Young's modulus [1]	4.56	MPa
Poisson ratio [2]	0.25	-
Density	1050	Kg/m^3
[1] HY-FIB Young Modulus was measured experimentally [**53**] [2] Poisson ratio value was taken in the literature [**62**].		

2.9. Statistical Analysis

The statistical analysis was conducted using GraphPad Prism software version 6.0 for Windows. The data collected from several experiments is presented as mean with standard deviation and assessed for statistical significance using ANOVA test for independent groups. Differences were considered statistically significant when $p \leq 0.05$ [**63**].

3. RESULTS

3.1. hBM-MSCs Cultivation in 2D Environment

hBM-MSCs were cultivated in a two-dimensional (2D) monolayer environment with medium supplemented with either 1.6 ng/mL or 100 ng/mL of inactive human Growth Differentiation Factor 5 (ihGDF-5) for up to 16 days. These two concentration conditions (two order of magnitude of difference) were chosen to ascertain absence of any effect of the inactive hGDF-5 form on cells expression of tenogenic markers (COL3A1, COL1A1, DCN, SCX-A and TNMD) and of cytokines (pro-inflammatory: IL-6, TNF, IL-12A, IL-1β; anti-inflammatory: IL-10, TGF-β1) by RT-qPCR (see **Figure 1**a–d).

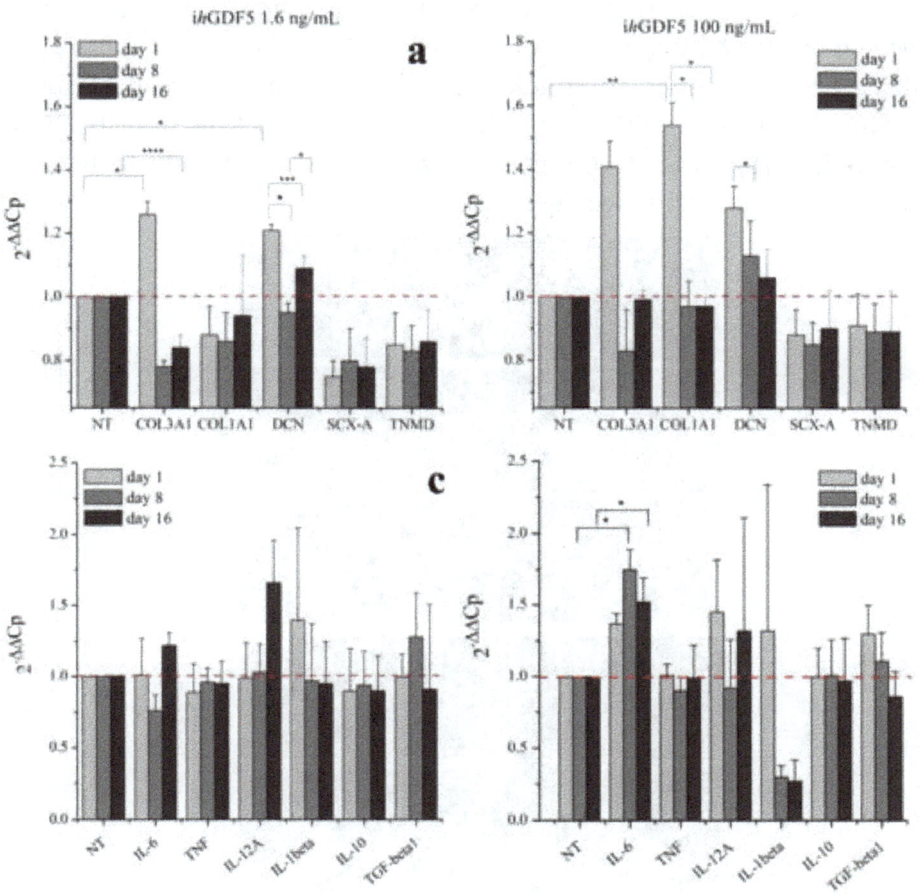

Figure 1. Gene expression profiles for tenogenic markers and pro-inflammatory and anti-inflammatory cytokines by hBM-MSCs treated with 1.6 ng/mL (a,c) and 100 ng/mL (b,d) of ihGDF-5 in monolayer 2D culture up to 16 days. mRNA levels of COL1A1, DCN, SCX-A, and TNMD were considered as tenogenic markers and COL3A1 selected as negative ones; pro-inflammatory (IL-6, TNF, IL-12A and IL-1β) and anti-inflammatory (IL-10 and TGF-β1) cytokines were monitored. ihGDF-5 not had significant impact on genes expression, especially at the lower concentration tested. Untreated cells for matched time-points were used as control. * ≤ 0.05; ** <0.01; * <0.005; **** <0.001 N = 3 (biological replicates); n = 3 (technical replicates).**

Transient and slight, though significant, upregulation of COL3A1 (0.4-fold), DCN (0.2-fold), and COL1A1 (0.5-fold) was observed at Day 1 in cultures supplemented with 100 ng/mL ihGDF-5 (**Figure 1**b). The reduced dose of 1.6 ng/mL induced low-level transient expression at Day 1 for only COL3A1 (0.3-fold) and DCN (0.2-fold) only (**Figure 1**a). No significant upregulation was noted for TNF, IL-12A, IL-1β, IL-10, or TGFβ at any time point or ihGDF-5 concentration tested (**Figure 1**c,d). Compared to controls, IL-6 displayed significant levels of elevation at Days 8 (0.8-fold) and 16

(0.5-fold) with 100 ng/mL ihGDF-5 (**Figure 1**d). Types 1 and 3 Collagen expression levels were monitored by immunofluorescence during the 16 day culture period, as illustrated in **Figure 2**a,b. Immunofluorescence quantitative data by image analysis were congruent with RT-qPCR outputs when 1.6 ng/mL ihGDF-5 was supplemented, in this case, both proteins signals were not significantly elevated, compared to untreated cells (see **Figure 2**c).

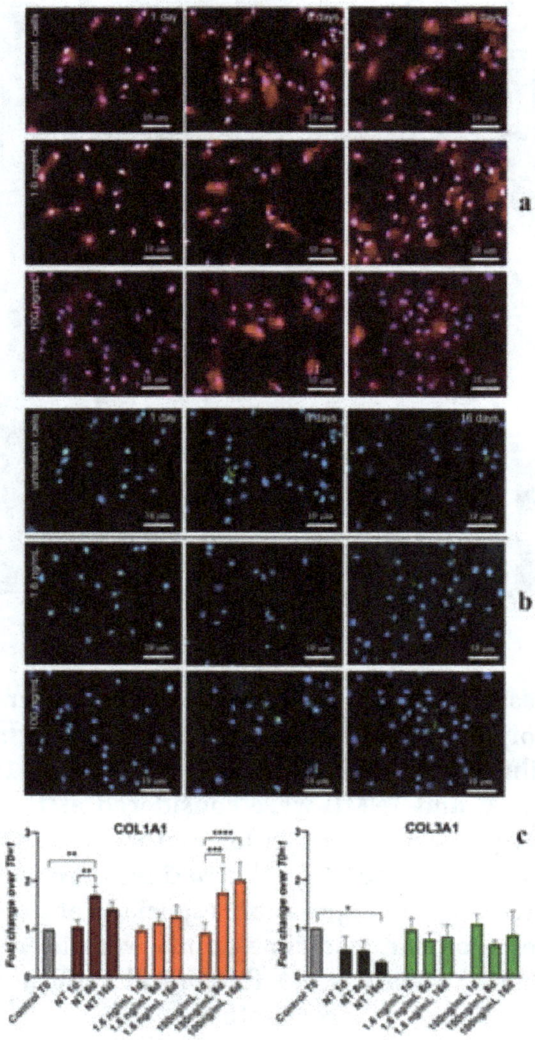

Figure 2. IF and quantitative-IF assays of type 1 Collagen (COL1A1) and type 3 Collagen (COL3A1) monitored along hBM-MSCs treatment with 1.6 ng/ and 100 ng/mL of ihGDF-5 for 16 days. Type 1 collagen was stained in red; type 3 collagen was stained in green; cell nuclei highlighted with DAPI in blue (a,b). Quantitative signal detection was performed via ImageJ software (c). A slight up-regulation of COL1A1 was observed when hBM-MSC were in routine culture for 16 days. Color intensity in each time point was normalized by the cell number. * ≤0.05; * *<0.01; * <0.005; **** <0.001. n = 10 (image fields for each time point).**

Quantitative image analysis displayed COL1A1 signal increase (1 fold) at Day 16 only with 100 ng/mL ihGDF-5 supplementation. This last data is in contrast with gene expression ones. COL1A1 and COL3A1 are the major components of the extracellular matrix in connective tissues, and their slight up-regulations was reported when hBM-MSC were in routine culture for 16 days [**64**]. However, in our case, ihGDF-5 seemed not to impact on their production, especially at the lower concentration tested. This preliminary information is important to confirm the inactivity of the biochemical input in regards to the gene expression and proteins that will be monitored in the 3D experiments.

3.2. PLGA-NCs Fabrication and ihGDF-5 Controlled Deliver

Poly-lactic-co-glycolic-acid nano-carriers (PLGA-NCs) displayed a spherical morphology with a mean size of 230 ± 80 nm (**Figure 3**a). PLGA-NCs had an ihGDF-5 loading of 350 ng/g and provided a daily released peptide mean concentration of 1.6 ng/mL/day (**Figure 3**b), when an amount of 100 mg were inserted within HY-FIB over 11 days of culture. As highlighted above, these ihGDF-5 concentration levels did not stimulate sustained impacts on hBM-MSCs gene expression in 2D monolayer culture (see **Figure 1**a,c).

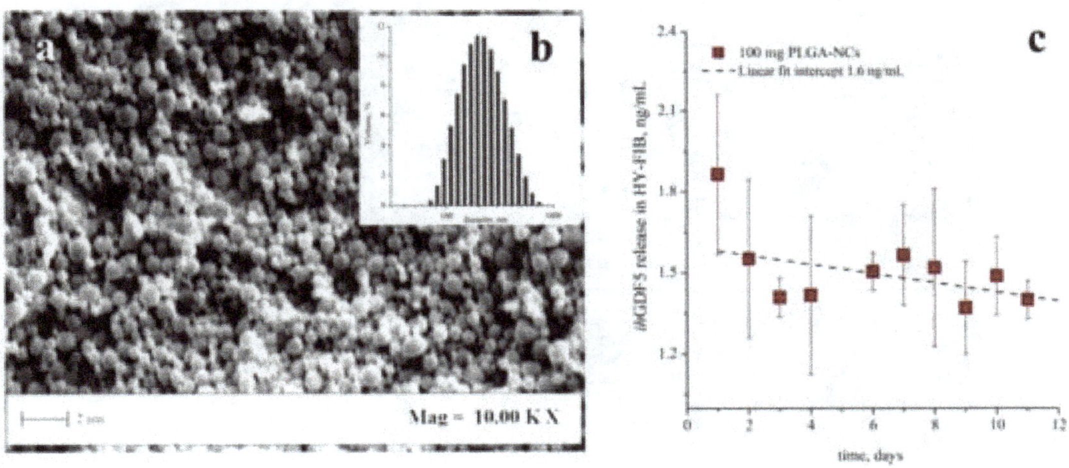

Figure 3. Poly-lactic-co-glycolic-acid (PLGA) transient carriers field emission-scanning electron microscopy (FE-SEM) image, particle size distribution, and ihGDF-5 release profile. FE-SEM images indicated spherical morphology of carriers (a); the size distribution set at 230 ± 80 nm their mean size (b). Release profiles performed in vitro at 37 °C indicated a ihGDF-5 mean concentration of 1.6 ng/mL/day released from the 100 mg of PLGA-NCs loaded within HY-FIB over 11 days of culture (c).

By eliminating any non-specific ihGDF-5 induction from the 3D scaffold by the NCs, we were able to monitor cell behaviors resulting from the HY-FIB microenvironment under static and dynamic settings.

3.3. hBM-MSCs Cultivation in HY-FIB 3D Microenvironment

The HY-FIB assembly featured a braided band (3 × 10cm) joined to a fibrin hydrogel (on a band surface of 6 cm^2) containing 8 × 10^5 hBM-MSCs and 100 mg of ihGDF-5/PLGA-NCs. The picture and schematic representation of the 3D system is shown (**Figure 4**a,b). Field Emission Scanning Electron Microscopy (FE-SEM) images of the scaffold illustrate hyaluronate fibers, embedded within a fibrin hydrogel (**Figure 4**c), which provided an entrapment surface for both NCs and hBM-MSCs (**Figure 4**d).

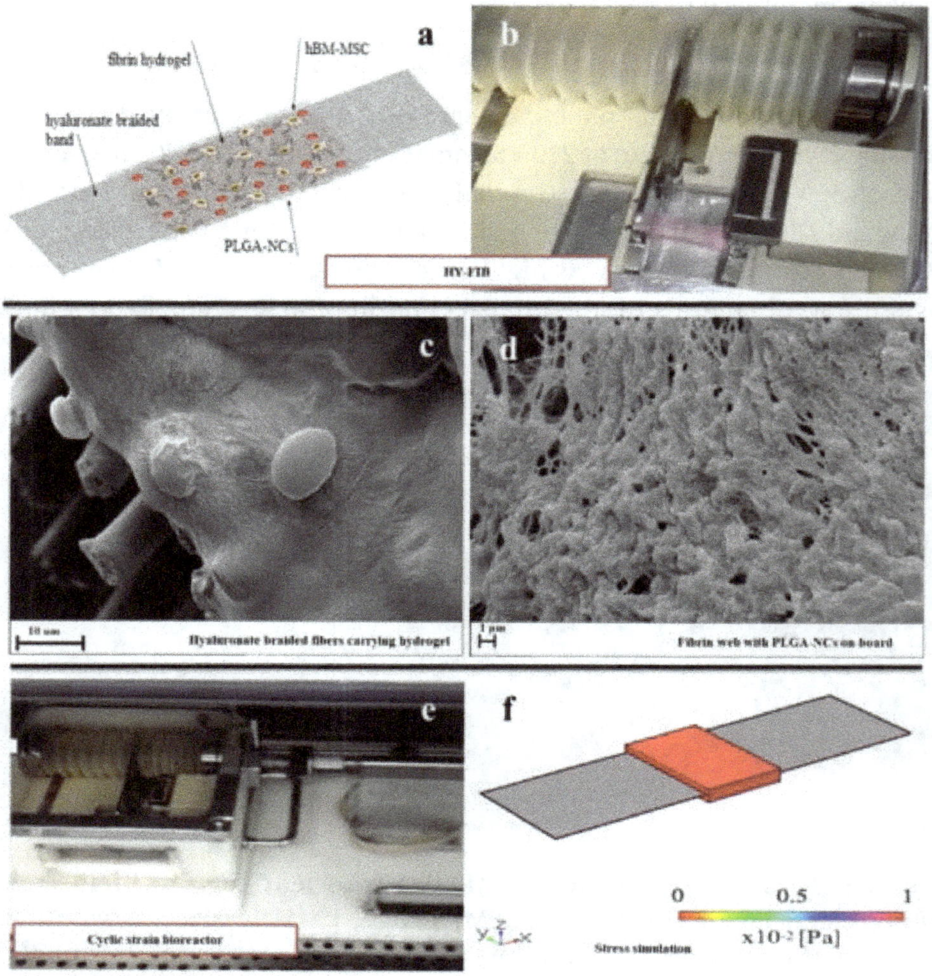

Figure 4. HY-FIB three-dimensional (3D) scaffold features and cyclic strain bioreactor. Schematic HY-FIB representation (a) and image of 3D scaffold (b). SEM images of hyaluronate braided fibers (10 µm mean diameter size) (c) joined to a fibrin web which entrapped both NCs and hBM-MSCs (d). Cyclic strain bioreactor (e) and in-silico study of stress distribution over HY-FIB upon mechanical strain of 10% (f). The simulation involved only the stress of the fibrin 3D environment, neglecting any further contribution.

HY-FIB was exposed to 10% deformation over a 1 Hz frequency for 4 h a day during the dynamic culture experiments via a cyclic strain bioreactor, illustrated in **Figure 4**e [**24**]. In greater detail, a HY-FIB braided band was held at one end by a motionless arm and at the other end by a sliding one. Motion was driven by a linear motor and transmitted through the braided band to cells embedded within the fibrin hydrogel. The motionless arm comprises a base, attached to the side wall of the culture chamber, housing the electronic components for load monitoring, and from which extended a cantilevered shelf whose deformation is measured by four strain gauges. The whole system was housed within an incubator to ensure the appropriate CO_2 gaseous environment to control the pH of the cell culture media and 37 °C operational temperature.

The stress delivered to the cells immobilized within the system was explored via computational analysis that estimated a mean shear stress value estimated at 9×10^{-2} Pa within the fibrin 3D environment (**Figure 4**f). This order of magnitude of stress value was reported for tenogenic induction [**30**]; larger deformation for longer times were excluded to focus the study on 3D environment assembled.

HY-FIB samples were collected at Day 1, 2, 5, and 11 to monitor tenogenic and cytokine marker expression. Time points at Day 1 and Day 2 were added for 3D culture to monitor the effect of HY-FIB on cells behavior alone or in combination with cyclic strain culture. Indeed, in static conditions COL1A1 and DCN both displayed significant upregulation of 3.8 fold (COL1A1) and 2.6-fold (DCN) at Days 1 and 2 before dropping progressively to elevated but non-significant levels (**Figure 5**a), confirming an HY-FIB effect on this gene expression in the first days of culture. In dynamic conditions, COL1A1 levels displayed responses similar to the static culture in the first two days but progressively rising thereafter to significant levels (2.9 fold) at Day 11, probably due to strain input. DCN expression levels in response to dynamic culture were to be elevated throughout, achieving significance at Day 11 (3-fold) (**Figure 5**b).

SCX-A displayed significant upregulation (~340-fold) in both static and dynamic conditions at Day 1, suggesting an effect of HY-FIB system, on this gene expression. SCX-A levels were substantially elevated in both static and dynamic condition at all following time points studied, even if a larger and significant increase was observed in dynamic condition; an increase of 800-fold in static and of 1600-fold in dynamic culture conditions was monitored at Day 11 (**Figure 5**a,b). Tenomodulin gene expression was also tested by RT-qPCR, but no expression was detected, probably because it is an event occurring during late differentiation [**65**]. Sustained, significant, downregulation of COL3A1 was observed in either static or dynamic conditions which instead either decreased progressively (static) or decreased through to Day 5 before reestablishing Day 0 levels at Day 11 (dynamic).

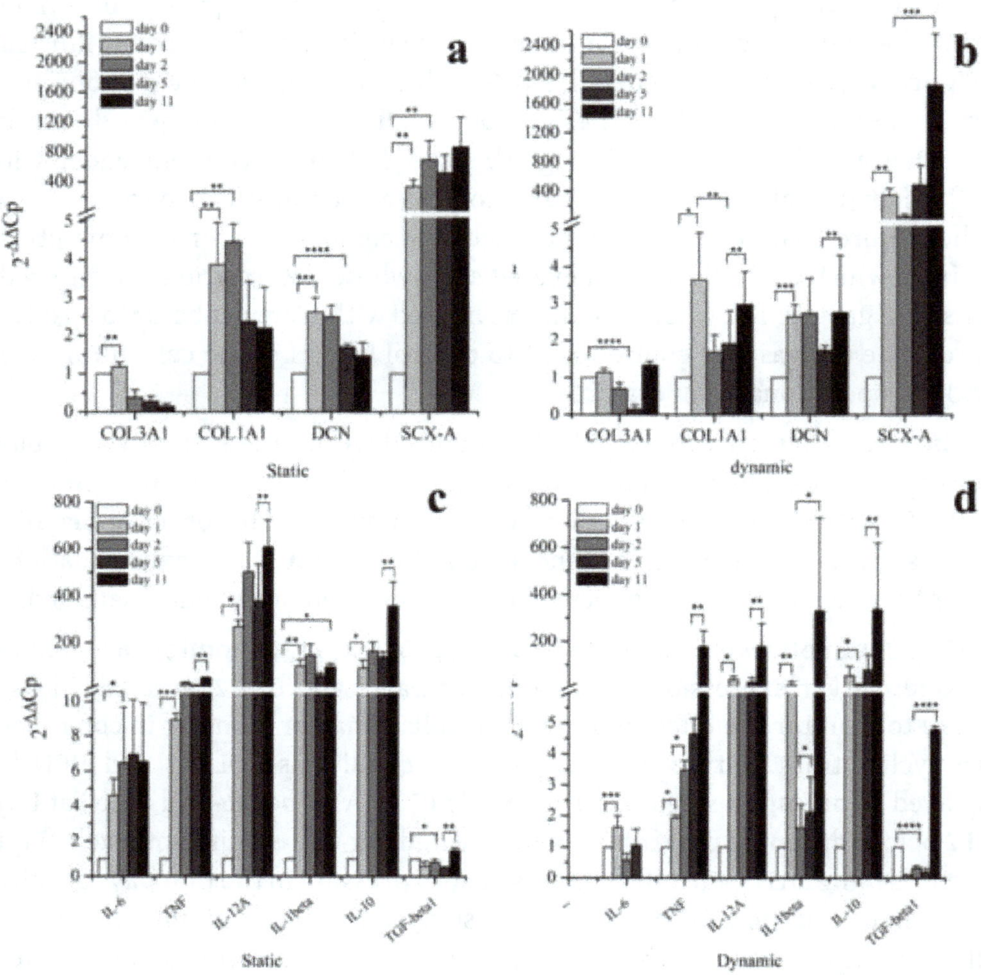

Figure 5. Gene expression profiles of tenogenic markers and pro-inflammatory and anti-inflammatory cytokines from hBM-MSCs within HY-FIB environment in static (a,c) and dynamic culture (b,d) up to 11 days. Days 1, 2, 5, and 11 were selected as time points to study the mRNA levels of positive tenogenic markers (COL1A1, DCN, SCX-A, and TNMD), negative ones (COL3A1) and pro-inflammatory (IL-6, TNF, IL-12A and IL-1β) and anti-inflammatory (IL-10 and TGF-β1) cytokines. Effect of HY-FIB environment on cells behavior was visible along the first two days of culture; a better over expression of tenogenic markers and anti-inflammatory cytokines was observed in dynamic culture at Day 11. hBM-MSCs within HY-FIB at time zero were used as control. * <0.05; ** <0.01; * <0.005; **** <0.001. N = 3 (biological replicates); n = 3 (technical replicates).**

The data suggested an overall effect of the 3D environment on cells behavior clearly visible along the first two days of culture; furthermore, a statistically significant COL1A1, DCN, and SCX-A over-expression was observed after 11 days when mechanical strain was provided.

Cytokine transcript expression data is illustrated in **Figure** 5c,d, for static and dynamic culture, respectively. HY-FIB system has an effect also on cytokines gene expression, as observed in all time points monitored with respect to Day 0, within static culture. Indeed, pro-inflammatory cytokines IL-6 (~6-fold), TNF (~10-fold), IL-12A (≤600-fold), and IL-1β (~200-fold) displayed rapid and significant upregulation that was maintained for the entirety of the experimental duration. Anti-inflammatory TGF-β1 on the other hand displayed either no change (Day 11) or significant down-regulation (other time points) while IL-10 exhibited an overall similar profile to Il-1β culminating in marked upregulation at day 11 (~300-fold) (**Figure** 5c).

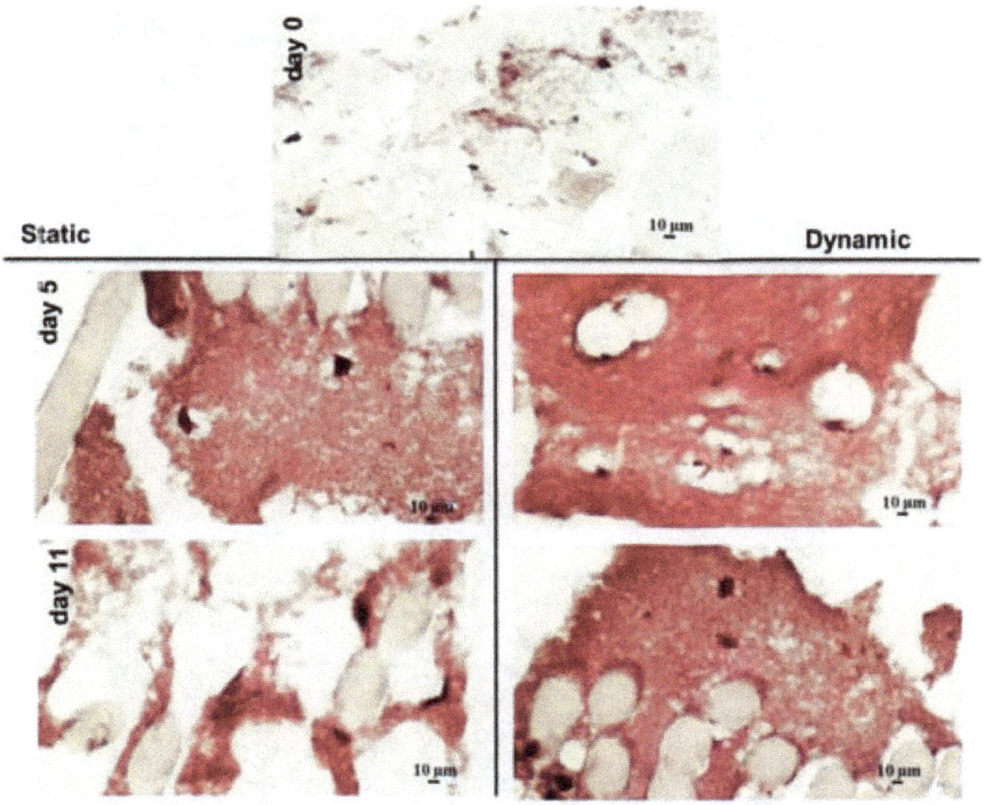

Figure 6. Histology characterization of the overall HY-FIB scaffold structure with Sirius Red staining. HY-FIB scaffolds in both static and dynamic culture at Days 5 and 11 are reported; the overall scaffold structure was stained with Sirius Red for collagen highlighting. Fibrin hydrogel was light pink stained in the sample collected at Day 0. Fibrin matrix was clearly stained in red at Day 5 and 11 in both samples from static and dynamic culture. Less homogeneous scaffold matrix structure and staining was observed in samples taken from static culture.

Dynamic culture conditions had a distinct and significant effect on IL-6 with expression levels achieving a peak upregulation of 1.5-fold at Day 1 and decreasing to undetectable levels by Day 11.

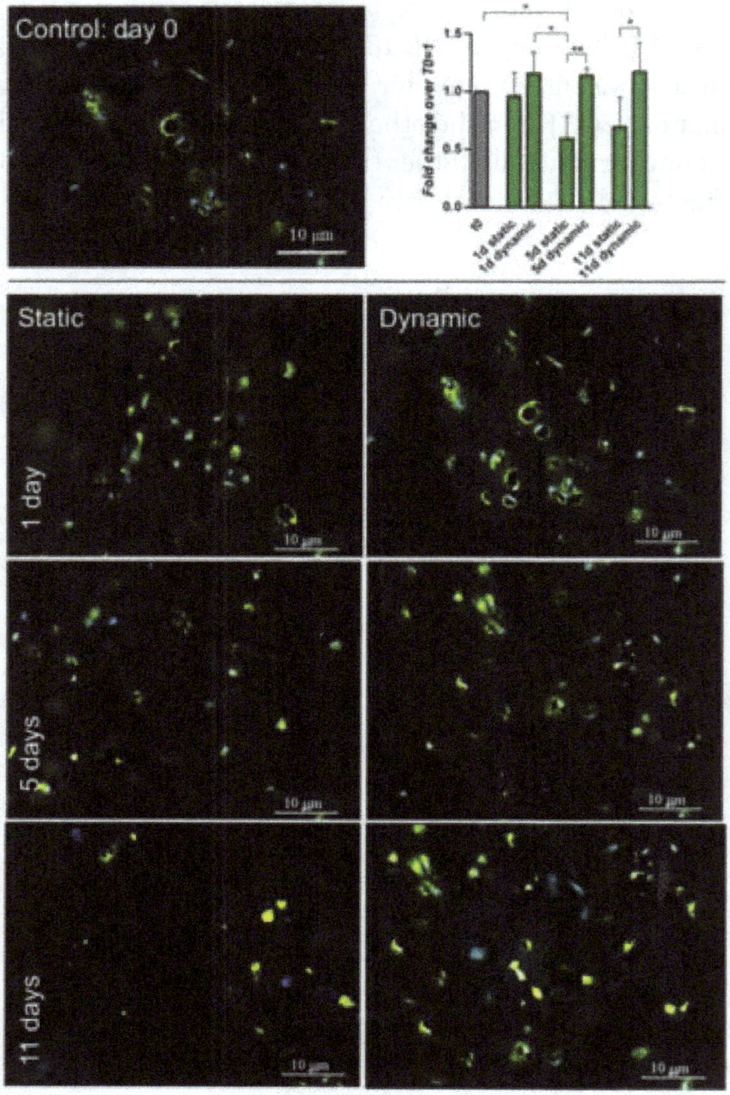

Figure 7. IF and quantitative-IF assays of type 1 Collagen (COL1A1) in 3D static and dynamic culture of hBM-MSCs for 11 days. At day 1, holes within the hydrogel structure are evident nearby cells surroundings. These areas were progressively filled by COL1A1 protein (stained in green) and it happened more uniformly during the dynamic cultivation (see day 11). Fluorescence quantification by ImageJ software, reported in the plot, confirmed the presence of more abundant signal (0.2–0.3 fold changes) in dynamic condition; signal intensity in each time point was normalized by cell number (e.g., by amount of cell nuclei revealed by DAPI staining). * ≤0.05; ** <0.01. N = 3 (biological replicates); n = 3 (technical replicates).

TNF and IL-1β were both gradually upregulated before achieving ~200-fold and ~300-fold, respectively, upregulations at day 11 (compared to 10-fold and 100-fold in static conditions). IL-12 displayed a similar profile of upregulation in dynamic vs. static culture conditions while achieving maximal levels that were 3X less in dynamic. Anti-inflammatory IL-10 expression levels were consistent across both dynamic and static conditions. In contrast to static culture, TGF-β1 was significantly downregulated until day 5, and it underwent a 5-fold increase at Day 11 in dynamic culture conditions (**Figure 5**d).

Histological characterization of HY-FIB scaffold in both static and dynamic culture at Days 5 and 11 are reported in **Figure 6**; the overall scaffold structure was stained with Sirius Red for collagen highlighting. Despite fibrin hydrogel matrix, collected at Day 0, was only light pink stained, the same matrix was clearly stained in red at Day 5 and 11 in both samples taken from static and dynamic culture. However, a less homogeneous matrix organization and staining was observed in the samples taken from static culture. This data is in agreement with gene expression indications and confirmed that both HY-FIB alone and HY-FIB plus cyclic strain had an effect on cells phenotype commitment.

The expression of type 1 Collagen, a tenogenic matrix-associated marker, was monitored by immunofluorescence over the culture time (see **Figure 7**). At day 1, empty areas surrounding the cells are present, probably due to absence of uniform fibrin hydrogel. These spaces were then progressively filled with the protein, presumably via secretion into the extracellular environment. The level of staining observed under static conditions decreased after Day 1 and was maintained at ~50% of original levels thereafter while levels were maintained consistent to Day 0 in dynamic culture. Moreover, in the dynamic condition a more uniform cells distribution was noted throughout the hydrogel matrix, especially at day 11.

4. DISCUSSION

The HY-FIB system is designed to facilitate the transportation of PLGA nanocarriers (PLGA-NCs) in the hydrogel matrix, allowing precise delivery of particular molecules in a 3D setting, such as medications or biological signals. A prior work examined the utilization of the active form of hGDF-5 encapsulated in PLGA-NCs for regulated release in a HY-FIB setting. We studied how the HY-FIB 3D environment impacts the gene expression of tenogenic and cytokine markers in hBM-MSCs under static and dynamic mechanical conditions. We implemented the prior HY-FIB setup using PLGA-NCs, however this time we administered an inactive version of hGDF5. By excluding the biochemical input from the growth factor, we kept the whole HY-FIB configuration to solely evaluate the impact of mechanical input.

HY-FIB braided fibers enabled a defined mechanical stimulation of 9×10^{-2} Pa provided to hBM-MSCs during the 4h/day dynamic culture regime. The mean shear stress was calculated by FEM modeling [**62**], assuming a system homogeneous behavior at a density of 1050 kg/m^3 and Young's modulus of 4.56 Mpa [**53**]. A Poisson ratio value of 0.25 was adopted as described elsewhere [**62**]. Further mechanical inputs with different intensities and durations were not investigated, not being the aim of the present work. Stress values resembling reduced physiological activity, similar that the ones used here, have been reported to direct stem cell commitment to a tenogenic phenotype [**31,36,66**].

COL1A1 is the major component of tendon tissue (75–85% of the dry mass of tendon), and is responsible for its mechanical strength [**64**]. In the static group, COL1A1 showed a ≥3-fold upregulation during the first and second day of cultivation. These data seem to suggest an overall effect of the 3D environment on cells behavior. COL1A1 expression was progressively reduced to a 2-fold upregulation at Day 11, in static environment. In dynamic conditions, its mRNA levels showed similar behavior during the first two days of cultivation (an increase up to 3-fold-changes, then reduced at Day 2). However, its expression was subsequently increased again to 2.8-fold at Day 11. Decorin (DCN), a small leucine-rich proteoglycan implicated in the regulation of fibrillogenesis, is a fundamental component of the tendon extracellular matrix (ECM) [**67**]. Compared to the static condition, a significant enhancement, up to 2.5-fold, of the mRNA level of DCN was shown when hBM-MSCs were cultured for 11 days with mechanical stimulation.

Scleraxis-A (SCX-A) is a neotendon marker, expressed in pro-tendon sites in the developing embryo. Specifically, SCX-A is a tendon-specific basic helix-loop-helix transcription factor responsible for the transition of MSCs into tendon progenitors [**68**]. We observed substantial increases in SCX-A expression, up to 800-fold in static and 1600-fold in dynamic conditions after 11 days, demonstrating a stimulatory effect via the 3D system organization and consistent with previous observations [**69,70,71**].

COL3A1 mRNA level seems to be downregulated after 2 days in the static group and after 5 days in the dynamic group. Its downregulation can be considered a positive indication of proper cell differentiation; indeed, it seems that COL3A1 is the main responsible of fibrotic and scarred tissue arrangement and has been consistently reported at the rupture site of human tendons. [**64**].

From both histology and immunofluorescence assays, we noted that the area surrounding the cells was progressively filled by type 1 Collagen and, at Day 11, the extracellular matrix seemed to undergo remodeling (**Figure 6** and **Figure 7**). Moreover, in dynamic conditions a more homogeneous cell distribution within the hydrogel matrix was observed in the IF images. These findings support the concept that 3D cultivation provides cues to the hBM-MSCs, and that dynamic signaling enables the adoption of a more uniform behavior including type 1 Collagen protein deposition in the externally available space of the fibrin hydrogel. A near total absence of type 3 Collagen was found, except for a very small fluorescence signal at day 1, in both static and dynamic conditions (data not shown). These data suggest that tenogenic commitment of hBM-MSCs cultured within HY-FIB environment may be enhanced when dynamic stretching is applied.

MSCs secrete a variety of cytokines and growth factors that promote cell recruitment, migration, proliferation, and differentiation. MSCs are also immunomodulatory, which may allow them to exert beneficial effects on the local immune cell population at the site of muscle injury [72]. To better understand the hBM-MSCs inflammatory response when cultured within HY-FIB, cytokine expression was monitored along the 11 days of culture. The balance between pro- and anti-inflammatory soluble factors in the tendon healing process exerts a major impact on successful resolution of inflammation [73]. Recent analysis of tendinopathy biopsies showed a distinct inflammatory infiltrate in the initial phase of tendinopathy with a high content of pro-inflammatory factors such as IL-6, TNF-α and IL-17 [74].

To exclude a role for ihGDF5 in cytokine expression induction we evaluated their expression in hBM-MSCs undergoing 2D planar cultivation as a negative control. Indeed, in disc degeneration models using in vitro three-dimensional cultures, human annulus cells display increased expression of pro-inflammatory cytokines, such as IL-1β and TNF-α, while exposure to TNF-α and IL-1β resulted in significant downregulation of GDF-5 [75]. Therefore, it is plausible that the GDF-5 may upregulate the expression of pro-inflammatory genes in hBM-MSCs leading to the maintenance of an autocrine feedback. However, when the ihGDF-5 was added, no statistically significant expression of pro-inflammatory cytokines was observed; therefore, ihGDF-5 did not exert any effect on cytokines expression.

The addition of PLGA-NCs enabled an informed analysis of the inductive role of the HY-FIB overall structure. Previous studies have noted that cytotoxicity of SEE-fabricated PLGA-NCs on blood mononucleate viability, monitored with MTT assay [76], was not affected after either 24 or 48 h. Here, the overall HY-FIB system (loaded with SEE fabricated NCs) does not evidence any toxic effect on hBM-MSC cultivated within it for 11 days, providing an indirect indication about SEE technology as suitable process for biomedical carriers production.

In general, we observed that pro-inflammatory gene expression was higher in static than in dynamic conditions at all-time points. On the contrary, the anti-inflammatory cytokines IL-10 was consistently upregulated in both static and dynamic conditions; while TGF-β1 was downregulated at all the time points tested except day 11, when, it showed a marked increase (4-fold) only in dynamic environment. The described behavior confirmed that MSCs respond to a variety of biophysical cues; indeed, as suggested by Qazi et al., 3D culture of MSCs on biomaterials can promote cell-cell interactions and enhance the paracrine effects of MSCs [77]. Moreover, as concluded by Ogle et al., historically, biomaterial-based therapies to promote tissue regeneration were designed to minimize the host inflammatory response. Recently, the roles that monocytes and macrophages can play in tissue repair have been highlighted. In this context, material properties and their possibility of specific biomolecule controlled delivery has been engineered to achieve a given biological response that can be tuned not only to a better integration with biological systems but also in regulating the inflammatory response [5].

The considerable imbalance of pro- and anti-inflammatory cytokines generated by cells highlights the relevance of dynamic culture in 3D in vitro model systems. IL-6, a versatile cytokine produced by tissues in response to various changes like exercise, infection, and injury, has been found to significantly impact the skeletal muscle environment. It affects the function and quality of cellular components during tissue regeneration, ultimately contributing to a fibrotic response. IL-6 gene expression was significantly decreased in hBM-MSCs that were subjected to dynamic 3D HY-FIB growth compared to those grown in a static environment in our 3D model system.

5. CONCISE SUMMARY

The 3D cell culture showed evidence of type 1 Collagen expression by both immunohistology and gene testing. When the 3D system was subjected to cyclic strain stimulation, there was a statistically significant increase in the expression of tenogenic markers compared to the 3D system cultured in a static environment. Future research could focus on exploring the connection between collagen type I production, cell commitment, and mechanical strain percentage or duration. The HY-FIB system could serve as a valuable tool for investigating this relationship. The 3D culture technique induced the expression of pro-inflammatory cytokines. When cyclic strain was applied, there was a better balance between the over-expression of pro-inflammatory cytokine genes by hBM-MSCs and the over-expression of anti-inflammatory cytokines. The involvement and immunomodulatory activity of hBM-MSCs, as well as the significance of implanted biomaterials in stimulating inflammatory reactions, still need to be identified. Local inflammation is considered a crucial factor in initiating repair processes in avascular tissues including cartilage and tendons. [5].

Alternatively, including PLGA-NCs into the fibrin hydrogel could provide the targeted release of particular biomolecules for investigating their potential in regulating inflammatory responses or enhancing regeneration and repair processes.

HY-FIB offers a strategic way to tackle various difficulties by implementing a closely monitored in vitro regimen. The 3D scaffold has the potential to control the continuous release of various biochemical signals. This offers promising opportunities for creating 3D bioengineered models to study the precise molecular and cellular makeup of damaged systems.

6. AT A GLANCE

We developed a (three-dimensional) 3D scaffold, we named HY-FIB, incorporating a force-transmission band of braided hyaluronate embedded in a cell localizing fibrin hydrogel and poly-lactic-co-glycolic acid (PLGA) nanocarriers as transient components for growth factor controlled delivery. The tenogenic supporting capacity of HY-FIB on human-Bone Marrow Mesenchymal Stem Cells (hBM-MSCs) was explored under static conditions and under bioreactor-induced cyclic strain conditions. HY-FIB elasticity enabled to deliver a mean shear stress of 0.09 Pa for 4 h/day. Tendon and cytokine marker expression by hBM-MSCs were studied. Results: hBM-MSCs embedded in HY-FIB and subjected to mechanical stimulation, resulted in a typical tenogenic phenotype, as indicated by type 1 Collagen fiber immunofluorescence. RT-qPCR showed an increase of type 1 Collagen, scleraxis, and decorin gene expression (3-fold, 1600-fold, and 3-fold, respectively, at day 11) in dynamic conditions. Cells also showed pro-inflammatory (IL-6, TNF, IL-12A, IL-1β) and anti-inflammatory (IL-10, TGF-β1) cytokine gene expressions, with a significant increase of anti-inflammatory cytokines in dynamic conditions (IL-10 and TGF-β1 300-fold and 4-fold, respectively, at day 11). Mechanical signaling, conveyed by HY-FIB to hBM-MSCs, promoted tenogenic gene markers expression and a pro-repair cytokine balance. The results provide strong evidence in support of the HY-FIB system and its interaction with cells and its potential for use as a predictive in vitro model.

REFERENCES

1. Ahmed, S.; Chauhan, V.M.; Ghaemmaghami, A.M.; Aylott, J.W. New generation of bioreactors that advance extracellular matrix modelling and tissue engineering. Biotechnol. Lett. 2019, 41, 1–25. [Google Scholar] [CrossRef] [PubMed] [Green Version]

2. Okamoto, M. The role of Scaffolds in Tissue Engineering. In Handbook of Tissue Engineering Scaffolds: Volume One; Elsevier: Amsterdam, The Netherlands, 2019; pp. 23–49. ISBN 978-0-08-102563-5. [Google Scholar]

3. D’Angelo, M.; Benedetti, E.; Tupone, M.G.; Catanesi, M.; Castelli, V.; Antonosante, A.; Cimini, A. The Role of Stiffness in Cell Reprogramming: A Potential Role for Biomaterials in Inducing Tissue Regeneration. Cells 2019, 8, 1036. [Google Scholar] [CrossRef] [PubMed] [Green Version]

4. Cipollaro, L.; Ciardulli, M.C.; Della Porta, G.; Peretti, G.M.; Maffulli, N. Biomechanical issues of tissue-engineered constructs for articular cartilage regeneration: In vitro and in vivo approaches. Br. Med. Bull. 2019, 132, 53–80. [Google Scholar] [CrossRef] [PubMed]

5. Ogle, M.E.; Segar, C.E.; Sridhar, S.; Botchwey, E.A. Monocytes and macrophages in tissue repair: Implications for immunoregenerative biomaterial design. Exp. Biol. Med. 2016, 241, 1084–1097. [Google Scholar] [CrossRef] [PubMed]

6. Vinhas, A.; Rodrigues, M.T.; Gomes, M.E. Exploring Stem Cells and Inflammation in Tendon Repair and Regeneration. In Cell Biology and Translational Medicine, Volume 2; Turksen, K., Ed.; Springer International Publishing: Cham, Germany, 2018; Volume 1089, pp. 37–46. ISBN 978-3-030-04169-4. [Google Scholar]

7. Rees, J.D.; Stride, M.; Scott, A. Tendons—Time to revisit inflammation. Br. J. Sports Med. 2014, 48, 1553–1557. [Google Scholar] [CrossRef] [PubMed] [Green Version]

8. Dakin, S.G.; Martinez, F.O.; Yapp, C.; Wells, G.; Oppermann, U.; Dean, B.J.F.; Smith, R.D.J.; Wheway, K.; Watkins, B.; Roche, L.; et al. Inflammation activation and resolution in human tendon disease. Sci. Transl. Med. 2015, 7, 311ra173. [Google Scholar] [CrossRef] [PubMed] [Green Version]

9. John, T.; Lodka, D.; Kohl, B.; Ertel, W.; Jammrath, J.; Conrad, C.; Stoll, C.; Busch, C.; Schulze-Tanzil, G. Effect of pro-inflammatory and immunoregulatory cytokines on human tenocytes. J. Orthop. Res. 2010, 28, 1071–1077. [Google Scholar] [CrossRef]

10. Manning, C.N.; Havlioglu, N.; Knutsen, E.; Sakiyama-Elbert, S.E.; Silva, M.J.; Thomopoulos, S.; Gelberman, R.H. The early inflammatory response after flexor tendon healing: A gene expression and histological analysis: Early inflammatory response after flexor tendon healing. J. Orthop. Res. 2014, 32, 645–652. [Google Scholar] [CrossRef]

11. Marsolais, D.; Coté, C.H.; Frenette, J. Neutrophils and macrophages accumulate sequentially following Achilles tendon injury. J. Orthop. Res. 2001, 19, 1203–1209. [Google Scholar] [CrossRef]

12. Chisari, E.; Rehak, L.; Khan, W.S.; Maffulli, N. The role of the immune system in tendon healing: A systematic review. Br. Med. Bull. 2020, 133, 49–64. [Google Scholar] [CrossRef]

13. Giordano, L.; Della Porta, G.; Peretti, G.M.; Maffulli, N. Therapeutic potential of microRNA in tendon injuries. Br. Med. Bull. 2020, 133, 79–94. [Google Scholar] [CrossRef] [PubMed]

14. Oryan, A.; Moshiri, A.; Meimandi Parizi, A.; Maffulli, N. Implantation of a Novel Biologic and Hybridized Tissue Engineered Bioimplant in Large Tendon Defect: An In Vivo Investigation. Tissue Eng. Part A 2013, 20, 447–465. [Google Scholar] [CrossRef] [PubMed] [Green Version]

15. Gaspar, D.; Spanoudes, K.; Holladay, C.; Pandit, A.; Zeugolis, D. Progress in cell-based therapies for tendon repair. Adv. Drug Deliv. Rev. 2015, 84, 240–256. [Google Scholar] [CrossRef] [PubMed]

16. Lui, P.P.Y.; Wong, O.T. Tendon stem cells: Experimental and clinical perspectives in tendon and tendon-bone junction repair. Muscles Ligaments Tendons J. 2012, 2, 163–168. [Google Scholar]

17. Chang, C.-H.; Chen, C.-H.; Liu, H.-W.; Whu, S.-W.; Chen, S.-H.; Tsai, C.-L.; Hsiue, G.-H. Bioengineered Periosteal Progenitor Cell Sheets to Enhance Tendon-Bone Healing in A Bone Tunnel. Biomedical 2012, 35, 473. [Google Scholar] [CrossRef]

18. Ito, R.; Matsumiya, T.; Kon, T.; Narita, N.; Kubota, K.; Sakaki, H.; Ozaki, T.; Imaizumi, T.; Kobayashi, W.; Kimura, H. Periosteum-derived cells respond to mechanical stretch and activate Wnt andBMP signaling pathways. Biomed. Res. 2014, 35, 69–79. [Google Scholar] [CrossRef] [Green Version]

19. Doroski, D.M.; Levenston, M.E.; Temenoff, J.S. Cyclic Tensile Culture Promotes Fibroblastic Differentiation of Marrow Stromal Cells Encapsulated in Poly(Ethylene Glycol)-Based Hydrogels. Tissue Eng. Part A 2010, 16, 3457–3466. [Google Scholar] [CrossRef] [Green Version]

20. Chaudhury, S. Mesenchymal stem cell applications to tendon healing. Muscles Ligaments Tendons J. 2012, 2, 222–229. [Google Scholar]

21. Youngstrom, D.W.; LaDow, J.E.; Barrett, J.G. Tenogenesis of bone marrow-, adipose-, and tendon-derived stem cells in a dynamic bioreactor. Connect. Tissue Res. 2016, 57, 454–465. [Google Scholar] [CrossRef]

22. Bi, Y.; Ehirchiou, D.; Kilts, T.M.; Inkson, C.A.; Embree, M.C.; Sonoyama, W.; Li, L.; Leet, A.I.; Seo, B.-M.; Zhang, L.; et al. Identification of tendon stem/progenitor cells and the role of the extracellular matrix in their niche. Nat. Med. 2007, 13, 1219–1227. [Google Scholar] [CrossRef]

23. Yang, G.; Rothrauff, B.B.; Lin, H.; Gottardi, R.; Alexander, P.G.; Tuan, R.S. Enhancement of tenogenic differentiation of human adipose stem cells by tendon-derived extracellular matrix. Biomaterials 2013, 34, 9295–9306. [Google Scholar] [CrossRef] [PubMed] [Green Version]

24. Govoni, M.; Lotti, F.; Biagiotti, L.; Lannocca, M.; Pasquinelli, G.; Valente, S.; Muscari, C.; Bonafè, F.; Caldarera, C.M.; Guarnieri, C.; et al. An innovative stand-alone bioreactor for the highly reproducible transfer of cyclic mechanical stretch to stem cells cultured in a 3D scaffold: A novel stand-alone bioreactor to induce cell muscle phenotype. J. Tissue Eng. Regen. Med. 2014, 8, 787–793. [Google Scholar] [CrossRef] [PubMed]

25. Lovecchio, J.; Gargiulo, P.; Vargas Luna, J.L.; Giordano, E.; Sigurjonsson, O.E. A standalone bioreactor system to deliver compressive load under perfusion flow to hBMSC-seeded 3D chitosan-graphene templates. Sci. Rep. 2019, 9, 16854. [Google Scholar] [CrossRef] [PubMed]

26. Barber, J.G.; Handorf, A.M.; Allee, T.J.; Li, W.-J. Braided Nanofibrous Scaffold for Tendon and Ligament Tissue Engineering. Tissue Eng. Part A 2013, 19, 1265–1274. [Google Scholar] [CrossRef] [PubMed]

27. Wang, T.; Lin, Z.; Day, R.E.; Gardiner, B.; Landao-Bassonga, E.; Rubenson, J.; Kirk, T.B.; Smith, D.W.; Lloyd, D.G.; Hardisty, G.; et al. Programmable mechanical stimulation influences tendon homeostasis in a bioreactor system. Biotechnol. Bioeng. 2013, 110, 1495–1507. [Google Scholar] [CrossRef]

28. Delaine-Smith, R.M.; Reilly, G.C. Mesenchymal stem cell responses to mechanical stimuli. Muscles Ligaments Tendons J. 2016, 2, 169–180. [Google Scholar]

29. Chen, Y.-J.; Huang, C.-H.; Lee, I.-C.; Lee, Y.-T.; Chen, M.-H.; Young, T.-H. Effects of Cyclic Mechanical Stretching on the mRNA Expression of Tendon/Ligament-Related and Osteoblast-Specific Genes in Human Mesenchymal Stem Cells. Connect. Tissue Res. 2008, 49, 7–14. [Google Scholar] [CrossRef]

30. Govoni, M.; Muscari, C.; Lovecchio, J.; Guarnieri, C.; Giordano, E. Mechanical Actuation Systems for the Phenotype Commitment of Stem Cell-Based Tendon and Ligament Tissue Substitutes. Stem Cell Rev. Rep. 2016, 12, 189–201. [Google Scholar] [CrossRef]

31. Youngstrom, D.W.; Rajpar, I.; Kaplan, D.L.; Barrett, J.G. A bioreactor system for in vitro tendon differentiation and tendon tissue engineering. J. Orthop. Res. 2015, 33, 911–918. [Google Scholar] [CrossRef] [Green Version]

32. Testa, S.; Costantini, M.; Fornetti, E.; Bernardini, S.; Trombetta, M.; Seliktar, D.; Cannata, S.; Rainer, A.; Gargioli, C. Combination of biochemical and mechanical cues for tendon tissue engineering. J. Cell. Mol. Med. 2017, 21, 2711–2719. [Google Scholar] [CrossRef]

33. Woon, C.Y.L.; Kraus, A.; Raghavan, S.S.; Pridgen, B.C.; Megerle, K.; Pham, H.; Chang, J. Three-Dimensional-Construct Bioreactor Conditioning in Human Tendon Tissue Engineering. Tissue Eng. Part A 2011, 17, 2561–2572. [Google Scholar] [CrossRef] [PubMed]

34. Rinoldi, C.; Fallahi, A.; Yazdi, I.K.; Campos Paras, J.; Kijeńska-Gawrońska, E.; Trujillo-de Santiago, G.; Tuoheti, A.; Demarchi, D.; Annabi, N.; Khademhosseini, A.; et al. Mechanical and Biochemical Stimulation of 3D Multilayered Scaffolds for Tendon Tissue Engineering. ACS Biomater. Sci. Eng. 2019, 5, 2953–2964. [Google Scholar] [CrossRef]

35. Nam, H.Y.; Pingguan-Murphy, B.; Abbas, A.A.; Merican, A.M.; Kamarul, T. Uniaxial Cyclic Tensile Stretching at 8% Strain Exclusively Promotes Tenogenic Differentiation of Human Bone Marrow-Derived Mesenchymal Stromal Cells. Stem Cells Int. 2019, 2019, 1–16. [Google Scholar] [CrossRef] [PubMed] [Green Version]

36. Grier, W.G.; Moy, A.S.; Harley, B.A. Cyclic tensile strain enhances human mesenchymal stem cell Smad 2/3 activation and tenogenic differentiation in anisotropic collagen-glycosaminoglycan scaffolds. Eur. Cell Mater. 2017, 33, 227–239. [Google Scholar] [CrossRef] [PubMed]

37. Kay, A.G.; Dale, T.P.; Akram, K.M.; Mohan, P.; Hampson, K.; Maffulli, N.; Spiteri, M.A.; El Haj, A.J.; Forsyth, N.R. BMP2 repression and optimized culture conditions promote human bone marrow-derived mesenchymal stem cell isolation. Regen. Med. 2015, 10, 109–125. [Google Scholar] [CrossRef]

38. Correia, S.I.; Pereira, H.; Silva-Correia, J.; Van Dijk, C.N.; Espregueira-Mendes, J.; Oliveira, J.M.; Reis, R.L. Current concepts: Tissue engineering and regenerative medicine applications in the ankle joint. J. R. Soc. Interface 2013, 11, 20130784. [Google Scholar] [CrossRef]

39. Keller, T.C.; Hogan, M.V.; Kesturu, G.; James, R.; Balian, G.; Chhabra, A.B. Growth/differentiation factor-5 modulates the synthesis and expression of extracellular matrix and cell-adhesion-related molecules of rat Achilles tendon fibroblasts. Connect. Tissue Res. 2011, 52, 353–364. [Google Scholar] [CrossRef]

40. Hogan, M.; Girish, K.; James, R.; Balian, G.; Hurwitz, S.; Chhabra, A.B. Growth differentiation factor-5 regulation of extracellular matrix gene expression in murine tendon fibroblasts. J. Tissue Eng. Regen. Med. 2011, 5, 191–200. [Google Scholar] [CrossRef]

41. Tan, S.-L.; Ahmad, R.E.; Ahmad, T.S.; Merican, A.M.; Abbas, A.A.; Ng, W.M.; Kamarul, T. Effect of Growth Differentiation Factor 5 on the Proliferation and Tenogenic Differentiation Potential of Human Mesenchymal Stem Cells in vitro. Cells Tissues Organs 2012, 196, 325–338. [Google Scholar] [CrossRef]

42. Lui, P.P. Stem cell technology for tendon regeneration: Current status, challenges, and future research directions. SCCAA 2015, 8, 163. [Google Scholar] [CrossRef] [Green Version]

43. MacLean, S.; Khan, W.S.; Malik, A.A.; Snow, M.; Anand, S. Tendon Regeneration and Repair with Stem Cells. Stem Cells Int. 2012, 2012, 1–6. [Google Scholar] [CrossRef] [PubMed]

44. Liu, L.; Hindieh, J.; Leong, D.J.; Sun, H.B. Advances of stem cell based-therapeutic approaches for tendon repair. J. Orthop. Transl. 2017, 9, 69–75. [Google Scholar] [CrossRef] [PubMed]

45. Caplan, A.I. Adult mesenchymal stem cells for tissue engineering versus regenerative medicine. J. Cell. Physiol. 2007, 213, 341–347. [Google Scholar] [CrossRef] [PubMed]

46. Akram, K.M.; Samad, S.; Spiteri, M.A.; Forsyth, N.R. Mesenchymal stem cells promote alveolar epithelial cell wound repair in vitro through distinct migratory and paracrine mechanisms. Respir. Res. 2013, 14, 9. [Google Scholar] [CrossRef] [Green Version]

47. Pontikoglou, C.; Deschaseaux, F.; Sensebé, L.; Papadaki, H.A. Bone Marrow Mesenchymal Stem Cells: Biological Properties and Their Role in Hematopoiesis and Hematopoietic Stem Cell Transplantation. Stem Cell Rev. Rep. 2011, 7, 569–589. [Google Scholar] [CrossRef]

48. Dominici, M.; Le Blanc, K.; Mueller, I.; Slaper-Cortenbach, I.; Marini, F.C.; Krause, D.S.; Deans, R.J.; Keating, A.; Prockop, D.J.; Horwitz, E.M. Minimal criteria for defining multipotent mesenchymal stromal cells. Cytotherapy 2006, 8, 315–317. [Google Scholar] [CrossRef]

49. Chamberlain, G.; Fox, J.; Ashton, B.; Middleton, J. Concise Review: Mesenchymal Stem Cells: Their Phenotype, Differentiation Capacity, Immunological Features, and Potential for Homing. Stem Cells 2007, 25, 2739–2749. [Google Scholar] [CrossRef] [Green Version]

50. Mosna, F.; Sensebé, L.; Krampera, M. Human Bone Marrow and Adipose Tissue Mesenchymal Stem Cells: A User's Guide. Stem Cells Dev. 2010, 19, 1449–1470. [Google Scholar] [CrossRef]

51. Kumar, D.; Gerges, I.; Tamplenizza, M.; Lenardi, C.; Forsyth, N.R.; Liu, Y. Three-dimensional hypoxic culture of human mesenchymal stem cells encapsulated in a photocurable, biodegradable polymer hydrogel: A potential injectable cellular product for nucleus pulposus regeneration. Acta Biomater. 2014, 10, 3463–3474. [Google Scholar] [CrossRef] [Green Version]

52. Bullough, R.; Finnigan, T.; Kay, A.; Maffulli, N.; Forsyth, N.R. Tendon repair through stem cell intervention: Cellular and molecular approaches. Disabil. Rehabil. 2008, 30, 1746–1751. [Google Scholar] [CrossRef]

53. Govoni, M.; Berardi, A.C.; Muscari, C.; Campardelli, R.; Bonafè, F.; Guarnieri, C.; Reverchon, E.; Giordano, E.; Maffulli, N.; Della Porta, G. An Engineered Multiphase Three-Dimensional Microenvironment to Ensure the Controlled Delivery of Cyclic Strain and Human Growth Differentiation Factor 5 for the Tenogenic Commitment of Human Bone Marrow Mesenchymal Stem Cells. Tissue Eng. Part A 2017, 23, 811–822. [Google Scholar] [CrossRef] [PubMed]

54. Della Porta, G.; Ciardulli, M.C.; Maffulli, N. Microcapsule Technology for Controlled Growth Factor Release in Musculoskeletal Tissue Engineering. Sports Med. Arthrosc. Rev. 2018, 26, e2–e9. [Google Scholar] [CrossRef] [PubMed]

55. Giordano, R.; Canesi, M.; Isalberti, M.; Isaias, I.; Montemurro, T.; Viganò, M.; Montelatici, E.; Boldrin, V.; Benti, R.; Cortelezzi, A.; et al. Autologous mesenchymal stem cell therapy for progressive supranuclear palsy: Translation into a phase I controlled, randomized clinical study. J. Transl. Med. 2014, 12, 14. [Google Scholar] [CrossRef] [PubMed]

56. Jensen, E.C. Quantitative Analysis of Histological Staining and Fluorescence Using ImageJ: Histological Staining/Fluorescence Using ImageJ. Anat. Rec. 2013, 296, 378–381. [Google Scholar] [CrossRef]

57. Rinoldi, C.; Costantini, M.; Kijeńska-Gawrońska, E.; Testa, S.; Fornetti, E.; Heljak, M.; Ćwiklińska, M.; Buda, R.; Baldi, J.; Cannata, S.; et al. Tendon Tissue Engineering: Effects of Mechanical and Biochemical Stimulation on Stem Cell Alignment on Cell-Laden Hydrogel Yarns. Adv. Healthc. Mater. 2019, 8, 1801218. [Google Scholar] [CrossRef]

58. Bustin, S.A.; Benes, V.; Garson, J.A.; Hellemans, J.; Huggett, J.; Kubista, M.; Mueller, R.; Nolan, T.; Pfaffl, M.W.; Shipley, G.L.; et al. The MIQE Guidelines: Minimum Information for Publication of Quantitative Real-Time PCR Experiments. Clin. Chem. 2009, 55, 611–622. [Google Scholar] [CrossRef] [Green Version]

59. Hellemans, J.; Mortier, G.; De Paepe, A.; Speleman, F.; Vandesompele, J. qBase relative quantification framework and software for management and automated analysis of real-time quantitative PCR data. Genome Biol. 2007, 8, R19. [Google Scholar] [CrossRef] [Green Version]

60. Della Porta, G.; Falco, N.; Reverchon, E. Continuous supercritical emulsions extraction: A new technology for biopolymer microparticles production. Biotechnol. Bioeng. 2011, 108, 676–686. [Google Scholar] [CrossRef]

61. Della Porta, G.; Falco, N.; Giordano, E.; Reverchon, E. PLGA microspheres by Supercritical Emulsion Extraction: A study on insulin release in myoblast culture. J. Biomater. Sci. Polym. Ed. 2013, 24, 1831–1847. [Google Scholar] [CrossRef]
62. Duong, H.; Wu, B.; Tawil, B. Modulation of 3D Fibrin Matrix Stiffness by Intrinsic Fibrinogen–Thrombin Compositions and by Extrinsic Cellular Activity. Tissue Eng. Part A 2009, 15, 1865–1876. [Google Scholar] [CrossRef]
63. De Winter, J.C.F. Using the Student's t-test with extremely small sample sizes. Pract. Assess Res. Eval. 2013, 18, 10. [Google Scholar]
64. Pajala, A.; Melkko, J.; Leppilahti, J.; Ohtonen, P.; Soini, Y.; Risteli, J. Tenascin-C and type I and III collagen expression in total Achilles tendon rupture. An immunohistochemical study. Histol. Histopathol. 2009, 24, 1207–1211. [Google Scholar] [CrossRef] [PubMed]
65. Shukunami, C.; Yoshimoto, Y.; Takimoto, A.; Yamashita, H.; Hiraki, Y. Molecular characterization and function of tenomodulin, a marker of tendons and ligaments that integrate musculoskeletal components. Jpn. Dent. Sci. Rev. 2016, 52, 84–92. [Google Scholar] [CrossRef] [PubMed] [Green Version]
66. Wang, T.; Thien, C.; Wang, C.; Ni, M.; Gao, J.; Wang, A.; Jiang, Q.; Tuan, R.S.; Zheng, Q.; Zheng, M.H. 3D uniaxial mechanical stimulation induces tenogenic differentiation of tendon-derived stem cells through a PI3K/AKT signaling pathway. FASEB J. 2018, 32, 4804–4814. [Google Scholar] [CrossRef] [Green Version]
67. Wagenhäuser, M.U.; Pietschmann, M.F.; Sievers, B.; Docheva, D.; Schieker, M.; Jansson, V.; Müller, P.E. Collagen type I and decorin expression in tenocytes depend on the cell isolation method. Bmc Musculoskelet. Disord. 2012, 13, 140. [Google Scholar] [CrossRef] [Green Version]
68. Alberton, P.; Popov, C.; Prägert, M.; Kohler, J.; Shukunami, C.; Schieker, M.; Docheva, D. Conversion of Human Bone Marrow-Derived Mesenchymal Stem Cells into Tendon Progenitor Cells by Ectopic Expression of Scleraxis. Stem Cells Dev. 2012, 21, 846–858. [Google Scholar] [CrossRef] [Green Version]
69. Bagchi, R.A.; Czubryt, M.P. Scleraxis: A New Regulator of Extracellular Matrix Formation. In Genes and Cardiovascular Function; Ostadal, B., Nagano, M., Dhalla, N.S., Eds.; Springer: Boston, MA, USA, 2011; pp. 57–65. ISBN 978-1-4419-7206-4. [Google Scholar]
70. Chen, X.; Yin, Z.; Chen, J.; Shen, W.; Liu, H.; Tang, Q.; Fang, Z.; Lu, L.; Ji, J.; Ouyang, H. Force and scleraxis synergistically promote the commitment of human ES cells derived MSCs to tenocytes. Sci. Rep. 2012, 2, 977. [Google Scholar] [CrossRef] [Green Version]

71. Scott, A.; Danielson, P.; Abraham, T.; Fong, G.; Sampaio, A.V.; Underhill, T.M. Mechanical force modulates scleraxis expression in bioartificial tendons. J. Musculoskelet Neuronal Interact 2011, 11, 124–132. [Google Scholar]

72. Gao, F.; Chiu, S.M.; Motan, D.A.L.; Zhang, Z.; Chen, L.; Ji, H.-L.; Tse, H.-F.; Fu, Q.-L.; Lian, Q. Mesenchymal stem cells and immunomodulation: Current status and future prospects. Cell Death Dis. 2016, 7, e2062. [Google Scholar] [CrossRef] [Green Version]

73. Sugg, K.B.; Lubardic, J.; Gumucio, J.P.; Mendias, C.L. Changes in macrophage phenotype and induction of epithelial-to-mesenchymal transition genes following acute Achilles tenotomy and repair. J. Orthop. Res. 2014, 32, 944–951. [Google Scholar] [CrossRef] [Green Version]

74. Millar, N.L.; Akbar, M.; Campbell, A.L.; Reilly, J.H.; Kerr, S.C.; McLean, M.; Frleta-Gilchrist, M.; Fazzi, U.G.; Leach, W.J.; Rooney, B.P.; et al. IL-17A mediates inflammatory and tissue remodelling events in early human tendinopathy. Sci. Rep. 2016, 6. [Google Scholar] [CrossRef] [PubMed]

75. Gruber, H.E.; Hoelscher, G.L.; Ingram, J.A.; Bethea, S.; Hanley, E.N. Growth and differentiation factor-5 (GDF-5) in the human intervertebral annulus cells and its modulation by IL-1ß and TNF-α in vitro. Exp. Mol. Pathol. 2014, 96, 225–229. [Google Scholar] [CrossRef] [PubMed]

76. Govoni, M.; Lamparelli, E.P.; Ciardulli, M.C.; Santoro, A.; Oliviero, A.; Palazzo, I.; Reverchon, E.; Vivarelli, L.; Maso, A.; Storni, E.; et al. Demineralized Bone Matrix Paste Formulated with biomimetic PLGA microcarriers for the Vancomycin Hydrochloride Controlled Delivery: Release Profile, Citotoxicity and Efficacy against S. aureus. Int. J. Pharm. 2020, 582, 119322. [Google Scholar] [CrossRef] [PubMed]

77. Qazi, T.H.; Mooney, D.J.; Duda, G.N.; Geissler, S. Biomaterials that promote cell-cell interactions enhance the paracrine function of MSCs. Biomaterials 2017, 140, 103–114. [Google Scholar] [CrossRef] [PubMed]

78. Forcina, L.; Miano, C.; Scicchitano, B.; Musarò, A. Signals from the Niche: Insights into the Role of IGF-1 and IL-6 in Modulating Skeletal Muscle Fibrosis. Cells 2019, 8, 232. [Google Scholar] [CrossRef] [Green Version]

06 SELF-ASSEMBLING SCAFFOLDS FACILITATED EXTENDED GROWTH OF HUMAN PRIMED EMBRYONIC STEM CELLS AND INCREASED THE EXPRESSION OF CORE AND NAÏVE PLURIPOTENT MARKERS

1. INTRODUCTION: AN OVERVIEW

Pluripotency is characterized by a cell's ability to develop into germline cells and all three germ layer [1,2]. Pluripotency in development starts from the epiblast formation and continues until gastrulation and lineage commitment, leading to a variety of pluripotent cell states within the cell population. [3,4]. Pluripotency in vitro is determined by the developmental stage from which the cell line is derived and by culture conditions [**5**,**6**,**7**,**8**] with distinct naïve and primed states of pluripotency corresponding to in vivo pre-implantation and post-implantation epiblast cells, respectively [**4**].

Embryonic stem cells (ESCs) have the ability to continuously renew themselves and transform into multiple cell types in a controlled environment, making them well-suited for creating cell-based therapies and regenerative medicine treatments [9]. However, the clinical use of ESCs requires a high quality and quantity of cells, which is limited by currently used culturing techniques [**10**]. ESCs are typically grown as a monolayer in two-dimensional (2-D) plastic culture plates coated with extracellular matrix (ECM) components (such as gelatin from porcine skin [**11**], matrigel [**12**], laminin [**13**], fibronectin [**14**], vitronectin [**15**], or collagen

[16]) or a mouse embryonic fibroblast (MEF) feeder layer to aid in attachment [17]. Monolayer culture also necessitates routine passaging and the removal of spontaneously differentiated colonies to maintain the self-renewal and potency of cells [18], which pose a major impediment to the large-scale expansion of cells. Generally, 2-D culturing methods often lead to heterogeneous cell populations as well as batch-to-batch variation.

Additionally, 2-D culture settings do not possess the complexities required to replicate the ESC niche, dynamic, and specialized three-dimensional (3-D) microenvironments, which are crucial for controlling cell destiny in living organisms. Moreover, native 3-D environments facilitate intricate spatial relationships among cells, extracellular matrix components, and gradients of nutrients, oxygen, and metabolic waste [19,20,21,22,23,24]. The microenvironment is important for the self-renewal of ESCs, since cell fate and function is affected by the composition and organization of the ECM [25,26,27] as well as mechanical forces generated between cells and attachment substrates [25,28,29,30,31]. Furthermore, mechanical forces generated by the expansion of the blastocoel have been shown to play an important role in blastocyst lineage formation, stimulating the generation of pluripotent cells [32]. These early morphogenic events in the mammalian embryo indicate a significant interaction between mechanical forces, cell polarity, and the regulation of gene expression in cell fate determination [33]. We hypothesized that 3-D culture would better mimic the in vivo microenvironment, promoting the proliferation and maintenance of human ESCs.

We have previously demonstrated that 3-D self-assembling scaffolds composed of thiolated dextran and 4-arm polyethylene glycol (PEG) functionalized with acrylate groups (Dex-SH/PEG-4-Acr) supported the growth and maintenance of naïve mouse ESCs [34]. However, these 3-D culture conditions failed to support the growth of human primed ESCs. Unlike mouse ESCs, human cells display poor viability and clonogenicity following single cell dissociation [9,10].

In this study, we describe 3-D hydrogel scaffolds that support the long-term growth and maintenance of human primed ESCs (H9). Chemically cross-linked hydrogels were formed by a Michael-type addition reaction by combining two 8-arm PEG polymers functionalized with either thiol (PEG-8-SH) or acrylate end groups (PEG-8-Acr). The PEG-8-SH/PEG-8-Acr scaffold provided a microenvironment that maintained self-renewal and pluripotency for an extended time period. Interestingly, H9 cells displayed an upregulation of core pluripotency markers during 3-D culture. However, the expression of core markers reverted to normal levels when 3-D grown cells were subcultured under 2-D culture conditions. Interestingly, 3-D cultured H9 cells also exhibited a significantly higher expression of naïve pluripotent markers when compared to human naïve ESCs (Elf1) cultured under 2-D conditions. Our results suggest the importance of the 3-D scaffold microenvironment in maintaining the stemness of ESCs.

2. MATERIALS AND METHODS

2.1. Maintenance of Human ESCs in 2-D culture

H9 cells, derived from a human blastocyst [**35**], obtained from WiCell (Madison, WI, USA) were maintained in the culture medium containing Knockout/F12 Dulbecco's Modified Eagle Media (DMEM; Life Technologies, Carlsbad, CA, USA) with 20% KnockOut serum replacement (Life Technologies), 0.1 mM 2-mercaptoehtanol (Life Technologies), 1% GlutaMax (Life Technologies), and 1% non-essential amino acid solution (Life Technologies), supplemented with 20 ng/mL of basic fibroblast growth factor (FGF2, Prospec, Ness Ziona, Israel) and 10 μM ROCK inhibitor, Y-27632 (Cayman Chemical, Ann Arbor, MI, USA) and subcultured by manual passaging. For dissociation into single cells, H9 were treated with Accutase (Thermo Fisher Scientific, Waltham, MA, USA) for 5 min, and then cells were centrifuged at 200 g for 5 min. The supernatant was aspirated, and the cell pellet was resuspended in H9 culture media for plating.

Elf1 cells, isolated from a cryopreserved 8-cell human embryo [**36**], were maintained in the culture medium containing KnockOut/F12 DMEM with GlutaMax (Life Technologies) with 20% KnockOut serum replacement (Life Technologies), 1 mM sodium pyruvate (Life Technologies), 0.1mM 2-mercaptoehtanol (Life Technologies), 1% non-essential amino acids (Life Technologies), and 0.2% penicillin–streptomycin solution (Life Technologies), supplemented with 12 ng/mL of FGF2 (Prospec), 1.5 μM CHIR99021 (Caymen Chemical), 0.4 μM PD03296501 (Caymen Chemical), and 0.01 μg/mL human LIF (Prospec) and cultured according to the published protocol [**36**].

2.2. Selection and Composition of Scaffolds for 3-D Culture of Human ESCs

Several polymers end functionalized with thiol and acrylate end groups were tested for their ability to self-assemble and form hydrogels scaffolds via a thiol-Michael addition reaction, allowing for the formation of covalent bonds by the addition of a nucleophile to a nucleophile acceptor containing an α,β-unsaturated carbonyl compound [**37**]. Then, the scaffolds were tested in various compositions to determine the optimal concentration, molar ratio, and degree of modification that would best support the growth of human ESCs. Our preliminary results showed that scaffolds made using 8-arm PEG polymers yielded optimal growth. These scaffolds were prepared using 8-arm PEG-thiol (PEG-8-SH, 20 kDa) and 8-arm PEG-acrylate (PEG-8-Acr, 20 kDa) purchased from JenKem Technology USA (Plano, TX, USA). Functionalized PEG polymers were stored at −20 °C and protected from light.

The preparation of scaffolds for the 3-D culture of ESCs is depicted in **Figure 1**. Briefly, PEG-8-SH and PEG-8-Acr polymers were dissolved at a concentration of 2.5 w/v % (dry weight of polymer per volume of culture medium), combined at a 1:1 molar ratio and mixed with cells. Then, the resulting mixture was transferred to a 1 cc syringe mold for polymerization. After self-assembly, scaffolds were placed in a 24-well culture plate (Fisher Scientific, Pittsburgh, PA, USA), supplemented with culture medium, and maintained in a 5% CO_2 incubator at 37 °C. The medium was changed daily or as needed. Cell growth in the scaffolds was monitored by phase-contrast microscopy.

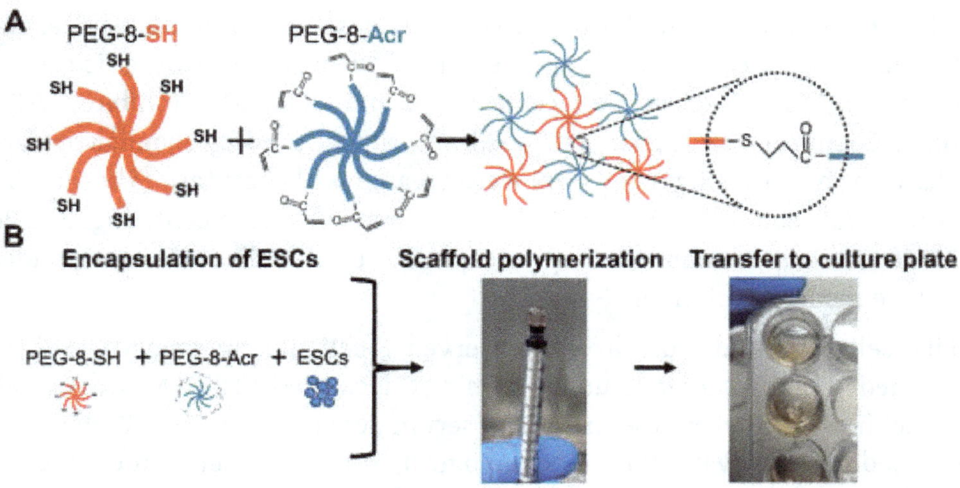

Figure 1. Schematic of self-assembling scaffolds. (A) Self-assembly of functionalized polymers, 8-arm polyethylene glycol functionalized with thiol (PEG-8-SH) and acrylate (PEG-8-Acr) via a thiol–Michael addition reaction. (B) The encapsulation of H9 cells human embryonic stem cells (ESCs), was achieved upon mixing with the self-assembling polymers in a syringe mold. Following polymerization, the scaffolds were then incubated in culture plates containing medium.

2.3. Cell Proliferation and Viability Assays

The growth rate of cells grown under 2-D and 3-D culture conditions were analyzed at various time intervals using a proliferation assay. Briefly, triplicate samples were treated with 5 mg/mL 3-(4,5-dimethylthiazol-2-yl)-2,5-diphenyltetrazolium bromide (MTT) reagent (Sigma, St. Louis, MO, USA), protected from light, and incubated at 37 °C for 4 h to obtain insoluble formazan, which was then solubilized using 15:1 isopropanol/hydrochloride. Then, the absorbance of the solubilized formazan was measured at 570 nm using an Epoch microplate reader (BioTek, Winooski, VT), and the background absorbance of the cells was subtracted from all measured values. The viability of encapsulated cells was determined by direct microscopic counts and trypan blue exclusion assay. Briefly, cells were counted using a hemocytometer and cells stained blue were considered non-viable.

2.4. Differentiation of Human ESCs

Germ layer differentiation was achieved by the spontaneous formation of embryoid bodies (EBs). ESCs were allowed to spontaneously aggregate for 3 days in non-adherent flat-bottomed 96-well plates in their respective ESC culture medium containing growth factors. Then, the resultant EBs were transferred to 0.1% gelatin-coated wells for adherent growth and grown in high-glucose DMEM supplemented with 10% fetal bovine serum (FBS). Spontaneous differentiation into all three germ layers was assessed by germ layer marker expression by quantitative real time-polymerase chain reaction (qRT-PCR) and immunocytochemistry.

2.5. Teratoma Assay

For teratoma formation, ESCs were harvested following accutase treatment, washed and resuspended in PBS, and mixed with an equal volume of matrigel (BD Biosciences, San Jose, CA, USA). Cells (1×10^6) were subcutaneously injected (20 µL) using a Hamilton syringe into 4-week-old male immune-compromised SCID (severe combined immunodeficient) Beige mice (Fox Chase SCID Beige, Charles River, Wilmington, MA, USA). Animals were monitored daily and humanely euthanized by CO_2 overdose after teratoma formation at 10–12 weeks. Teratomas were explanted, and teratoma tissue was either fixed for histological analysis or flash frozen in liquid nitrogen for RNA isolation. Teratoma assays were performed in triplicate. All the procedures involving animals were reviewed and approved by the Institutional Animal Care and Use Committee of Oakland University (IACUC protocol number: 17031).

2.6. Gene Expression Analysis

Transcriptional analysis was performed by qRT-PCR. Briefly, cells, scaffolds, and teratoma tissue (100–250 mg) were harvested and total cellular mRNA was isolated following the manufacturer's instructions using the GeneJET RNA purification kit (Thermo Fisher Scientific) and RNeasy Midi kit (Qiagen, Germantown, MD, USA), respectively. cDNA was synthesized with the iScript kit (BioRad, Hercules, CA, USA). qRT-PCR was performed using SsoAdvanced SYBR Green Supermix (Bio-Rad) and the CFX90 Real-Time PCR system. The primers (IDT Technologies, Coralville, IA, USA) used in this study are in **Table 1**. All reactions were prepared in triplicate and normalized to reference genes, HMBS, GAPDH, and β-ACTIN.

Table 1. List of human primer sequences used in qRT-PCR.

Gene	Primer Sequence Forward (5'-3')	Reverse (5'-3')	Product Length
ACTIN	AATCTGGCACCACACCTTCTAC	ATAGCACAGCCTGGATAGCAAC	170
BRACHYURY	TGCTTCCCTGAGACCCAGTT	GATCACTTCTTTCCTTTGCATCAAG	121
DNMT3L	CTGCTCCATCTGCTGCTCC	ATCCACACACTCGAAGCAGT	85
DPPA3	AGACCAACAAACAAGGAGCCT	CCCATCCATTAGACACGCAGA	88
ESRRB	GACATTGCCTCTGGCTACCA	CTCCGTTTGGTGATCTCGCA	131
FGF4	CGTGGTGAGCATCTTCGGC	GTAGGACTCGTAGGCGTTGT	145
FOXA2	GGGAGCGGTGAAGATGGA	TCATGTTGCTCACGGAGGAGTA	89
FOXF1	AAGCCGCCCTATTCCTACATC	GCGCTTGGTGGGTGAACT	63
GAPDH	ACAACTTTGGTATCGTGGAAGG	GCCATCACGCCACAGTTTC	101
GATA4	TCCCTCTTCCCTCCTCAAAT	TCAGCGTGTAAAGGCATCTG	194
GATA6	CCCACAACACAACCTACAGC	GCGAGACTGACGCCTATGTA	131
GDF3	GTCTCCCGAGACTTATGCTACG	AGTAGAGGAGCTTCTGCAGGCA	136
GP130	GGAGTGAAGAAGCAAGTGGGA	AGGCAATGTCTTCCACACGA	128
HMBS	AGGAGTTCAGTGCCATCATCCT	CACAGCATACATGCATTCCTCA	104
ITGA2	TTGCGTGTGGACATCAGTCT	GCTGGTATTTGTCGGACATCT	158
ITGA5	GCCGATTCACATCGCTCTCAA	GTCTTCTCCACAGTCCAGCAA	139
ITGA6	CGAAACCAAGGTTCTGAGCCC	CTTGGATCTCCACTGAGGCAG	151
ITGAV	AGGAGAAGGTGCCTACGAAGC	GCACAGGAAAGTCTTGCTAAGG	105
ITGB1	GGATTCTCCAGAAGGTGGTTT	TGCCACCAAGTTTCCCATCT	143
ITGB3	CATGGATTCCAGCAATGTCCTC	TTGAGGCAGGTGGCATTGAAG	126
ITGB5	GCCTTTCTGTGAGTGCGACAA	CCGATGTAACCTGCATGGCAC	111
KLF17	TCAGGAAGGGACTGGTAGAA	GTACCCGCATATGTCGTCTAAG	206
KLF2	CCAAGAGTTCGCATCTGAAGG	CCGTGTGCTTTCGGTAGTG	132
KLF4	CGAACCCACACAGGTGAGAA	TACGGTAGTGCCTGGTCAGTTC	75
KLF5	ACCCTGGTTGCACAAAAGTT	CAGCCTTCCCAGGTACACTT	100
LATS1	CTCTGCACTGGCTTCAGATG	TCCGCTCTAATGGCTTCAGT	145
LATS2	ACATTCACTGGTGGGGACTC	GTGGGAGTAGGTGCCAAAAA	147
LIFR	CACCTTCCAAAATAGCGAGTATGG	ATGGTTCCGACCGAGACGAGTT	159
MIXL1	CCGAGTCCAGGATCCAGGTA	CTCTGACGCCGAGACTTGG	58
NANOG	AAAGAATCTTCACCTATGCC	GAAGGAAGAGGAGAGACAGT	110
N-CADHERIN	TGTTTGGCCTGGCGTTCTTT	AGGAGACAGAAACGAAGCCA	156
NCAM	AGGAGACAGAAACGAAGCCA	GGTGTTGGAAATGCTCTGGT	161
OCT4	CCCCTGGTGCCGTGAA	GCAAATTGCTCGAGTTCTTTCTG	97
PAX6	CTTTGCTTGGGAAATCCGAG	AGCCAGGTTGCGAAGAACTC	103

Gene	Primer Sequence Forward (5'-3')	Reverse (5'-3')	Product Length
PRDM14	CCTTGTGTGGTATGGAGACTGC	CTTTCACATCTGTAGCCTTCTGC	126
RAC1	ATGTCCGTGCAAAGTGGTATC	CTCGGATCGCTTCGTCAAACA	249
RHOA	CATCCGGAAGAAACTGGT	TCCCACAAAGCCAACTC	168
ROCK1	GGTGGTCGGTTGGGGTATTTT	CGCCCTAACCTCACTTCCC	196
SALL2	GGCTTGCCTTATGGTATGTCCG	TGGCACTGAGTGCTGTTGTGGA	115
SOCS3	ATTCGGGACCAGCCCCC	AAACTTGCTGTGGGTGACCA	121
SOX11	CGACGACCTAATGTTCGACC	GACAGGGATAGGTTCCCCG	105
SOX17	CGCACGGAATTTGAACAGTA	GGATCAGGGACCTGTCACAC	182
SOX2	TTGCTGCCTCTTTAAGACTAGGA	CTGGGGCTCAAACTTCTCTC	75
SOX7	ACGCCGAGCTCAGCAAGAT	TCCACGTACGGCCTCTTCTG	73
STAT3	CTTTGAGACCGAGGTGTATCAC	GGTCAGCATGTTGTACCACAG	133
TAZ	GAGGGTGTATGGTGGAGATAAA	CCAACTGTAGCAAACAGGATTAG	86
TBX3	GGACACTGGAAATGGCCGAAG	GCTGCTTGTTCACTGGAGGAC	123
TBX3	CGGACATACTTGTTCCCCGA	GCAGGGTGAGCTGTTTTCTTTT	154
TEAD4	CCAAGCTCTGGATGTTGGAGTTC	GATGTCCACGGCTTCGAGGTA	161
TFCP2L1	TTTGTGGGACCCTGCGAAG	TGCTTAAACGTGTCAATCTGGA	129
TUJ1	GGCCAAGTTCTGGGAAGTCA	CGAGTCGCCCACGTAGTTG	70
YAP	GCTGCCACCAAGCTAGATAA	GTGCATGTGTCTCCTTAGATCC	101
ZFP42	CGCAATCGCTTGTCCTCAGA	GCTCTCAACGAACGCTTTCC	130
ZIC2	CGCTCCGAGAACCTCAAGAT	CCCTCAAACTCACACTGGAA	71

2.7. Immunocytochemical Analysis

Protein expression was determined by immunocytochemical staining using selected antibodies. H9 cells grown under 2-D culture conditions on coverslips, H9 cells encapsulated in the self-assembling scaffolds, and harvested teratoma tissue were fixed in 4% paraformaldehyde for 10 min, 30 min, and overnight, respectively. Subsequently, teratoma tissue and scaffolds were embedded and frozen in optimal cutting temperature (O.C.T) compound and cryosectioned into 10 μm sections. For immunochemical analysis, fixed cells and cryosections were permeabilized with 0.5% Triton X-100 (Sigma) for 10 min and blocked with 2% bovine serum albumin (BSA; Sigma) for 1 h at room temperature. Next, samples were incubated with primary antibodies (1:100 dilution) overnight at 4 °C. Primary antibody-treated samples were washed three times with phosphate buffer saline (PBS), stained with secondary antibody at 1:200 dilutions for 2 h at 37 °C, and counterstained with 1 mg/mL 4′,6-diamidino-2-phenylindole (DAPI; Life Technologies). The stained samples were visualized by using confocal microscopy. The antibodies used are listed in **Table 2**.

Table 2. List of primary and secondary antibodies used in immunocytochemical staining.

BRACHYURY	Rabbit Polyclonal	Anti-Rabbit Alexa Fluor 488
GATA4	Mouse Polyclonal	Anti-Mouse-Cy3
NANOG	Rabbit Polyclonal	Anti-Rabbit Alexa Fluor 488
OCT4	Rabbit Polyclonal	Anti-RabbitAlexa Fluor 488
SOX2	Rabbit polyclonal	Anti-Mouse Alexa Fluor 488
TUJ1	Mouse Polyclonal	Anti-Mouse-Cy3
YAP	Rabbit Polyclonal	Anti-Rabbit Alexa Fluor 488

2.8. Effect of YAP Inhibitor on Human ESCs Grown in 3-D Self-Assembling Scaffolds

For analysis of yes-associated protein (YAP) signaling in 3-D culture, human ESCs were grown in self-assembling scaffolds for 7 days, and then treated with 2 µM YAP inhibitor (YAPi), Verteporfin (VP, R&D Systems, Minneapolis, MN), for an additional 7 days. Cell growth in the scaffolds was monitored by light microscopy. Embryonic stem cells cultivated in three-dimensional self-assembling structures were collected after 14 days of incubation, with and without YAP inhibitor therapy for comparison. Cells were collected for RNA and immunocytochemical examination.

2.9. Statistical analysis

Data are presented as mean ± standard error of the mean (SE). One-way ANOVA analysis was performed and analyzed for unequal variances using post hoc tests for multiple comparisons. Results with a p-value less than 0.05 were considered to be significant (* $p < 0.05$ and ** $p < 0.01$). All analyses were performed using SPSS version 26 (SPSS Inc., Chicago, IL., USA).

3. RESULTS

3.1. Cultivation and Analysis of H9 Cells in a 3-Dimensional Environment

H9 cells encapsulated in self-assembling scaffolds composed of PEG-8-SH and PEG-8-Acr polymers grew for extended periods without requiring routine passaging or manipulation. The optimal growth of ESCs was achieved by using a concentration of 2.5 w/v % (dry weight of polymer per volume of culture medium) at a 1:1 molar ratio of PEG-8-SH and PEG-8-Acr. The results depicted in **Figure 2** show steady cell growth up to 21 days as observed by light microscopy (**Figure** 2A–D). Cells grew clonally in a time-dependent manner. Visual observations were consistent with the results obtained by MTT assay.

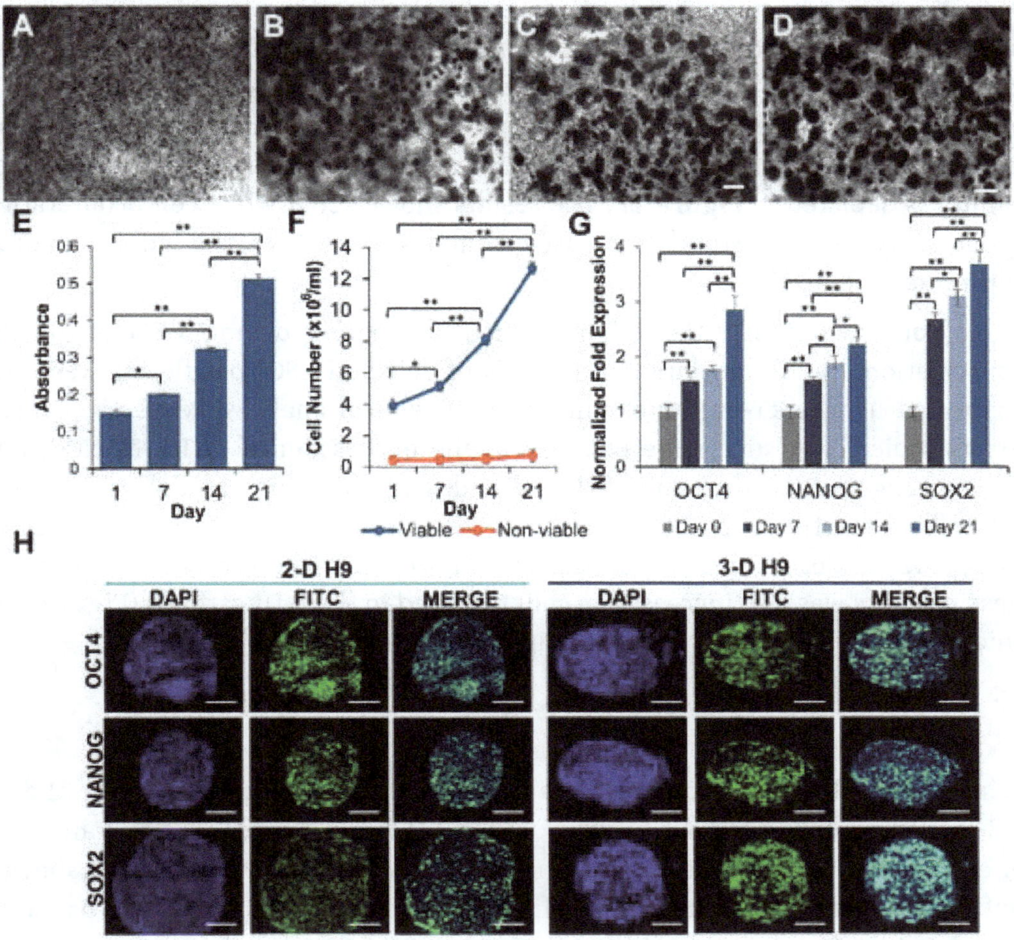

Figure 2. Growth of pluripotent human ESCs in 3-D self-assembling scaffolds. (A–D) Clonal growth of ESCs (H9 cells) encapsulated in PEG-8-SH/PEG-8-Acr scaffolds and incubated in culture medium was observed by light microscopy at 0, 7, 14, and 21 days. (E) Quantitative determination of cell proliferation by 3-(4,5-dimethylthiazol-2-yl)-2,5-diphenyltetrazolium bromide (MTT) assay using microplate reader. Results were expressed as the absorbance ± standard error (SE) with a significant increase in cell number. (F) Growth of ESCs encapsulated in 3-D scaffolds was assayed by direct counts using a hemocytometer, and cell viability was determined by trypan blue exclusion assay at various time intervals. Data presented as cell number (×10^6 cells/mL) ± SE. (G) Expression of selected pluripotency markers, OCT4, NANOG, and SOX2, in ESCs cultured in self-assembling scaffolds for 0, 7, 14, and 21 days as determined by qRT-PCR. The expression of genes at day 0 was set to 1 and results were expressed as the fold expression ± SE normalized to reference genes HMBS, GAPDH, and β-ACTIN (* $p < 0.05$ and ** $p < 0.01$). (H) Confocal images (20X) of 2-D and 3-D grown ESCs displaying the expression of pluripotent proteins, OCT4, NANOG, and SOX2. All scale bars represent 100 μm.

A significant and continuous increase in the proliferation of cells was observed during day 7 to 21. However, cells grew more rapidly between day 14 and 21 than between day 1 and 14 (**Figure 2**E), suggesting that the growth of ESCs required a longer acclimation period in 3-D self-assembling scaffolds compared to 2-D culture conditions. The viability of 3-D cultured ESCs was further validated by direct cell counts, as depicted in **Figure 2**F. The results showed that while cell proliferation significantly and consistently increased from day 1 to day 21, the number of dead cells remained low.

To confirm whether H9 cells remained pluripotent during 3-D culture, the transcriptional and translational analysis of selected ESC-specific markers was performed using qRT-PCR and immunocytochemical analysis, respectively. The results indicated a successive increase in the expression of OCT4, NANOG, and SOX2 throughout the duration of the 3-D culture, which increased 2.85, 2.23, and 3.69-fold, respectively in ESCs grown in 3-D scaffolds for 21 days as compared to cells grown under 2-D culture conditions (**Figure 2**G). The protein expression of these markers was also increased in cells cultured in the 3-D scaffolds (**Figure 2**H), which was consistent with the transcriptional upregulation.

3.2. Preservation of Pluripotency in H9 Cells Cultivated in 3-Dimensional Environment

To investigate if the 3-D grown H9 cells maintained their pluripotency after 21 days in 3-D culture, cells were subcultured under 2-D culture conditions and analyzed for cell morphology and the expression of pluripotent markers. The results showed that there were no morphological differences between cells that were passaged from 3-D to 2-D culture conditions and the initial ESCs used for encapsulation in the 3-D self-assembling scaffolds (**Figure 3**A–C). When H9 cells grown in 3-D self-assembling scaffolds for 21 days were subsequently subcultured under 2-D culture conditions, the expression of core pluripotent markers, OCT4 and NANOG, was statistically similar to that of initial 2-D grown cells, while the expression of SOX2 (1.55 fold) was slightly upregulated (**Figure 3**D). Apparently, repeated the subculturing of 3-D grown cells in 2-D culture conditions reverted the expression of these markers back to the normal level of expression. Despite the high expression of key pluripotent markers, it was prudent to further investigate the 3-D grown cells for the maintenance of their differentiation potential both in in vitro and in vivo.

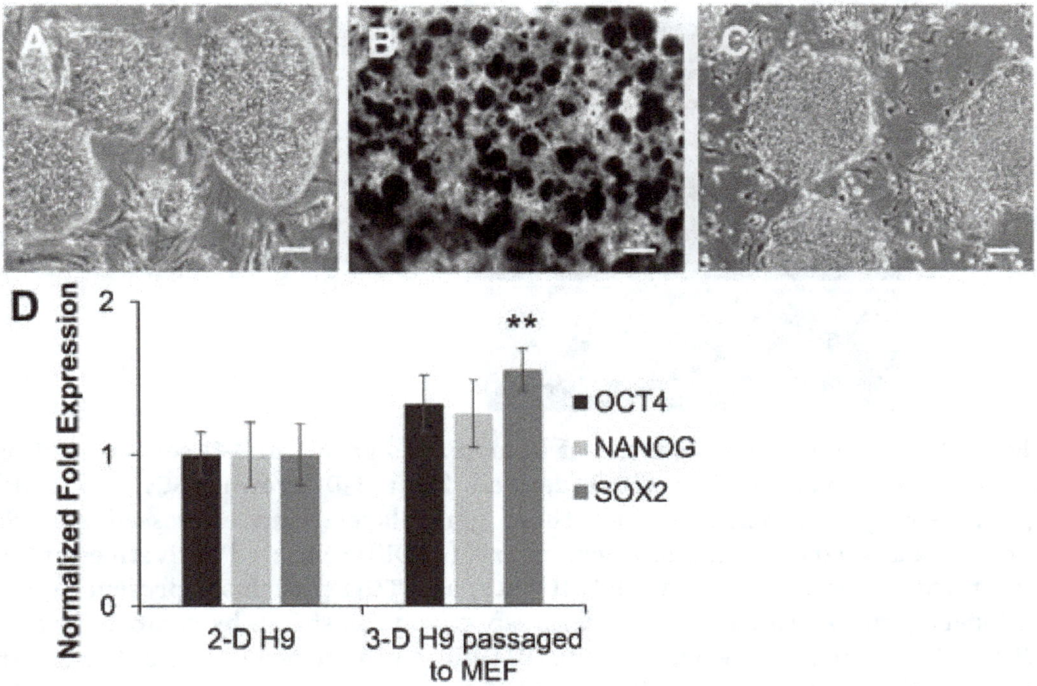

Figure 3. Self-renewal and pluripotency of ESCs were maintained following extended culture in 3-D scaffolds. (A–C) Cell morphology of ESCs (H9 cells) grown in 2-D cultures prior to encapsulation, in self-assembling scaffolds for 3-D culture for 21 days, and then subsequently subcultured back to 2-D culture conditions, respectively, as determined by light microscopy. All scale bars represent 100 µm. (D) Comparison of expression of OCT4, NANOG, and SOX2 in ESCs grown in 2-D conditions and first in 3-D self-assembling scaffolds, and then passaged in 2-D culture conditions as determined by qRT-PCR. Results were expressed as the fold expression ± SE normalized to reference genes HMBS, GAPDH, and β-ACTIN (* $p < 0.05$ and ** $p < 0.01$).

3.3. Differentiation of H9 Cells Grown in 3-D Self-Assembling Scaffolds

The preservation of the pluripotency of 3-D cultured H9 cells was examined by inducing differentiation into three germ layers after forming embryoid bodies (EB). The results presented in **Figure 4** show that EBs from 3-D grown cells spontaneously differentiated into endoderm, mesoderm, and ectoderm germ layers, as evident by the protein expression of specific markers, GATA4, BRACHYURY, and TUJ1, respectively (**Figure** 4A). Transcriptional analysis also confirmed that differentiated derivatives of 3-D grown cells expressed markers of all three germ layers, including SOX7 and GATA6, BRACHYURY and MIXL1, and PAX6 and NCAM, representing the endoderm, mesoderm, and ectoderm, respectively (**Figure** 4B).

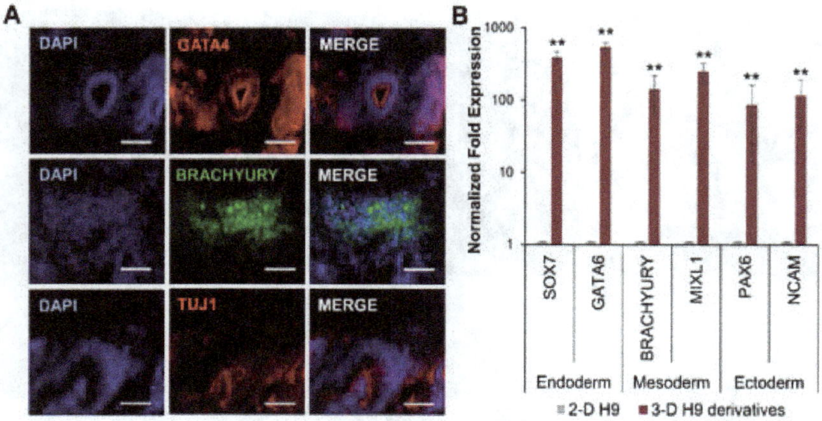

Figure 4. Differentiation potential of human ESCs grown in 3-D self-assembling scaffolds. Embryoid bodies (EBs) derived from 3-D grown ESCs (H9 cells) spontaneously differentiated into three germ layers and expressed specific proteins analyzed by immunocytochemistry. (A) Differentiated derivatives of 3-D grown ESCs expressed GATA4, BRACHYURY, and TUJ1 proteins representing the endoderm, mesoderm, and ectoderm, respectively, as shown by confocal images (20X). All scale bars represent 100 μm. (B) Differentiated derivatives of 3-D grown ESCs expressed germ layer-specific genes SOX7 and GATA6 (endoderm), BRACHYURY and MIXL1 (mesoderm), and PAX6 and NCAM (ectoderm) as determined by qRT-PCR. Results are expressed as the fold expression ± SE normalized to reference genes HMBS, GAPDH, and β-ACTIN (* $p < 0.05$ and ** $p < 0.01$).

Next, the pluripotency of 3-D grown H9 cells was validated in vivo by an analysis of teratoma formation. The results showed that the 3-D grown cells injected into SCID Beige mice formed teratomas (**Figure 5**). An analysis of teratoma tissue showed the expression of GATA4, BRACHYURY, and TUJ1 proteins, indicating that teratoma tissue had cells representing the endoderm, mesoderm, and ectoderm, respectively (**Figure 5**C). The transcriptional analysis of teratoma tissues also showed the expression of genes of all three germ layers: the endoderm (SOX7, and SOX17), mesoderm (BRACHYURY, and MIXL1), and ectoderm (PAX6, and TUJ1) (**Figure 5**D). Taken together, these results indicated that H9 cells grown in 3-D self-assembling scaffolds maintained their pluripotency and differentiation potential.

3.4. Naïve pluripotent markers in H9 cells were examined under 3-D culture conditions and the impact of YAP inhibition was studied.

Since a significant upregulation of core pluripotent markers, OCT4, NANOG, and SOX2, was observed in ESCs cultured in the 3-D scaffolds, we also assessed the expression of both primed and naïve pluripotent markers. A comparative transcriptional analysis of H9 cells grown in 3-D scaffolds and 2-D cultured H9 and Elf1 cells (representing primed and naïve ESC lines, respectively) is depicted in **Figure 6**.

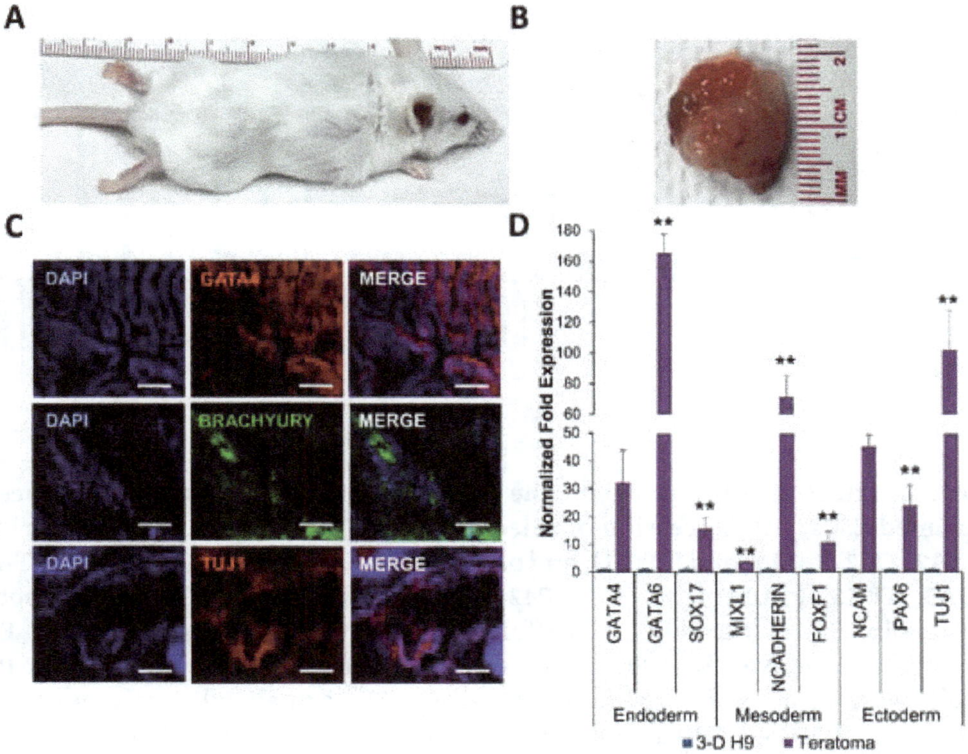

Figure 5. Teratoma formation by 3-D grown human ESCs in severe combined immunodeficient (SCID) Beige mice. (A) Tumor growth was observed in all mice (n = 3) injected with 3-D grown ESCs (H9 cells). (B) Explanted tumor at 4 weeks showed encapsulated, lobular, and well-circumscribed gross morphology consistent with teratoma growth. (C) Expression of GATA4, BRACHYURY, and TUJ1 proteins representing the endoderm, mesoderm, and ectoderm, respectively in excised teratomas, as shown by confocal images (20X). All scale bars represent 100 μm. (D) Expression of germ layer-specific genes, SOX7 and GATA6 (endoderm), BRACHYURY and MIXL1 (mesoderm), and PAX6 and NCAM (ectoderm) in excised teratomas, as determined by qRT-PCR. Results are expressed as the fold expression ± SE normalized to reference genes HMBS, GAPDH, and β-ACTIN (* $p < 0.05$ and ** $p < 0.01$).

Expected primed pluripotent markers (FOXA2, ZIC2, SALL2, and SOX11) were expressed at higher levels in H9 than Elf1 cells cultured under 2-D conditions. Interestingly, the expression of primed pluripotent markers was significantly decreased in H9 cells grown in 3-D scaffolds to levels comparable to Elf1 cells grown under 2-D conditions. More strikingly, 3-D grown H9 cells expressed significantly higher levels of naïve markers (KLF2, ESRRB, DNMT3L, KLF17, STAT3, DPPA3, TBX3, PRDM14, KLF5, ZFP42, TFCP2L1, FGF4, and GDF3) in comparison to 2-D cultured Elf1 cells, suggesting that the 3-D scaffold microenvironment modulated gene expression.

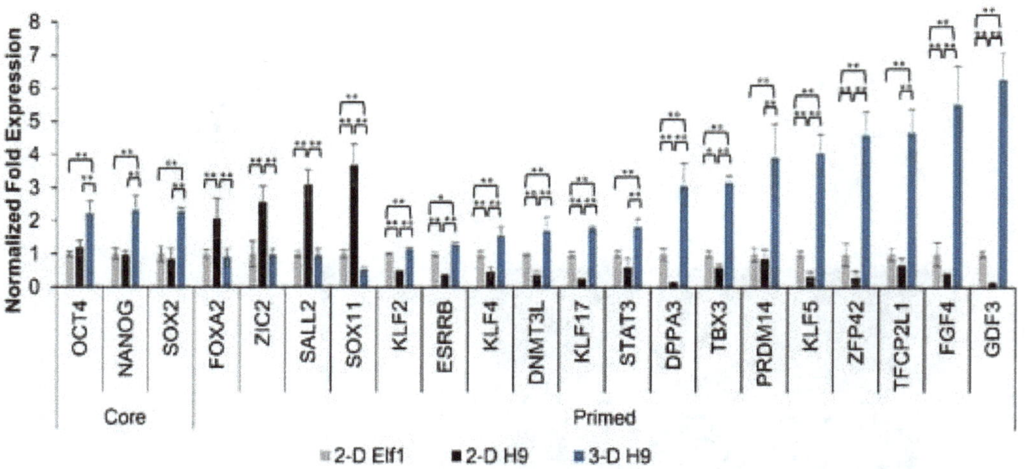

Figure 6. Effect of 3-D culture on the expression of naïve pluripotent markers in primed ESCs. (A) Expression of select core (OCT4, NANOG, and SOX2), primed (FOXA2, ZIC2, SALL2, and SOX11), and naïve (KLF2, ESRRB, DNMT3L, KLF17, STAT3, DPPA3, TBX3, PRDM14, KLF5, ZFP42, TFCP2L1, FGF4, and GDF3) pluripotent markers in ESCs cultured in 3-D scaffolds for 21 days and 2-D grown primed ESCs (H9 cells) and naïve ESCs (Elf1 cells, set to control) was analyzed by qRT-PCR. Results were expressed as the fold expression ± SE normalized to reference genes HMBS, GAPDH, and β-ACTIN (* $p < 0.05$ and ** $p < 0.01$).

Many reports have stated that 3-D scaffolds induce differential gene expression due to mechanical and biological stimuli [**10,38,39**]. Since the overexpression of YAP has been shown to induce the naïve state of pluripotency in primed ESCs [**40**], we investigated the effect of YAP in 3-D cultured H9 cells using VP, which is a YAP inhibitor (YAPi). Our results in **Figure** 7A showed that mechanosensitive genes, YAP and TAZ, were upregulated in H9 cells grown in 3-D scaffolds in comparison to 2-D cultured cells. In contrast, YAP and TAZ expression significantly decreased when 3-D grown H9 cells were subjected to YAPi. A similar trend was observed at a translational level, where it appears that the immunofluorescence signal for YAP in 3-D grown H9 cells was brighter than in 2-D cultured cells. Moreover, an increased signal for YAP was observed in the cytoplasm of 3-D grown cells treated with YAPi (**Figure** 7B).

The incubation of YAP also affected the clonal growth of H9 cells encapsulated in 3-D scaffolds, with YAPi-treated H9 cells exhibiting a significantly smaller colony size in comparison to untreated cells (**Figure** 7C). Interestingly, YAPi treatment also abrogated the upregulation of core (OCT4, NANOG, and SOX2), and naïve (ESRRB, KLF4, DNMT3L, KLF17, DPPA3, KLF5, ZFP42, TFCP2L1, and FGF4) pluripotent markers in 3-D cultured cells (**Figure** 7D). In addition, a concurrent decrease in the expression of core pluripotent proteins, OCT4, NANOG, and SOX2 was observed when compared with the untreated 3-D grown cells (**Figure** 7E).

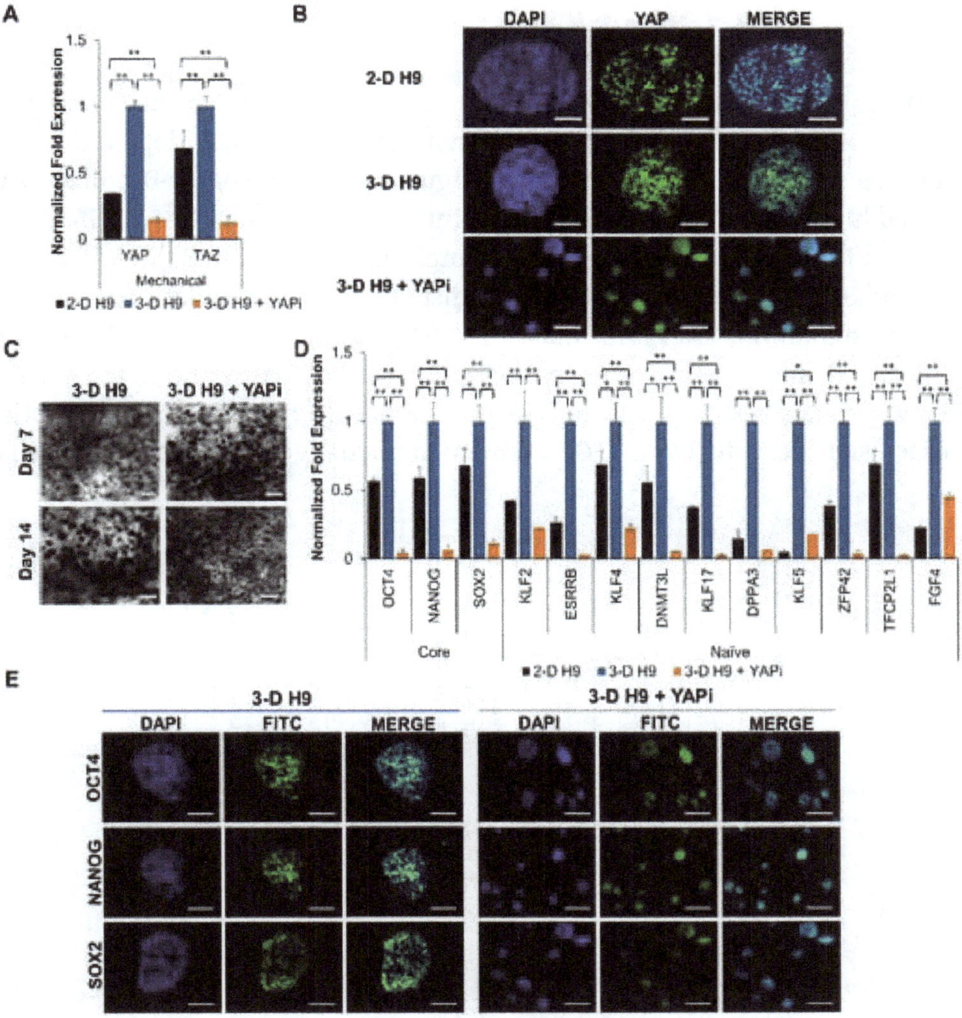

Figure 7. Effect of Yes-associated protein (YAP) inhibition (YAPi) on cell growth and expression of pluripotent markers in human ESCs cultured under 3-D conditions. ESCs (H9 cells) were grown under 3-D culture conditions for 14 days and incubated in the absence (control) or presence of a YAPi. (A) The effect of YAPi on the expression of mechanosensitive markers, YAP and TAZ, in H9 cells grown in 2-D and 3-D culture conditions as determined by qRT-PCR. (B) Merged confocal images (20X) showing YAP protein expression in 2-D and 3-D grown H9 cells. (C) Light micrographs depicting the cell morphology and colony size of 3-D grown H9 cells incubated in the presence or absence of YAPi. (D) Comparison of relative gene expression of core and naïve pluripotent markers in H9 cells grown under 2-D, 3-D, and 3-D + YAPi conditions as determined by qRT-PCR. Results were expressed as the fold expression ± SE normalized to reference genes HMBS, GAPDH, and β-ACTIN (* $p < 0.05$ and ** $p < 0.01$). (E) Merged confocal images (20X) of 3-D H9 cells with and without YAPi treatment for the protein expression of OCT4, NANOG, and SOX2. All scale bars represent 100 μm.

3.5. Mechanism of Regulation of Pluripotent Genes in H9 Cells Grown under 3-D Culture Conditions

Concurrent increase in LIF signaling led to the increase in naïve pluripotent markers in H9 cells cultured in 3-D self-assembling scaffolds, as depicted in Figure 8B. (**Figure 8**). The results depicted in **Figure 8**A show that 3-D cultured cells expressed higher levels of genes encoding integrin subunits, ITGA5, ITGA6, ITGAV, ITGB1, and ITGB3 as well as G-coupled protein receptors (GCPRs), LPAR1, LPAR2, S1PR1, and S1PR3. In addition, these cells displayed the upregulation of RHOA and RAC1 (Rho signaling), YAP, TAZ, and TEAD4 (Hippo signaling), LIFR, GP130, SOCS3, and TBX3 (LIF signaling). However, the expression of ITGA2, ROCK1, LATS1, and LATS2, which is associated with integrin, Rho, and Hippo signaling, respectively, decreased significantly, while ITGB5 remained unchanged in 3-D cultured cells.

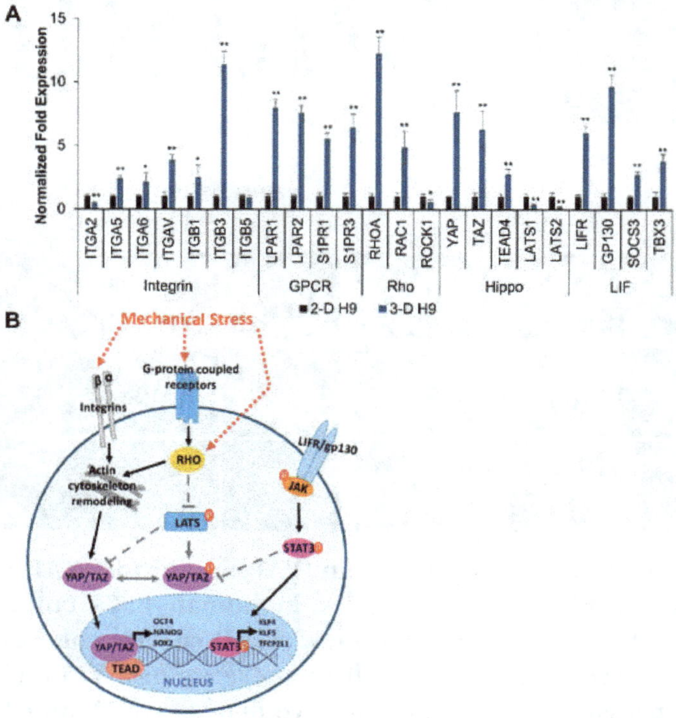

Figure 8. Molecular mechanism of upregulation of pluripotent markers in human ESCs grown in 3-D scaffolds. (A) The effect of 3-D culture of ESCs (H9 cells) on the expression of markers associated with integrin (ITGA2, ITGA5, ITGA6, ITGAV, ITGB1, ITGB3, and ITGB5) and G-coupled protein receptors (GCPRs; LPAR1, LPAR2, S1PR1, and S1PR3), Hippo (YAP, TAZ, TEAD4, LATS1, and LATS2), Rho (RHOA, RAC1, and ROCK1), and LIF (LIFR, GP130, SOCS3, and TBX3) signaling pathways as determined by qRT-PCR. Results were expressed as the fold expression ± SE normalized to reference genes HMBS, GAPDH, and β-ACTIN (* $p < 0.05$ and ** $p < 0.01$). (B) Proposed pathway involved in the induction of naïve pluripotency in primed human ESCs (H9 cells) encapsulated in 3-D self-assembling scaffolds.

These results further indicate that 3-D self-assembling scaffolds stimulated mechanosensitive signaling resulting in the upregulation of integrin receptors and GPCRs, thus promoting the activation of Rho signaling, which is associated with actin cytoskeleton remodeling; in turn, this led to the upregulation of mechanosensitive YAP/TAZ signaling. Activated YAP/TAZ act as transcription factors in the nucleus assisted by transcription co-factor, TEAD4, which binds to the DNA, to stimulate the expression of pluripotent genes. Concurrent increase in LIF signaling led to the increase in naïve pluripotent markers in H9 cells cultured in 3-D self-assembling scaffolds, as depicted in Figure 8B.

4. DISCUSSION

Cultivating human embryonic stem cells in 2-D culture methods is complex and involves frequent handling and transferring of cell colonies through enzymatic dissection. Cultivating human ESCs in 2-D culture using standard procedures is complex and involves regular manipulation and passaging using enzymatic or non-enzymatic approaches. [**41,42,43**]. These manipulations can result in poor viability, large batch-to-batch variation, and spontaneous differentiation. We theorized that utilizing a 3-D culture could more accurately replicate the natural environment of ESCs, perhaps enhancing their long-term development and viability. Our study investigated the effect of the microenvironment in stemness by developing 3-D scaffolds made of two functionalized PEG polymers that self-assembled via a Michael addition reaction. When ESCs were included in the polymer mixtures, they were encapsulated upon self-assembly of the scaffolds. It has been previously reported that fully hydrated hydrogels mimic the 3-D native microenvironment, which allow nutrient diffusion and promote the growth of cells [**44**]. We have previously shown that soft 3-D scaffolds composed of Dex-SH and PEG-4-Acr self-assembling polymers were capable of supporting mouse ESC pluripotency for over 6 weeks [**34**]. Several other studies have also reported that mouse ESC self-renewal could be maintained on soft and low stiffness substrates in 2-D culture [**45,46,47**]. In addition, mechanically stiffer prefabricated scaffolds have been shown to promote the differentiation of mouse ESCs [**48**], while softer 3-D scaffolds supported the differentiation of human adult stem cells [**49**]. The culture of H9 cells in soft scaffolds did not support the viability of encapsulated cells, and growth was severely curtailed. This is consistent with previous studies, which showed that stiffer substrates promoted the maintenance of human ESCs [**22,50,51**]. Consequently, we created more rigid scaffolds using modified PEG polymers.

We experimented with many self-assembling polymers at different concentrations to enhance scaffold polymerization, encapsulation, and proliferation of H9 cells in our initial research (unpublished data). These studies showed that scaffolds made of PEG-8-SH and PEG-8-Acr prepared at 2.5% w/v improved the clonal growth of H9 cells in comparison to scaffolds with lower cross-linking densities and higher swelling ratios (i.e., Dex-SH/PEG-4-Acr and PEG-4-SH/PEG-4-Acr). These results were in line with other the reported studies performed using scaffolds made of multi-arm PEG functionalized with vinyl sulfone (VS) **[52]**. In these studies, H9 cells grew upon encapsulation in scaffolds made of VS functionalized 4-arm and 8-arm but not 3-arm PEG hydrogels **[52]**. However, this study was performed using clumps of H9 cells and not single cells for encapsulation. Whereas, in our study, PEG-8-SH/PEG-8-Acr scaffolds supported cell viability, allowing for even dispersal and clonal growth of H9 cells encapsulated as single cells. This has important implications because the growth of single cell inoculations and the generation of homologous populations of pluripotent cells is necessary for cell-based therapeutics **[53]**. Furthermore, the maintenance and growth of H9 cells was achieved using PEG-8-SH/PEG-8-Acr self-assembling scaffolds for long-term 3-D culture without passaging or manipulation. The pluripotency of the 3-D grown H9 cells was further demonstrated by their ability to differentiate into three germ layers and teratoma formation in vitro and in vivo, respectively. Additionally, core pluripotent markers, OCT4, NANOG, and SOX2, were upregulated during growth in the self-assembling scaffolds, showing significantly higher expression on day 21 of 3-D culture as compared to cells grown in 2-D culture. When 3-D grown H9 cells were passaged back to 2-D culture conditions, they exhibited undifferentiated morphology, and the expression of pluripotent markers decreased to levels similar to the 2-D cultured cells, suggesting that the encapsulated cells cultured under 3-D conditions were not altered. Changes in the expression of core and naïve pluripotent markers in H9 cells cultured in 3-D self-assembling scaffolds can be attributed to multiple factors, including matrix dimensionality, stiffness, and/or bioinductive signaling **[10]**. While the incorporation of natural biomaterials has been shown to increase biological signaling, synthetic biomaterials lack biological activities minimizing batch-to-batch variation, but still allow for biophysical modifications, including pore size and mechanical stiffness **[54]**. Scaffolds composed of natural polymers including hyaluronic acid **[55]**, chitosan, and alginate **[56]** have been shown to support human ESC self-renewal without a significant change in pluripotent marker expression. Whereas thermoresponsive synthetic hydrogels composed of PEG functionalized with poly-N-isopropylacrylamide allowed for the continuous 3-D culture of cells for 60 passages but only yielded cells 95% positive for OCT4 **[57]**. We noticed an increase in the expression of OCT4, NANOG, and SOX2 when maintaining human ESCs in 3-D scaffolds.

Earlier research on mouse ESCs found that the varying increase in pluripotent markers in 3-D culture was influenced by the composition and rigidity of the scaffold. **[34,58]**. A recent study using single cell inoculation and the expansion of human ESCs in large-scale bioreactors resulted in the maintenance of OCT4 levels but the upregulation of SOX2 in 3-D grown ESC aggregates [**59**]. In another study, a 3-D culture of H9 clumps in VS functionalized PEG scaffolds resulted in upregulated gene expression of SOX2 and KLF4 but not OCT4 and NANOG when compared to 2-D cultured cells [**52**]. Interestingly, we observed that primed ESCs, H9 cells, encapsulated in the 3-D self-assembling scaffolds exhibited a decreased expression of primed pluripotency markers, FOXA2, ZIC2, SALL2, and SOX11, which is characteristic of post-implantation epiblast cells [**60,61**], to levels comparable to naïve Elf1 cells. Furthermore, a 3-D culture of H9 cells resulted in an increase in the expression of naïve pluripotent markers, (KLF2, ESRRB, DNMT3L, KLF17, STAT3, DPPA3, TBX3, PRDM14, KLF5, ZFP42, TFCP2L1, FGF4, and GDF3), which was associated with naïve pre-implantation epiblast cells [**7,60,61,62,63,64,65,66**]. Recent studies have shown that traditionally derived primed human ESC lines can be reprogrammed to naïve pluripotency using the ectopic expression of select genes and specific media conditions containing inhibitor cocktails [**67,68**]. In one study, a transcriptomic comparison of primed and reprogrammed naïve human demonstrated the differential expression of certain genes such as KLF2, KLF4, GDF3, SOCS3, STAT3, and TBX3 expressed at higher levels in naïve than primed cells [**63**]. However, the expression of core pluripotent markers OCT4 and NANOG remained unchanged, while SOX2 levels decreased upon reversion to naïve pluripotency [**63**]. An increase in core and naïve pluripotent markers was noted during 3-D culture, likely due to the influence of the 3-D scaffold microenvironment.

Research has shown that biophysical signals such as substrate stiffness, cell-cell interactions, and mechanical pressures can affect the destiny and self-renewal of human embryonic stem cells in 2-D culture. [**39**]. The interplay between external and internal mechanical stresses of cells and their ECM play important roles in tensional homeostasis of tissues in vivo [**69**]. The impact of 3-D culture on the regulation of ESCs' pluripotency has not been well investigated.

Physical contacts with cells or the extracellular matrix can be converted into biological signals and impact actin dynamics through mechanosensitive receptors like integrin receptors and GPCRs. [**70**]. Evidence has shown that integrin heterodimers, $\alpha5\beta1$, $\alpha6\beta1$, and $\alpha v\beta3$, mediate interactions between ESCs and various ECM substrates [**13,71,72,73**]; they also play an important role in the maintenance of pluripotency [**74**], and matrix stiffness regulates integrin binding [**75**]. Whereas GPCRs, including lysophosphatidic acid receptors (LPARs) and sphingosine-1-phosphate receptors (S1PRs), play a role in the YAP signaling axis. In response to LPA and S1P ligand binding, the dephosphorylation of YAP and TAZ allows them to enter the nucleus to activate transcription [**76**]. Treatment with exogenous LPA has been shown to aid in the reversion of primed pluripotency to naïve pluripotency in ESCs due to the role that both YAP and LPA serve in suppressing differentiation associated with GSK3 inhibition [**40**]. However, the transduction of mechanical signals has also been shown to activate G-protein signaling independent of ligand binding [**77**]. We noticed an increase in various integrin subunits, LPARs, and S1PRs in H9 cells cultured in a 3-D environment. This indicates that the 3-D scaffolds enhanced mechanical signaling pathways in H9 cells, but further research is needed to identify how these receptors are triggered.

Substrate stiffness can activate Rho signaling, which controls actin cytoskeleton organization, resulting in higher levels of F-actin and YAP and TAZ moving into the cell nucleus. [**78**]. YAP is a mechanosensitive transcription factor in the Hippo signaling pathway, which plays a crucial role in cancer, regeneration, and the regulation of organ size [**79**]. In addition, Hippo signaling regulates the first cell fate specification to the trophoectoderm and the inner cell mass (ICM) of early blastocysts via mechanically sensitive pathways [**80**]. YAP is mostly retained in the cytoplasm in the ICM of early blastocysts, but becomes active during epiblast specification with a strong nuclear signal [**64**]. YAP and its transcription cofactor, TAZ, act as major downstream effectors in the Rho signaling pathway and have been shown to control the pluripotent state, allowing for the long-term survival and expansion of human ESCs in vitro [**81**].Furthermore, cell culture on stiffer substrates has also been shown to increase the nuclear function of YAP/TAZ in human ESCs [**82**]. TAZ itself is required for the maintenance of self-renewal marker expression in ESCs, and the loss of TAZ leads to the inhibition of transforming growth factor beta (TGFβ) signaling and differentiation into a neuroectoderm lineage [**83**]. Similarly, reducing YAP levels leads to a decrease in pluripotency in mouse embryonic stem cells, while introducing YAP artificially inhibits the process of differentiation [**84**].

In the nucleus, YAP mediates transcriptional enhanced associate domain (TEAD) transcription, and YAP/TAZ complexes associate with TEAD to regulate pluripotency by activating OCT4 expression [**85**]. Pluripotency is determined by an autoregulatory core transcriptional circuitry comprised of OCT4, NANOG, and SOX2, which inhibits lineage specification genes [**86**]. The phosphorylation of YAP by LATS kinases prevents interaction with TEAD and results in cytoplasmic retention and the inactivation of YAP [**87**]. In contrast, YAP overexpression has been shown to promote the reversion of primed pluripotency into naïve pluripotency [**40**]. When 3-D grown H9 cells were cultured with a YAPi (VP), the upregulation of core and naïve pluripotent markers was abrogated. VP acts to inhibit the interaction of YAP and TEAD, disrupting downstream transcriptional activation, and sequestering YAP in the cytoplasm for inactivation [**88**]. Therefore, we postulate that mechanical forces in 3-D scaffolds stimulated the upregulation of mechanosensitive receptors, including integrins and GPCRs, leading to enhanced Rho signaling and higher levels of YAP/TAZ. In addition, the mechanical forces generated by the expansion of cells may also have contributed to the inhibition of phosphorylated LATS kinases [**87**], which in turn allowed YAP/TAZ to enter the nucleus, activating the transcription of pluripotent genes. This was concurrent with the observed increase in LIF signaling receptors and downstream naïve pluripotent target genes including KLF4, KLF5, and TFCP2L1 [**89**]. While LIF/STAT3 signaling fails to maintain the self-renewal of primed human ESCs [**90**], naïve ESCs are dependent on LIF signaling [**63**].

The 3-D scaffolds created from PEG-8-SH/PEG-8-Acr facilitate the clonal proliferation of primed ESCs and promote increased expression of core and naïve pluripotency markers. This indicates that the scaffold offers a conducive environment for inducing a naïve-like state of pluripotency. The 3-D culture method we developed is strong, straightforward, and requires less effort for the extended growth of uniform populations of ESCs, potentially enhancing their utilization in research and medical treatments.

5. AT A GLANCE

Cultivating and growing human embryonic stem cells (ESCs) in two-dimensional (2-D) culture is difficult and involves regular handling and transferring. We created 3-D scaffolds to imitate the natural environment for stem cell growth. The scaffolds were constructed from two 8-arm polyethylene glycol (PEG) polymers modified with thiol (PEG-8-SH) and acrylate (PEG-8-Acr) end groups, which assembled spontaneously by a Michael addition process. Primed ESCs (H9 cells) were encapsulated and cultured with PEG polymers for a prolonged duration, preserving their vitality, self-renewal capacity, and ability to differentiate in both laboratory settings and living organisms. Cells cultured on a three-dimensional self-assembling scaffold showed increased expression of key pluripotency genes: OCT4, NANOG, and SOX2. Primed markers' expression dropped, but naïve markers' expression significantly increased. Notably, the mechanosensitive genes YAP and TAZ were also increased in expression. Verteporfin inhibited YAP, preventing the upregulation of YAP/TAZ and core and naïve pluripotent markers. The 3-D culture conditions clearly caused an increase in markers linked to a naïve state of pluripotency in the primed cells. Our 3-D culture technique facilitated the growth of a uniform population of ESCs, which could be beneficial for furthering their application in cell therapy and regenerative medicine.

REFERENCES

1. Reubinoff, B.E.; Pera, M.F.; Fong, C.Y.; Trounson, A.; Bongso, A. Embryonic stem cell lines from human blastocysts: Somatic differentiation in vitro. Nat. Biotech. 2000, 18, 399–404. [Google Scholar] [CrossRef]

2. Takahashi, K.; Yamanaka, S. Induction of pluripotent stem cells from mouse embryonic and adult fibroblast cultures by defined factors. Cell 2006, 126, 663–676. [Google Scholar] [CrossRef] [Green Version]

3. Nakamura, T.; Okamoto, I.; Sasaki, K.; Yabuta, Y.; Iwatani, C.; Tsuchiya, H.; Seita, Y.; Nakamura, S.; Yamamoto, T.; Saitou, M. A developmental coordinate of pluripotency among mice, monkeys and humans. Nature 2016, 537, 57–62. [Google Scholar] [CrossRef]

4. Nichols, J.; Smith, A. Naive and primed pluripotent states. Cell Stem Cell 2009, 4, 487–492. [Google Scholar] [CrossRef] [Green Version]

5. Gafni, O.; Weinberger, L.; Mansour, A.A.; Manor, Y.S.; Chomsky, E.; Ben-Yosef, D.; Kalma, Y.; Viukov, S.; Maza, I.; Zviran, A.; et al. Derivation of novel human ground state naive pluripotent stem cells. Nature 2013, 504, 282–286. [Google Scholar] [CrossRef]

6. Morgani, S.; Nichols, J.; Hadjantonakis, A.-K. The many faces of pluripotency: In vitro adaptations of a continuum of in vivo states. BMC Dev. Biol. 2017, 17, 7. [Google Scholar] [CrossRef] [PubMed] [Green Version]

7. Theunissen, T.W.; Powell, B.E.; Wang, H.; Mitalipova, M.; Faddah, D.A.; Reddy, J.; Fan, Z.P.; Maetzel, D.; Ganz, K.; Shi, L.; et al. Systematic identification of culture conditions for induction and maintenance of naive human pluripotency. Cell Stem Cell 2014, 15, 471–487. [Google Scholar] [CrossRef] [PubMed] [Green Version]

8. Ying, Q.L.; Wray, J.; Nichols, J.; Batlle-Morera, L.; Doble, B.; Woodgett, J.; Cohen, P.; Smith, A. The ground state of embryonic stem cell self-renewal. Nature 2008, 453, 519–523. [Google Scholar] [CrossRef] [PubMed] [Green Version]

9. Wu, J.; Yamauchi, T.; Izpisua Belmonte, J.C. An overview of mammalian pluripotency. Development 2016, 143, 1644–1648. [Google Scholar] [CrossRef] [PubMed] [Green Version]

10. McKee, C.; Chaudhry, G.R. Advances and challenges in stem cell culture. Colloids Surf. B Biointerfaces 2017, 159, 62–77. [Google Scholar] [CrossRef] [PubMed]

11. Li, Y.; Lin, C.; Wang, L.; Liu, Y.; Mu, X.; Ma, Y.; Li, L. Maintenance of human embryonic stem cells on gelatin. Chin. Sci. Bull. 2009, 54, 4214. [Google Scholar] [CrossRef]

12. Xu, C.; Inokuma, M.S.; Denham, J.; Golds, K.; Kundu, P.; Gold, J.D.; Carpenter, M.K. Feeder-free growth of undifferentiated human embryonic stem cells. Nat. Biotechnol. 2001, 19, 971–974. [Google Scholar] [CrossRef] [PubMed]

13. Rodin, S.; Domogatskaya, A.; Strom, S.; Hansson, E.M.; Chien, K.R.; Inzunza, J.; Hovatta, O.; Tryggvason, K. Long-term self-renewal of human pluripotent stem cells on human recombinant laminin-511. Nat. Biotechnol. 2010, 28, 611–615. [Google Scholar] [CrossRef] [PubMed] [Green Version]

14. Kalaskar, D.M.; Downes, J.E.; Murray, P.; Edgar, D.H.; Williams, R.L. Characterization of the interface between adsorbed fibronectin and human embryonic stem cells. J. R. Soc. Interface 2013, 10, 20130139. [Google Scholar] [CrossRef] [Green Version]

15. Braam, S.R.; Zeinstra, L.; Litjens, S.; Ward-van Oostwaard, D.; van den Brink, S.; van Laake, L.; Lebrin, F.; Kats, P.; Hochstenbach, R.; Passier, R.; et al. Recombinant vitronectin is a functionally defined substrate that supports human embryonic stem cell self-renewal via alphavbeta5 integrin. Stem Cells 2008, 26, 2257–2265. [Google Scholar] [CrossRef]

16. Richards, M.; Fong, C.Y.; Chan, W.K.; Wong, P.C.; Bongso, A. Human feeders support prolonged undifferentiated growth of human inner cell masses and embryonic stem cells. Nat. Biotechnol. 2002, 20, 933–936. [Google Scholar] [CrossRef]

17. Jozefczuk, J.; Drews, K.; Adjaye, J. Preparation of mouse embryonic fibroblast cells suitable for culturing human embryonic and induced pluripotent stem cells. J. Vis. Exp. 2012. [Google Scholar] [CrossRef] [Green Version]

18. Kent, L. Culture and maintenance of human embryonic stem cells. J. Vis. Exp. 2009. [Google Scholar] [CrossRef]

19. Akhmanova, M.; Osidak, E.; Domogatsky, S.; Rodin, S.; Domogatskaya, A. Physical, spatial, and molecular aspects of extracellular matrix of in vivo niches and artificial scaffolds relevant to stem cells research. Stem Cells Int. 2015, 2015, 35. [Google Scholar] [CrossRef] [Green Version]

20. Cosson, S.; Lutolf, M.P. Chapter 7—Microfluidic patterning of protein gradients on biomimetic hydrogel substrates. In Methods in Cell Biology; Piel, M., Théry, M., Eds.; Academic Press: Cambridge, MA, USA, 2014; Volume 121, pp. 91–102. [Google Scholar]

21. Infantes, E.C.; Prados, A.B.H.; Contreras, I.D.; Cahuana, G.M.; Hmadcha, A.; Bermudo, F.M.; Soria, B.; Huamán, J.R.T.; Bergua, F.J.B. Nitric oxide and hypoxia response in pluripotent stem cells. Redox Biol. 2015, 5, 417–418. [Google Scholar] [CrossRef] [Green Version]

22. Musah, S.; Morin, S.A.; Wrighton, P.J.; Zwick, D.B.; Jin, S.; Kiessling, L.L. Glycosaminoglycan-binding hydrogels enable mechanical control of human pluripotent stem cell self-renewal. ACS Nano 2012, 6, 10168–10177. [Google Scholar] [CrossRef] [PubMed] [Green Version]

23. Peerani, R.; Rao, B.M.; Bauwens, C.; Yin, T.; Wood, G.A.; Nagy, A.; Kumacheva, E.; Zandstra, P.W. Niche-mediated control of human embryonic stem cell self-renewal and differentiation. EMBO J. 2007, 26, 4744–4755. [Google Scholar] [CrossRef] [PubMed] [Green Version]
24. Szablowska-Gadomska, I.; Zayat, V.; Buzanska, L. Influence of low oxygen tensions on expression of pluripotency genes in stem cells. Acta Neurobiol. Exp. 2011, 71, 86–93. [Google Scholar]
25. Burdick, J.A.; Vunjak-Novakovic, G. Engineered microenvironments for controlled stem cell differentiation. Tissue Eng. Part A 2009, 15, 205–219. [Google Scholar] [CrossRef]
26. Janmey, P.A.; Miller, R.T. Mechanisms of mechanical signaling in development and disease. J. Cell Sci. 2011, 124, 9–18. [Google Scholar] [CrossRef] [Green Version]
27. Provenzano, P.P.; Keely, P.J. Mechanical signaling through the cytoskeleton regulates cell proliferation by coordinated focal adhesion and rho gtpase signaling. J. Cell Sci. 2011, 124, 1195–1205. [Google Scholar] [CrossRef] [Green Version]
28. Baker, B.M.; Chen, C.S. Deconstructing the third dimension: How 3d culture microenvironments alter cellular cues. J. Cell Sci. 2012, 125, 3015–3024. [Google Scholar] [CrossRef] [Green Version]
29. Lund, A.W.; Yener, B.; Stegemann, J.P.; Plopper, G.E. The natural and engineered 3d microenvironment as a regulatory cue during stem cell fate determination. Tissue Eng. Part B Rev. 2009, 15, 371–380. [Google Scholar] [CrossRef]
30. Lutolf, M.P.; Gilbert, P.M.; Blau, H.M. Designing materials to direct stem-cell fate. Nature 2009, 462, 433–441. [Google Scholar] [CrossRef] [Green Version]
31. Saha, K.; Pollock, J.F.; Schaffer, D.V.; Healy, K.E. Designing synthetic materials to control stem cell phenotype. Curr. Opin. Chem. Biol. 2007, 11, 381–387. [Google Scholar] [CrossRef] [Green Version]
32. Mammoto, A.; Mammoto, T.; Ingber, D.E. Mechanosensitive mechanisms in transcriptional regulation. J. Cell Sci. 2012, 125, 3061–3073. [Google Scholar] [CrossRef] [PubMed] [Green Version]
33. Krupinski, P.; Chickarmane, V.; Peterson, C. Simulating the mammalian blastocyst—Molecular and mechanical interactions pattern the embryo. PLOS Comput. Biol. 2011, 7, e1001128. [Google Scholar] [CrossRef] [PubMed] [Green Version]
34. McKee, C.; Perez-Cruet, M.; Chavez, F.; Chaudhry, G.R. Simplified three-dimensional culture system for long-term expansion of embryonic stem cells. World J. Stem Cells 2015, 7, 1064–1077. [Google Scholar] [PubMed]

35. Thomson, J.A.; Itskovitz-Eldor, J.; Shapiro, S.S.; Waknitz, M.A.; Swiergiel, J.J.; Marshall, V.S.; Jones, J.M. Embryonic stem cell lines derived from human blastocysts. Science 1998, 282, 1145–1147. [Google Scholar] [CrossRef] [Green Version]
36. Ware, C.B.; Nelson, A.M.; Mecham, B.; Hesson, J.; Zhou, W.; Jonlin, E.C.; Jimenez-Caliani, A.J.; Deng, X.; Cavanaugh, C.; Cook, S.; et al. Derivation of naive human embryonic stem cells. Proc. Natl. Acad. Sci. USA 2014, 111, 4484–4489. [Google Scholar] [CrossRef] [Green Version]
37. Nair, D.P.; Podgórski, M.; Chatani, S.; Gong, T.; Xi, W.; Fenoli, C.R.; Bowman, C.N. The thiol-michael addition click reaction: A powerful and widely used tool in materials chemistry. Chem. Mater. 2014, 26, 724–744. [Google Scholar] [CrossRef]
38. Antoni, D.; Burckel, H.; Josset, E.; Noel, G. Three-dimensional cell culture: A breakthrough in vivo. Int. J. Mol. Sci. 2015, 16, 5517–5527. [Google Scholar] [CrossRef]
39. Kraehenbuehl, T.P.; Langer, R.; Ferreira, L.S. Three-dimensional biomaterials for the study of human pluripotent stem cells. Nat. Methods 2011, 8, 731–736. [Google Scholar] [CrossRef]
40. Qin, H.; Hejna, M.; Liu, Y.; Percharde, M.; Wossidlo, M.; Blouin, L.; Durruthy-Durruthy, J.; Wong, P.; Qi, Z.; Yu, J.; et al. Yap induces human naive pluripotency. Cell Rep. 2016, 14, 2301–2312. [Google Scholar] [CrossRef] [Green Version]
41. Beers, J.; Gulbranson, D.R.; George, N.; Siniscalchi, L.I.; Jones, J.; Thomson, J.A.; Chen, G. Passaging and colony expansion of human pluripotent stem cells by enzyme-free dissociation in chemically defined culture conditions. Nat. Protoc. 2012, 7, 2029–2040. [Google Scholar] [CrossRef]
42. Chen, G.; Gulbranson, D.R.; Hou, Z.; Bolin, J.M.; Ruotti, V.; Probasco, M.D.; Smuga-Otto, K.; Howden, S.E.; Diol, N.R.; Propson, N.E.; et al. Chemically defined conditions for human ipsc derivation and culture. Nat. Methods 2011, 8, 424–429. [Google Scholar] [CrossRef] [PubMed] [Green Version]
43. Nie, Y.; Walsh, P.; Clarke, D.L.; Rowley, J.A.; Fellner, T. Scalable passaging of adherent human pluripotent stem cells. PLoS ONE 2014, 9, e88012. [Google Scholar] [CrossRef] [PubMed] [Green Version]
44. Lee, J.; Cuddihy, M.J.; Kotov, N.A. Three-dimensional cell culture matrices: State of the art. Tissue Eng. Part B Rev. 2008, 14, 61–86. [Google Scholar] [CrossRef] [PubMed] [Green Version]
45. Chowdhury, F.; Li, Y.; Poh, Y.C.; Yokohama-Tamaki, T.; Wang, N.; Tanaka, T.S. Soft substrates promote homogeneous self-renewal of embryonic stem cells via downregulating cell-matrix tractions. PLoS ONE 2010, 5, e15655. [Google Scholar] [CrossRef]

46. Chowdhury, F.; Na, S.; Li, D.; Poh, Y.C.; Tanaka, T.S.; Wang, F.; Wang, N. Material properties of the cell dictate stress-induced spreading and differentiation in embryonic stem cells. Nat. Mater. 2010, 9, 82–88. [Google Scholar] [CrossRef] [Green Version]

47. Higuchi, S.; Watanabe, T.M.; Kawauchi, K.; Ichimura, T.; Fujita, H. Culturing of mouse and human cells on soft substrates promote the expression of stem cell markers. J. Biosci. Bioeng. 2014, 117, 749–755. [Google Scholar] [CrossRef]

48. McKee, C.; Hong, Y.; Yao, D.; Chaudhry, G.R. Compression induced chondrogenic differentiation of embryonic stem cells in three-dimensional polydimethylsiloxane scaffolds. Tissue Eng. Part A 2017, 23, 426–435. [Google Scholar] [CrossRef]

49. McKee, C.; Beeravolu, N.; Brown, C.; Perez-Cruet, M.; Chaudhry, G.R. Mesenchymal stem cells transplanted with self-assembling scaffolds differentiated to regenerate nucleus pulposus in an ex vivo model of degenerative disc disease. Appl. Mater. Today 2019. [Google Scholar] [CrossRef]

50. Keung, A.J.; Asuri, P.; Kumar, S.; Schaffer, D.V. Soft microenvironments promote the early neurogenic differentiation but not self-renewal of human pluripotent stem cells. Integr. Biol. 2012, 4, 1049–1058. [Google Scholar] [CrossRef] [Green Version]

51. Sun, Y.; Villa-Diaz, L.G.; Lam, R.H.W.; Chen, W.; Krebsbach, P.H.; Fu, J. Mechanics regulates fate decisions of human embryonic stem cells. PLoS ONE 2012, 7, e37178. [Google Scholar] [CrossRef]

52. Jang, M.; Lee, S.T.; Kim, J.W.; Yang, J.H.; Yoon, J.K.; Park, J.C.; Ryoo, H.M.; van der Vlies, A.J.; Ahn, J.Y.; Hubbell, J.A.; et al. A feeder-free, defined three-dimensional polyethylene glycol-based extracellular matrix niche for culture of human embryonic stem cells. Biomaterials 2013, 34, 3571–3580. [Google Scholar] [CrossRef] [PubMed]

53. Chen, K.G.; Mallon, B.S.; McKay, R.D.G.; Robey, P.G. Human pluripotent stem cell culture: Considerations for maintenance, expansion, and therapeutics. Cell Stem Cell 2014, 14, 13–26. [Google Scholar] [CrossRef] [PubMed] [Green Version]

54. Kharkar, P.M.; Kiick, K.L.; Kloxin, A.M. Designing degradable hydrogels for orthogonal control of cell microenvironments. Chem. Soc. Rev. 2013, 42, 7335–7372. [Google Scholar] [CrossRef] [PubMed] [Green Version]

55. Gerecht, S.; Burdick, J.A.; Ferreira, L.S.; Townsend, S.A.; Langer, R.; Vunjak-Novakovic, G. Hyaluronic acid hydrogel for controlled self-renewal and differentiation of human embryonic stem cells. Proc. Natl. Acad. Sci. USA 2007, 104, 11298–11303. [Google Scholar] [CrossRef] [PubMed] [Green Version]

56. Li, Z.; Leung, M.; Hopper, R.; Ellenbogen, R.; Zhang, M. Feeder-free self-renewal of human embryonic stem cells in 3d porous natural polymer scaffolds. Biomaterials 2010, 31, 404–412. [Google Scholar] [CrossRef]

57. Lei, Y.; Schaffer, D.V. A fully defined and scalable 3d culture system for human pluripotent stem cell expansion and differentiation. Proc. Natl. Acad. Sci. USA 2013, 110, E5039–E5048. [Google Scholar] [CrossRef] [Green Version]

58. Wei, J.; Han, J.; Zhao, Y.; Cui, Y.; Wang, B.; Xiao, Z.; Chen, B.; Dai, J. The importance of three-dimensional scaffold structure on stemness maintenance of mouse embryonic stem cells. Biomaterials 2014, 35, 7724–7733. [Google Scholar] [CrossRef]

59. Li, X.; Ma, R.; Gu, Q.; Liang, L.; Wang, L.; Zhang, Y.; Wang, X.; Liu, X.; Li, Z.; Fang, J.; et al. A fully defined static suspension culture system for large-scale human embryonic stem cell production. Cell Death Dis. 2018, 9, 892. [Google Scholar] [CrossRef]

60. Collier, A.J.; Panula, S.P.; Schell, J.P.; Chovanec, P.; Plaza Reyes, A.; Petropoulos, S.; Corcoran, A.E.; Walker, R.; Douagi, I.; Lanner, F.; et al. Comprehensive cell surface protein profiling identifies specific markers of human naive and primed pluripotent states. Cell Stem Cell 2017, 20, 874–890. [Google Scholar] [CrossRef] [Green Version]

61. Rostovskaya, M.; Stirparo, G.G.; Smith, A. Capacitation of human naïve pluripotent stem cells for multi-lineage differentiation. Development 2019, 146, dev172916. [Google Scholar] [CrossRef] [Green Version]

62. Guo, G.; von Meyenn, F.; Santos, F.; Chen, Y.; Reik, W.; Bertone, P.; Smith, A.; Nichols, J. Naive pluripotent stem cells derived directly from isolated cells of the human inner cell mass. Stem Cell Rep. 2016, 6, 437–446. [Google Scholar] [CrossRef] [PubMed] [Green Version]

63. Hanna, J.; Cheng, A.W.; Saha, K.; Kim, J.; Lengner, C.J.; Soldner, F.; Cassady, J.P.; Muffat, J.; Carey, B.W.; Jaenisch, R. Human embryonic stem cells with biological and epigenetic characteristics similar to those of mouse escs. Proc. Natl. Acad. Sci. USA 2010, 107, 9222–9227. [Google Scholar] [CrossRef] [PubMed] [Green Version]

64. Hashimoto, M.; Sasaki, H. Epiblast formation by tead-yap-dependent expression of pluripotency factors and competitive elimination of unspecified cells. Dev. Cell 2019, 50, 139–154. [Google Scholar] [CrossRef]

65. Kilens, S.; Meistermann, D.; Moreno, D.; Chariau, C.; Gaignerie, A.; Reignier, A.; Lelièvre, Y.; Casanova, M.; Vallot, C.; Nedellec, S.; et al. Parallel derivation of isogenic human primed and naive induced pluripotent stem cells. Nat. Commun. 2018, 9, 360. [Google Scholar] [CrossRef] [PubMed]

66. Takashima, Y.; Guo, G.; Loos, R.; Nichols, J.; Ficz, G.; Krueger, F.; Oxley, D.; Santos, F.; Clarke, J.; Mansfield, W.; et al. Resetting transcription factor control circuitry toward ground-state pluripotency in human. Cell 2014, 158, 1254–1269. [Google Scholar] [CrossRef] [Green Version]

67. Sim, Y.J.; Kim, M.S.; Nayfeh, A.; Yun, Y.J.; Kim, S.J.; Park, K.T.; Kim, C.H.; Kim, K.S. 2i maintains a naive ground state in escs through two distinct epigenetic mechanisms. Stem Cell Rep. 2017, 8, 1312–1328. [Google Scholar] [CrossRef] [Green Version]

68. Van der Jeught, M.; Taelman, J.; Duggal, G.; Ghimire, S.; Lierman, S.; Chuva de Sousa Lopes, S.M.; Deforce, D.; Deroo, T.; De Sutter, P.; Heindryckx, B. Application of small molecules favoring naive pluripotency during human embryonic stem cell derivation. Cell. Reprogramming 2015, 17, 170–180. [Google Scholar] [CrossRef] [Green Version]

69. Zhang, Y.; Liao, K.; Li, C.; Lai, A.C.K.; Foo, J.J.; Chan, V. Progress in integrative biomaterial systems to approach three-dimensional cell mechanotransduction. Bioengineering 2017, 4, 72. [Google Scholar] [CrossRef] [Green Version]

70. Finch-Edmondson, M.; Sudol, M. Framework to function: Mechanosensitive regulators of gene transcription. Cell. Mol. Biol. Lett. 2016, 21, 28. [Google Scholar] [CrossRef]

71. Baxter, M.A.; Camarasa, M.V.; Bates, N.; Small, F.; Murray, P.; Edgar, D.; Kimber, S.J. Analysis of the distinct functions of growth factors and tissue culture substrates necessary for the long-term self-renewal of human embryonic stem cell lines. Stem Cell Res. 2009, 3, 28–38. [Google Scholar] [CrossRef]

72. Mei, Y.; Saha, K.; Bogatyrev, S.R.; Yang, J.; Hook, A.L.; Kalcioglu, Z.I.; Cho, S.W.; Mitalipova, M.; Pyzocha, N.; Rojas, F.; et al. Combinatorial development of biomaterials for clonal growth of human pluripotent stem cells. Nat. Mater. 2010, 9, 768–778. [Google Scholar] [CrossRef] [PubMed] [Green Version]

73. Vitillo, L.; Kimber, S.J. Integrin and fak regulation of human pluripotent stem cells. Curr. Stem Cell Rep. 2017, 3, 358–365. [Google Scholar] [CrossRef] [PubMed] [Green Version]

74. Lee, S.T.; Yun, J.I.; Jo, Y.S.; Mochizuki, M.; van der Vlies, A.J.; Kontos, S.; Ihm, J.E.; Lim, J.M.; Hubbell, J.A. Engineering integrin signaling for promoting embryonic stem cell self-renewal in a precisely defined niche. Biomaterials 2010, 31, 1219–1226. [Google Scholar] [CrossRef] [PubMed]

75. Sun, Y.; Chen, C.S.; Fu, J. Forcing stem cells to behave: A biophysical perspective of the cellular microenvironment. Annu. Rev. Biophys. 2012, 41, 519–542. [Google Scholar] [CrossRef] [Green Version]

76. Yu, F.X.; Zhao, B.; Panupinthu, N.; Jewell, J.L.; Lian, I.; Wang, L.H.; Zhao, J.; Yuan, H.; Tumaneng, K.; Li, H.; et al. Regulation of the hippo-yap pathway by g-protein-coupled receptor signaling. Cell 2012, 150, 780–791. [Google Scholar] [CrossRef] [Green Version]

77. Lam, R.M.; Chesler, A.T. Shear elegance: A novel screen uncovers a mechanosensitive gpcr. J. Gen. Physiol. 2018, 150, 907. [Google Scholar] [CrossRef] [Green Version]

78. Varelas, X. The hippo pathway effectors taz and yap in development, homeostasis and disease. Development 2014, 141, 1614–1626. [Google Scholar] [CrossRef] [Green Version]

79. Elosegui-Artola, A.; Andreu, I.; Beedle, A.E.M.; Lezamiz, A.; Uroz, M.; Kosmalska, A.J.; Oria, R.; Kechagia, J.Z.; Rico-Lastres, P.; Le Roux, A.L.; et al. Force triggers yap nuclear entry by regulating transport across nuclear pores. Cell 2017, 171, 1397–1410. [Google Scholar] [CrossRef]

80. Sasaki, H. Roles and regulations of hippo signaling during preimplantation mouse development. Dev. Growth Differ. 2017, 59, 12–20. [Google Scholar] [CrossRef]

81. Ohgushi, M.; Minaguchi, M.; Sasai, Y. Rho-signaling-directed yap/taz activity underlies the long-term survival and expansion of human embryonic stem cells. Cell Stem Cell 2015, 17, 448–461. [Google Scholar] [CrossRef] [Green Version]

82. Hsiao, C.; Lampe, M.; Nillasithanukroh, S.; Han, W.; Lian, X.; Palecek, S.P. Human pluripotent stem cell culture density modulates yap signaling. Biotechnol. J. 2016, 11, 662–675. [Google Scholar] [CrossRef] [PubMed] [Green Version]

83. Varelas, X.; Sakuma, R.; Samavarchi-Tehrani, P.; Peerani, R.; Rao, B.M.; Dembowy, J.; Yaffe, M.B.; Zandstra, P.W.; Wrana, J.L. Taz controls smad nucleocytoplasmic shuttling and regulates human embryonic stem-cell self-renewal. Nat. Cell Biol. 2008, 10, 837. [Google Scholar] [CrossRef] [PubMed]

84. Lian, I.; Kim, J.; Okazawa, H.; Zhao, J.; Zhao, B.; Yu, J.; Chinnaiyan, A.; Israel, M.A.; Goldstein, L.S.; Abujarour, R.; et al. The role of yap transcription coactivator in regulating stem cell self-renewal and differentiation. Genes Dev. 2010, 24, 1106–1118. [Google Scholar] [CrossRef] [PubMed] [Green Version]

85. Papaspyropoulos, A.; Bradley, L.; Thapa, A.; Leung, C.Y.; Toskas, K.; Koennig, D.; Pefani, D.E.; Raso, C.; Grou, C.; Hamilton, G.; et al. Rassf1a uncouples wnt from hippo signalling and promotes yap mediated differentiation via p73. Nat. Commun. 2018, 9, 424. [Google Scholar] [CrossRef]

86. Young, R.A. Control of the embryonic stem cell state. Cell 2011, 144, 940–954. [Google Scholar] [CrossRef] [Green Version]

87. Meng, Z.; Moroishi, T.; Guan, K.L. Mechanisms of hippo pathway regulation. Genes Dev. 2016, 30, 1–17. [Google Scholar] [CrossRef] [Green Version]

88. Wang, C.; Zhu, X.; Feng, W.; Yu, Y.; Jeong, K.; Guo, W.; Lu, Y.; Mills, G.B. Verteporfin inhibits yap function through up-regulating 14-3-3σ sequestering yap in the cytoplasm. Am. J. Cancer Res. 2015, 6, 27–37. [Google Scholar]

89. Onishi, K.; Zandstra, P.W. Lif signaling in stem cells and development. Development 2015, 142, 2230. [Google Scholar] [CrossRef] [Green Version]

90. Daheron, L.; Opitz, S.L.; Zaehres, H.; Lensch, M.W.; Andrews, P.W.; Itskovitz-Eldor, J.; Daley, G.Q. Lif/stat3 signaling fails to maintain self-renewal of human embryonic stem cells. Stem Cells 2004, 22, 770–778. [Google Scholar] [CrossRef]

07

REATING SPECIALIZED AND LONG-LASTING INTESTINAL STRUCTURES THAT MIRROR THE VARIED CELL TYPES FOUND IN THE CANINE INTESTINE.

1. INTRODUCTION: AN OVERVIEW

Gastrointestinal illnesses such inflammatory bowel disease (IBD), infection-induced GI disorders, and cancer significantly affect human health and place a substantial financial strain on healthcare systems. Young children's second biggest cause of death is infectious diarrhea[1] and GI cancers are the third most common cancer type worldwide, with one million newly diagnosed cases per year [**2**]. Potentially lethal GI diseases also affect livestock and companion animals, with enterotoxic bacteria and enteropathogenic viruses being frequently involved in disease onset and progression [**3**]. Although considerable efforts are made to establish new therapies for human and veterinary GI diseases, mortality rates remain high, because translation of biomedical research into clinical practice is hampered by the lack of epithelial models that reliably mimic the organ and recapitulate disease in patients [**4**,**5**,**6**]. Early attempts to bring the intestinal epithelium to in vitro culture were mostly short-lived, as exemplified by explanted biopsies and epithelial cells, which disintegrated after 72 h and two weeks, respectively [**7**,**8**,**9**]. To establish culture systems for long-lived homogenous cell populations tissue explants were either cultivated in collagen gels or on 3T3 feeder layers on an air-liquid interface [**10**,**11**]. However, growth factor-providing (myo)fibroblasts, which are prerequisites for prolonged cultivation in these systems, made them susceptible to inconsistencies from one experiment to another. A major step to overcome these limitations was the establishment of three-dimensional (3D) murine intestinal organoids derived from adult intestinal stem cells [**12**]. These organoids contained long-lived stem cells that differentiated into the main cell types of murine small intestine such as Paneth cells, enterocytes, enteroendocrine cells and goblet cells. Establishment of this innovative in vitro model was achieved by using a laminin-rich extracellular matrix (Matrigel) and growth media supplemented with epithelial growth factor (EGF), Noggin, and R-spondin as reviewed in detail by Date and Sato [**13**]. For the cultivation of human intestinal organoids, growth medium had to be supplemented with Wnt3a, gastrin, p38-MAPK inhibitor, nicotinamide and ALK4/5/7 inhibitor, thereby preventing the differentiation into goblet and enteroendocrine cells and retaining enterocytes in a premature state [**14**]. Withdrawing nicotinamide and p38-MAPK inhibitor induced de novo differentiation, thus shortening the lifespan of the intestinal stem cell pool and rendering this system into an endpoint assay. Further improvement of human 3D intestinal organoid models was achieved by microscaffolds that mimic the size and distance between crypts in transwell assays [**15**]. Differentiation was promoted by using a growth factor gradient system based on (i) intestinal stem cell-supporting expansion medium in lower wells, and (ii) addition of differentiation medium to upper wells, thereby inducing differentiation of migrating cells to goblet cells, enteroendocrine cells and enterocytes along the modeled crypt/villus axis. However, this technique is unsuitable for, e.g., high-throughput screenings because it is very labor-intensive, time-consuming and hampers down-stream analysis. An approach characterizing receptor tyrosine kinase signaling between the crypt base and its niche managed to omit nicotinamide and p38-MAPK inhibitor usage by a combination of two ligands, i.e., insulin-like growth factor 1 (IGF1) and basic fibroblast growth factor (FGF2). This combination sustains stem cell growth and allows simultaneous differentiation into enteroendocrine and goblet cells, mimicking corresponding natural epithelia more authentically with minimal effort.

Organoid technology has been incorporated into veterinary research in recent years, although to a limited degree. Current animal organoid systems primarily comprise stem and undifferentiated cells that necessitate customized species-specific conditions for differentiation. Dogs and their owners share similar settings, diet, and exposure to carcinogens, leading to the development of comparable gastrointestinal disorders such as GI cancer, infectious diseases, and inflammatory bowel disease (IBD) [23]. Dogs, with their limited genetic diversity in most breeds, serve as a valuable natural model for studying gastrointestinal diseases in humans. To fully utilize canine intestine organoids for correctly mimicking the corresponding organ, it is essential to achieve a balance between the self-renewal and differentiation of stem cells in order to create a system that is physiologically relevant. We describe the development of a new culture system for canine intestinal organoids, which is founded on the recent discoveries made by Fujii et al. [25]. This system effectively promotes the continuous growth of stem cells derived from the duodenum, jejunum, and colon, and facilitates their transformation into secretory lineage cells.

2. MATERIALS AND METHODS

2.1. Isolating and growing canine intestinal organoids

Three dogs, two males and one female, were euthanized due to non-intestinal illness, and tissue samples were taken from their duodenum, jejunum, and colon. Additionally, duodenal samples were collected from a solitary dog as part of a routine gastroduodenal endoscopic surgery. The institutional ethics committee approved tissue sampling in accordance with Good Scientific Practice guidelines and Austrian regulations. The University's "owner's consent for treatment" allows for the use of tissue samples obtained during therapeutic excision or post mortem, in accordance with the institutional ethics committee regulations, signed by all patient owners. Intestinal crypts were isolated from tissue samples and biopsies using established protocols[**12**]. In short, tissue was incubated with 5 mM EDTA (Sigma-Aldrich, St. Louis, MO, USA) in order to dissociate crypts for 30 min to one hour depending on bowel segment, followed by vigorous shaking until crypts were released. After two washing steps with PBS and Advanced Dulbecco's modified Eagle's medium/F12 (DMEM/F12, Invitrogen, Thermo Fisher Scientific, Waltham, MA, USA) 500 crypts were resuspended in 50 µL Matrigel (BD Biosciences, Franklin Lakes, NJ, USA) and seeded per well of a 24-well plate. Following Matrigel polymerization expansion medium was added. Canine intestinal growth media were prepared as indicated in **Table 1**.

Penicillin/streptomycin, HEPES, Glutamax, B27 (with Vitamin A) and N2 supplement were obtained from Invitrogen, Thermo Fisher Scientific. N-acetylcysteine, gastrin and nicotinamide were purchased from Sigma-Aldrich. EGF was provided by Thermo Fisher Scientific. ALK5 kinase inhibitor (A83-01) was obtained from Tocris Bioscience, Bristol, UK. p38 MAPK inhibitor (SB202190) was purchased from Selleck Chemicals, Houston, TX, USA. Human hepatocyte growth factor (HGF), human Noggin, human IGF1 and human FGF2 were provided by PeproTech, Rocky Hill, NJ, USA. Cultrex R-spondin1 cells were obtained from Trevigen, Gaithersburg, MD, USA. Expansion medium was supplemented with 10 µM Rock inhibitor (Y-27632, Selleck Chemicals) for the first two days after isolation, then medium was changed to not-supplemented expansion medium. For isolations using refined medium, EGF and 10 µM Y-27632 were additionally added only for the first two days. Growth medium was changed every two to three days. For weekly passaging at 1:4 to 1:8 split ratios, organoids were harvested, mechanically disrupted using a flame-polished Pasteur pipette. Depending on the splitting ratio, the corresponding quantity of organoid fragments were then embedded in 50 µL fresh Matrigel, seeded per well of a 24-well plate and cultured with either expansion or refined growth medium. Organoids were moved from expansion medium to differentiation medium to stimulate differentiation and then evaluated after 4 days. Derivation efficiency in expansion and refined medium was assessed by counting organoids 10 days after first isolation and calculating projected area using ImageJ64 (NIH).

Table 1. List of media compositions used in this study. Basal medium consists of Advanced DMEM/F12, 2 mM GlutaMAX, 10 mM HEPES, 1x B27, 1 mM N-acetylcystein. Final concentrations are given.

Reagent	Expansion Medium	Differentiation Medium	Refined Medium
basal medium	+	+	+
N2	1x	1x	-
EGF	50 ng/mL	50 ng/mL	– [a]
Noggin	100 ng/mL	100 ng/mL	100 ng/mL
Rspo1	10% *v/v*	10% *v/v*	10% *v/v*
Wnt3a	43% *v/v*	43% *v/v*	50% *v/v*
Nicotinamide	10 mM	–	–
Gastrin	10 nM	10 nM	10 nM
A83-01	500 nM	500 nM	500 nM
SB202190	10 µM	-	-
HGF	50 ng/mL	50 ng/mL	50 ng/mL
IGF1	-	-	100 ng/mL
FGF2	-	-	50 ng/mL

2.2. Gene Expression Analysis

Total RNA was purified from duodenal, jejunal and colonic organoids in expansion, differentiation and refined medium and from corresponding intestinal epithelium that was harvested during crypt isolation using ReliaPrep™ RNA Tissue Miniprep System (Promega, Madison, WI, USA) according to instructions of the manufacturer. Individual RNA concentrations were determined spectrophotometrically (Nanodrop One C, Thermo Fisher Scientific) and RNA integrity was checked using Agilent Tape Station 4200 (Agilent, Santa Clara, CA, USA). 500 ng RNA was reverse-transcribed to cDNA with oligo-dT and random hexamer primers according to recommendations of the manufacturer (GoScript™ Reverse Transcription System, Promega). Subsequently, qPCR reactions were carried out using GoTaq® qPCR Master Mix (Promega). Amplification conditions were as follows: 2 min of initial denaturation at 95 °C, 40 cycles of 15 s of denaturation at 95 °C, 60 s of annealing/extension at 60 °C and a read step, followed by 10 s of dissociation at 95 °C and a melting curve from 65 °C to 95 °C in 5 s per 0.5 °C increments. Data analysis was performed according to Pfaffl et al. [26] taking PCR efficiency into account. Relative quantification was accomplished by normalizing results to the consistently expressed canine housekeeping gene hypoxanthine phosphoribosyl transferase

(HPRT). Heat maps were created by using Excel's conditional formatting on log2 fold changes.

2.3. Periodic Acid-Schiff Reaction of Organoid and Tissue Sections

For the generation of formalin-fixed paraffin-embedded (FFPE) samples, organoids were fixed using 2% v/v paraformaldehyde (PFA, Merck, Darmstadt, Germany) for 15 min at room temperature, cast in 1.5% w/v agarose and dehydrated prior to embedding in paraffin (Sigma-Aldrich). 2.5 µm FFPE sections of organoids derived from duodenum, jejunum and colon and corresponding tissue were stained using PAS-Reaction staining kit and counterstained with Haematoxylin acidic after Mayer according to manufacturer's instructions (Morphisto, Frankfurt am Main, Germany). Images were acquired with a DMi8 microscope and LASX software (Leica, Wetzlar, Germany).

2.4. Transmission Electron Microscopy of Organoids

Samples were fixed in 3% v/v buffered glutaraldehyde (pH 7.4, Merck, Darmstadt, Germany), pre-embedded in 1.5% w/v agarose (Invitrogen, Thermo Fisher Scientific), washed three times in 0.1 M phosphate buffer (Soerensen, pH 7.4) afterwards and post-fixed in 1% v/v osmium tetroxide (Electron Microscopy Sciences, Hatfield, USA) for 2 h at room temperature. Dehydration was performed in a series of graded ethanol solutions (70%, 80%, 96% and 100%), subsequently infiltrated with propylene oxide (Sigma-Aldrich), followed by increasing ratios of epoxy resin-propylene oxide and finally pure resin (Serva, Mannheim, Germany). After an additional change, the resin was polymerized at 60 °C for 48 h. Semi-thin sections were cut at 0.8 µm and stained with toluidine blue, ultra-thin sections were cut at 70 nm, mounted on copper grids (Gröpl, Tulln, Austria) and stained with uranyl acetate (Fluka Chemie AG, Buchs, CH) and lead citrate (Merck, Darmstadt, Germany). Transmission electron micrographs were made with an EM900 (Zeiss, Oberkochen, Germany).

2.5. Proliferation Assay

In order to assess cell proliferation, the Click-iT® EdU Imaging Kit (Invitrogen, Thermo Fisher Scientific) was used. Canine intestinal organoids cultivated in expansion and refined medium were incubated with 5-ethynyl-2'deoxyuridine (EdU) at a final concentration of 10 µM for one hour at 37 °C and were then fixed with 2% v/v PFA for 15 min at room temperature. Staining procedure was carried out according to manufacturer's instructions. DNA was counterstained using 4′,6-Diamidine-2′-phenylindole dihydrochloride (DAPI, Sigma-Aldrich). Confocal images were taken using an LSM 880 (Zeiss). For 3D reconstruction of z-stack images, the Arivis 3D plugin of Zen 2.3 lite (Zeiss) was used.

2.6. Viability and Apoptosis Assays

Viability and apoptosis of organoids in the three media compositions were assessed using the RealTime-Glo MT Cell Viability Assay (Promega) and RealTime-Glo Annexin V Apoptosis Assay (Promega). Organoids were trypsinized for 2 min and seeded in 24-well plates with expansion or refined medium, both supplemented with Y-27632 inhibitor. After 2 days in culture, organoids were harvested, counted and 50 organoids were seeded in six wells of white 96-well plate for each condition and assay. Detection reagents were prepared according to manufacturer and added to the different culture media before overlaying the organoids with either expansion, differentiation or refined medium. Luminescence was measured 0 h, 24 h, 48 h and 72 h after adding the substrates using a GloMax plate reader (Promega). Six wells without organoids, but with medium, served as background controls.

2.7. Statistical Evaluation

Data were analyzed and plotted in Prism5 (GraphPad, San Diego, CA, USA). Using a t-test for independent samples (two tailed, unpaired) p-values ≤ 0.05 were considered statistically significant. qPCR data were analyzed by two-way ANOVA (factors are growth medium and individual dogs) and Tukey multiple comparison test using R (version 3.3.1). *** $p < 0.001$ ** $p < 0.01$ * $p < 0.05$. $p < 0.1$.

3. RESULTS

3.1. Expansion Medium Does Not Support Expression of Secretory Lineage Differentiation Markers

Canine intestinal organoids derived from duodenal, jejunal and colonic tissue were generated and cultivated in expansion medium. Initial cell isolates representing the intestinal epithelium after separation from the underlying tissue, as well as low- (≤5) and high-passage (≥10) organoids derived therefrom, were quantitatively assessed for expression of selected cell markers using RT-qPCR.

The stem cell marker LGR5 displayed similar expression levels in low- and high-passage organoids, except high-passage duodenal organoids, which exhibited significant up-regulation of LGR5 in comparison to their low-passage and initial cell isolate counterparts (**Figure 1**A). The enterocyte marker villin 1 (VIL1) exhibited significantly reduced expression in duodenal, jejunal and colonic organoids in low- and high-passage organoids compared to the initial cell isolates. Enteroendocrine cell marker chromogranin A (CHGA) [**27**] and goblet cell marker mucin 2 (MUC2) [**28,29**] transcripts were barely detectable in organoids when kept in expansion medium throughout passages (**Figure 1**A).

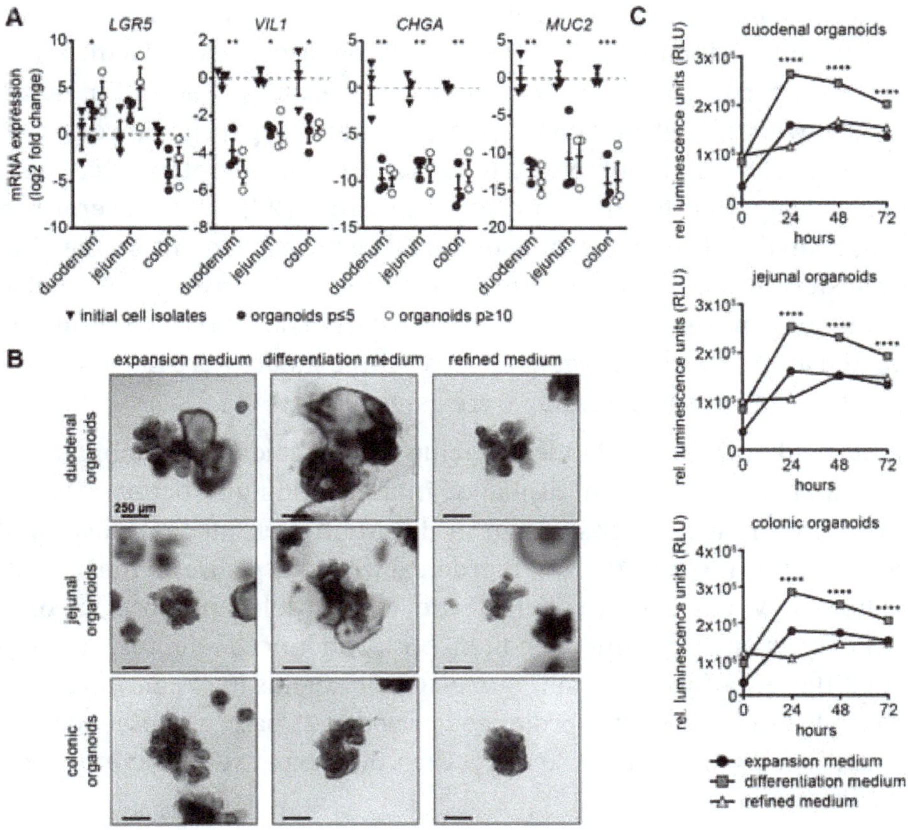

Figure 1. Establishment of new culture conditions for canine intestinal organoids. (A) RT-qPCR analysis of initial cell isolates (triangles), organoids with up to five passages (dark circles) and organoids with 10 or more passages (light circles) isolated from duodenum, jejunum or colon using LGR5, VIL1, CHGA and MUC2 primer. log2 fold changes normalized to expression of initial cell isolates are shown with scatter dot plots; mean is shown; whiskers present SEM; * $p < 0.05$, ** $p < 0.01$ and *** $p < 0.001$, statistical analysis given in detail in Supplementary Tables S2–S4; n = 3 individual dogs. (B) Light microscopic images of organoids derived from duodenum, jejunum and colon cultivated in expansion, differentiation and refined medium four days after seeding; scale bars represent 250 µm. (C) Mean activity of Annexin V-induced luciferase is shown for 0, 24, 48 and 72 h after addition of substrate to duodenal, jejunal and colonic organoids in expansion (circle), differentiation (square) and refined medium (triangle); whiskers represent SEM; **** $p < 0.0001$; 50 organoids seeded per replicate; n = 6 replicates.

3.2. Canine Intestinal Organoids Grow Efficiently in Refined Medium

To best reflect the in vivo situation and thus allow for downstream applications including drug and toxicity assessment, microbiome studies and modelling of infectious disease, intestinal organoids should harbor stem cells, undifferentiated transit-amplifying cells and differentiated cells. Three different media were compared to identify the ideal medium composition supporting such a scenario: (i) an expansion medium for the culture of canine organoids; (ii) a differentiation medium characterized by omission of nicotinamide and p38-MAPK inhibitor [**14**]; and (iii) a novel refined medium based on canine expansion medium without nicotinamide, p38-MAPK inhibitor, N2 and EGF, but supplemented with IGF1 and FGF2 as suggested for human organoid culture [**25**]. After several passages, duodenal, jejunal and colonic canine organoids grown in expansion medium were partly transferred to refined medium for long-term cultivation. For experiments, expansion medium-grown organoids where partly transferred to differentiation medium and after four days, organoids in all three media were harvested. Growth characteristics and gene expression were assessed.

Bright field images of duodenal, jejunal and colonic organoids grown in expansion and refined medium displayed intact, budding structures (**Figure 1**B). In contrast, all organoid types grown in differentiation medium displayed dark and necrotic areas (**Figure 1**B). In accordance with these observations, luciferase-based Annexin V assay revealed low and comparable apoptosis in organoids grown in expansion and refined medium, but pronounced apoptosis in organoids grown in differentiation medium (**Figure 1**C). Organoids in expansion and refined medium could be cultivated for prolonged period of 25 passages after adaptation of growth medium (**Figure S1C**). Taken together, only expansion and refined medium supported organoid growth.

3.3. Refined Medium Promotes Expression of Cell Differentiation Markers in Canine Intestinal Organoids

We next aimed at defining the cellular composition of organoids with respect to the different culture conditions. To this end, total RNA isolated from initial cell isolates and from the three different organoid types cultured in the three different media were subjected to gene expression analysis of stem cell and differentiation markers using RT-qPCR.

In general, a heat map representing log2 fold changes of organoids to respective initial cell isolates showed that transcription of stem cell markers was up-regulated in intestinal organoids grown in all three media. Conversely, transcription of differentiation markers was exclusively up-regulated in intestinal organoids grown in differentiation or refined medium (**Figure 2**A).

In more detail, duodenal organoids displayed significant up-regulation of stem cell marker LGR5 [**30,31**] gene expression irrespective of culture conditions (**Figure 2**B). Culture of duodenal organoids in differentiation and refined medium enhanced mRNA expression of the differentiation markers NEUROG3 (enteroendocrine progenitor cells) [**32,33**], CHGA (enteroendocrine cells) and MUC2 (Goblet cells).

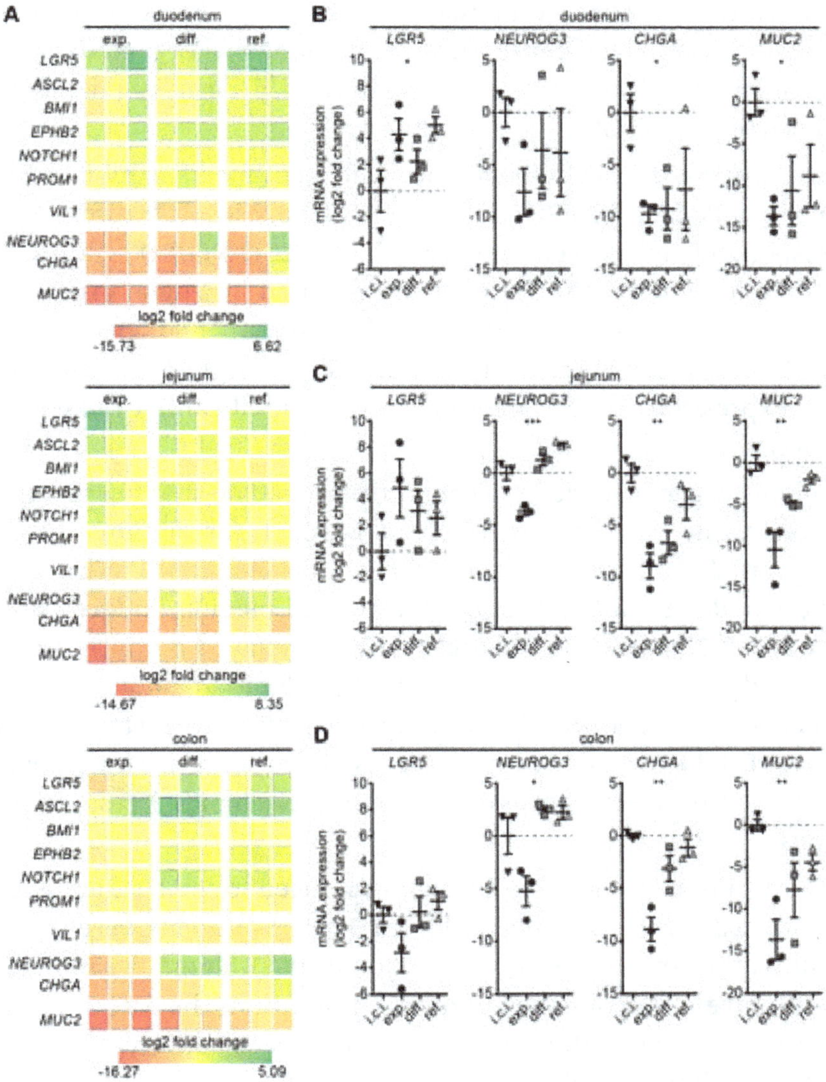

Figure 2. Refined medium and differentiation medium show elevated marker expression of enteroendocrine and goblet cells. (A) Heat map of log2 fold changes derived from RT-qPCR data of duodenal, jejunal and colonic organoids cultivated four days in expansion, differentiation and refined medium normalized to initial cell isolates (i.c.i. = 0); data from three individuals are shown in side-by-side columns. (B–D) Individual scatter dot plots of gene expression data from (A) shown for stem cell marker LGR5, secretory lineage precursor marker NEUROG3, enteroendocrine cell marker CHGA and goblet cell marker MUC2 for organoids derived from duodenum (B), jejunum (C) and colon (D) four days after seeding; mean is shown, whiskers are SEM; * $p < 0.05$, ** $p < 0.01$, *** $p < 0.001$, statistical analysis given in detail in Supplementary Tables S5–S7; n = 3 dogs; i.c.i., initial cell isolates; exp., expansion medium; diff., differentiation medium; ref., refined medium.

Transcription of stem cell markers ASCL2, EPHB2, BMI1, NOTCH1 and PROM1 [**30,31**] did not vary significantly throughout duodenal organoids analyzed, while enterocyte marker VIL1 mRNA was significantly down-regulated in duodenal organoids irrespective of culture conditions.

Jejunal organoids grown in the three different media exhibited no significant difference in LGR5, ASCL2, EPHB2, BMI1, NOTCH1 or PROM1 transcription compared to corresponding initial cell isolates (**Figure 2**C). NEUROG3, CHGA and MUC2 gene expression was significantly down-regulated in jejunal organoids grown in expansion medium. Transcription of differentiation markers NEUROG3, CHGA, and MUC2 mRNA was up-regulated when culturing jejunal organoids in refined medium. Expression of VIL1 was slightly, but significantly, reduced throughout jejunal organoids.

In colonic organoids, medium compositions had no significant impact on LGR5 expression, while NEUROG3, CHGA and MUC2 transcription was significantly down-regulated in organoids kept in expansion medium (**Figure 2**D). Culturing colonic organoids in differentiation and refined medium induced an increase of CHGA and MUC2 expression almost to levels displayed by initial cell isolates. In contrast to duodenal and jejunal organoids, colonic organoids showed aberrant ASCL2, EPHB2, BMI1 and PROM1 transcription in comparison to initial cell isolates, whereas NOTCH1 expression remained grossly unchanged. VIL1 transcription was generally slightly lower expressed in colonic organoids irrespective of culture conditions.

Marker transcription levels in organoids varied to some extent with respect to the individual dog they were derived from. These variations were less pronounced when cultivating organoids—notably jejunal and colonic organoids—in refined medium (**Figure 2**). Despite these individual variations the presented data indicate that differentiation and refined medium supported cell differentiation to secretory lineage cells within organoids.

3.4. Refined and Differentiation Medium Both Support Organoid Differentiation

The detection of markers for goblet and enteroendocrine cells by RT-qPCR prompted us to confirm and localize these cells within organoids. Therefore, periodic-acid Schiff (PAS) reaction and transmission electron microscopy (TEM) were used. PAS reaction of mucin as revealed by a purple signal demonstrated the presence of goblet cells that were evenly distributed in duodenal and jejunal tissue sections along the crypt-villus axis, and at higher frequency around the crypt base in colon tissue sections (**Figure 3**A). In organoid culture, expansion medium failed to induce differentiation into goblet cells, while growth in differentiation and refined medium gave rise to goblet cells irrespective of the intestinal segment.

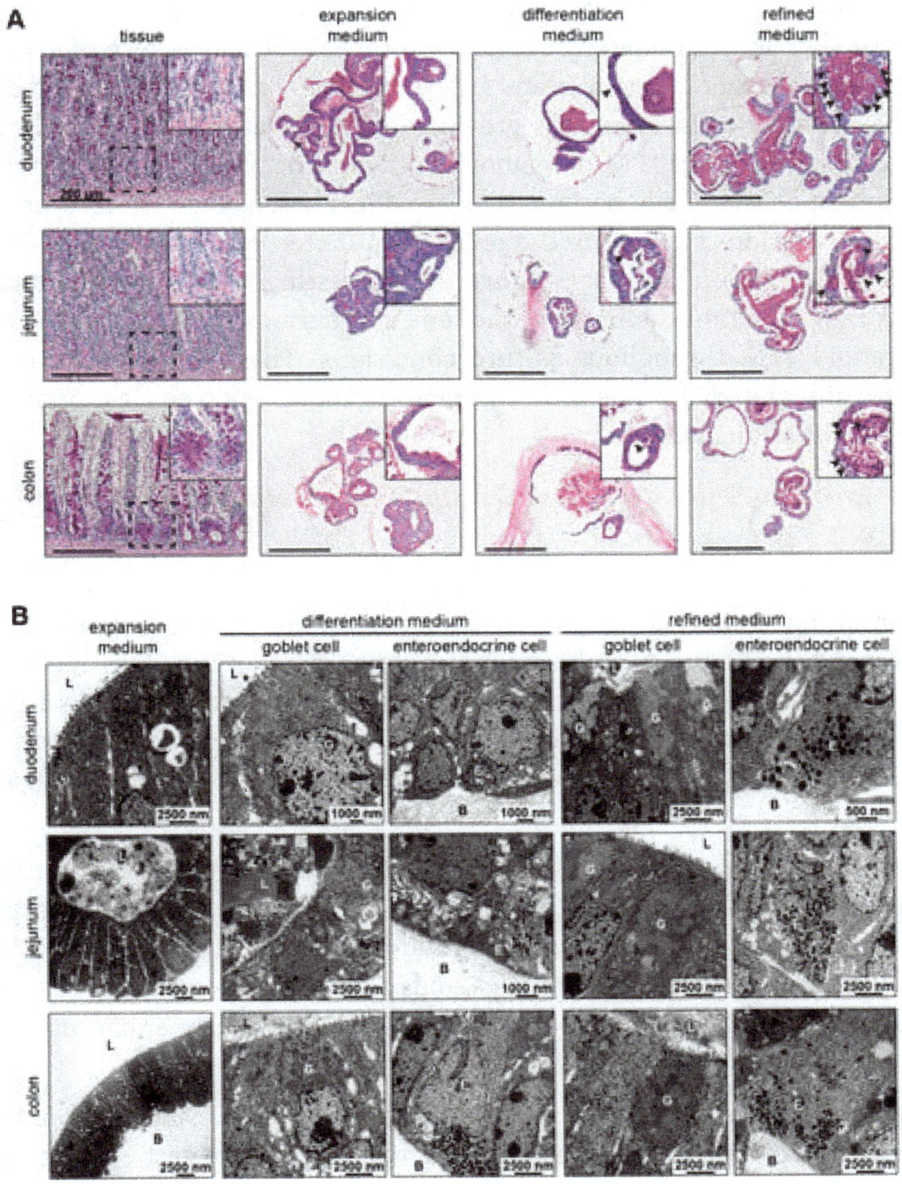

Figure 3. Goblet and enteroendocrine cells are present in organoids upon cultivation in differentiation and refined medium, but not in expansion medium. (A) PAS reaction in FFPE sections of canine intestinal tissue or organoids in expansion, differentiation and refined medium derived from duodenum, jejunum and colon; counterstained with Hematoxylin, images of duodenal and jejunal tissue were cropped in order to visualize crypts; scale bars 200 µm, inset depicts higher magnification; arrow heads indicate PAS positive goblet cells; one representative image is shown. (B) TEM images of duodenal, jejunal and colonic organoids in expansion, differentiation and refined medium; scale bars are indicated; L, lumen; B, basal lamina; G, goblet cell; E, enteroendocrine cell.

These observations were in accordance with MUC2 transcription data (see **Figure 2**) and further substantiated by TEM, which revealed the presence of goblet cells with apical large mucin granules and enteroendocrine cells characterized by small dark basal granules in organoids grown in differentiation and refined medium (**Figure 3**B). In contrast, TEM of organoids cultivated in expansion medium revealed uniformly appearing cells harboring microvilli. These cells were also present in all other conditions suggesting the presence of enterocytes, which is correlating with VIL1 expression data (see **Figure 2**). Interestingly, cell-to-cell interactions such as tight junctions, adherens junctions and desmosomes could be visualized by organoid TEM throughout culture conditions. These data demonstrate the presence of secretory lineage cells in canine organoids upon cultivation in refined and differentiation medium.

3.5. Refined Medium Supports Continuous Growth and Derivation of Organoids

So far, we have been able to verify that organoids in refined medium were differentiating similarly or even better than organoids in differentiation medium (see **Figure 2** and **Figure 3**) without concomitant induction of apoptosis (see **Figure 1**B,C). Therefore, we conclude that a refined medium composition is beneficial over the use of a separate differentiation medium. In a next step we assessed the effectiveness of refined versus expansion medium on the continuous growth of organoids.

Importantly, all organoid types showed a similar proliferation pattern, as revealed by a scattered distribution of single, EdU-positive cells within organoids when exposed to the two different medium conditions (**Figure 4**A). However, viability of duodenal and jejunal organoids in expansion medium was reduced compared to colonic organoids, which could be significantly enhanced by using refined medium (**Figure 4**B).

To assess the suitability of refined medium for the establishment of new organoid lines, duodenal biopsies were taken during routine gastroduodenoscopy. Following isolation, starting cell material was cultured either with expansion medium containing Rock inhibitor, or with EGF- and Rock inhibitor-supplemented refined medium for the first two days, then changed to unsupplemented expansion and refined medium. After 10 days in culture, an almost 4-fold higher number of organoids had grown in refined medium compared to in expansion medium (**Figure 4**C). Organoids exposed to refined medium also displayed a higher projected area compared to organoids formed in expansion medium, indicating that refined medium allows for easier adaption of canine intestinal cells to in vitro culture conditions.

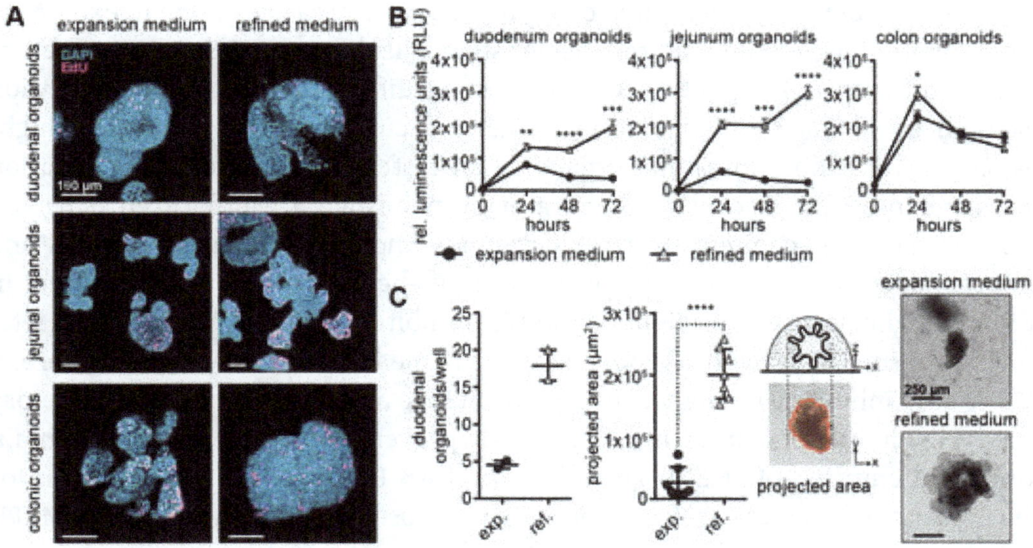

Figure 4. Derivation of organoids is more efficient using refined medium conditions. (A) 3D reconstruction of confocal z-stack images from duodenal, jejunal and colonic organoids in expansion and refined medium; staining for EdU after one hour labeling (magenta); organoids counterstained using DAPI (blue); scale bar represents 100 µm. (B) Relative luciferase activity of cell viability assay is shown for serial measurements at 0, 24, 48 and 72 h after addition of substrate to duodenal, jejunal and colonic organoids in expansion (circle) and refined medium (triangle); mean is shown; whiskers represent SEM; * $p < 0.05$, ** $p < 0.01$, *** $p < 0.001$ and **** $p < 0.0001$; 50 organoids seeded per replicate; n = 6 replicates. (C) Organoid number is shown for freshly isolated duodenal biopsies seeded in expansion and refined medium, in scatter dot plots with mean and range indicated by whiskers, n = 2 wells; projected area of organoids is depicted with mean and SEM defined by whiskers, **** $p < 0.0001$, n = 7 organoids; bright field images of representative organoids are shown, scale bar represents 250 µm.

4. DISCUSSION

Since the first reports on the derivation of organoids from murine and subsequently from human intestine, the establishment of canine intestinal organoids was a matter of time. Particularly as dogs develop GI diseases like cancer, infectious disease and IBD naturally [23], thereby representing a faithful model system for the corresponding human diseases. In early 2017 our group [17], Kingsbury et al. [34], and Powel and Behnke [16] reported on the successful derivation of canine intestinal organoids. We then focused on advancing organoid cultivation to bring them a step closer to the in vivo situation.

In the presented study, we found that expansion medium does not support stem cell commitment in the secretory lineage using transcription profiling. This finding is supported by reports on human intestinal organoids, which usually harbor only a limited number of differentiated cell types, because they are grown in expansion media that allow for the maintenance of stem cells but do not support secretory lineage differentiation [**14,17**]. This absence of differentiated cells in expansion medium could not be overcome by prolonged cultivation: low- (≤5) and high-passage (≥10) canine intestinal organoids all tested negative for differentiation marker expression. Recently, Chandra et al. published a well-written paper on the derivation of canine intestinal organoids and the presence of goblet and enteroendocrine cells [**35**]. The formulation of the expansion medium differs in a 5-fold higher concentration of p38-MAPK inhibitor and the addition of 8% fetal bovine serum FBS (Chandra) compared to the medium formulation used herein. p38-MAPK inhibitor in human organoid culture is used to suppress secretory lineage commitment of intestinal stem cells to prevent their depletion and maintain long-term culture [**14,36,37**]. The addition of 8% FBS is a likely explanation for the presence of secretory cells, potentially via subsequent activation of p38-MAPK signaling. To create a culture system with defined components, the culture medium used in the study presented herein corresponds to a widely used human organoid medium without FBS [**14**] that was only supplemented with HGF to allow for the cultivation of over 50 passages. These variations in medium additives may explain the differences between both studies.

To further develop canine intestinal organoid culture, we focused on optimizing the growth medium to obtain a more in vivo-like cell composition with stem cells, enterocytes, goblet and enteroendocrine cells. Recently, a newly composed medium was shown to enable stem cells of human intestinal organoids to undergo differentiation, while concomitantly preserving the stem cell pool [**25**]. To overcome the intrinsic limitations of classical expansion medium, we adapted our canine intestinal expansion medium based on the suggestions of Fujii et al. [**25**] by (i) withdrawal of nicotinamide, p38-MAPK inhibitor, N2 and EGF; and (ii) addition of IGF1 and FGF2. This medium termed "refined medium" promoted stem cell growth and differentiation of canine intestinal organoids simultaneously for over 6 months of cultivation (data not shown). To assess the benefits and limitations of this refined medium in regard to organoid growth and lineage commitment, canine intestinal organoids grown in expansion, differentiation or refined medium were comparatively characterized.

While duodenal, jejunal and colonic organoids displayed a viable morphology upon culture in expansion and refined medium, differentiation medium induced apoptosis in all three intestinal segments. Interestingly, apoptosis peaked as early as 24 h after transfer to differentiation medium, indicating that programmed cell death was initiated by differentiation-unrelated factors. This assumption is supported by previous reports on the promoting effect of nicotinamide on cell survival in human pluripotent stem cells [**38**], on proliferation of aged murine organoids [**39**] and on inducing apoptosis via reduced intracellular NAD concentrations upon its withdrawal [**40**]. Taken together, differentiation medium induced apoptosis, thus not supporting long-term culture of canine intestinal organoids. This induction of cell death by the medium formulation is unfavorable when differentiation, proliferation or even apoptosis are investigated upon compound treatment for drug development. In addition, differentiation of organoids in expansion medium must be repeated for every individual experiment making them susceptible to fluctuations between media batches, illustrating the need for a better culture system.

Refined medium induced similar levels of differentiation or even outperformed differentiation medium in this regard. Duodenal, jejunal and colonic organoids grown in refined medium revealed enhanced expression of markers indicating the presence of secretory lineage precursors, enteroendocrine and goblet cells. Interestingly, organoids in refined medium expressed comparable or even higher levels of stem cell marker compared to organoids in expansion medium. Organoids irrespective of the intestinal segment or media composition expressed the enterocyte marker VIL1. These data confirm findings reported for human intestinal organoids grown in niche-inspired culture media that supported expression of enteroendocrine, goblet and stem cell markers [**25**] and data reported for villin1 positive enterocytes in murine intestinal organoids [**12**]. However, expression of the differentiation markers CHGA, MUC2 and VIL1 in differentiation and refined medium reached the levels of the i.c.i. only to a certain extent. While an in vitro culture model cannot fully reproduce the complex in vivo situation, our data show that growth conditions in refined medium are more similar compared to those in expansion medium.

Since only a limited number of specific antibodies were available for reliable characterization of canine cells, we used two well-established alternative methods, PAS reaction and TEM, for the detection of goblet cells and enteroendocrine cells. These results supported our RT-qPCR data, substantiating that only organoids grown in differentiation and refined medium harbored enteroendocrine and goblet cells. These findings are in accordance with data obtained for human intestinal organoids grown in differentiation [**14**] or niche-inspired medium [**25**]. Furthermore, the presence of enterocytes in organoids cultivated in expansion, differentiation and refined medium of all segments was supported by microvilli bearing cells as reported for murine intestinal organoids [**12**], indicating that enterocytes are present irrespective of culture condition.

So far, our data provided evidence that cultivation of canine intestinal organoids in refined medium is preferable to the use of differentiation medium, since it promotes stem cell growth and differentiation simultaneously, allows long-term growth without fluctuations between media batches and does not induce apoptosis. Therefore, further analysis focused on comparison of organoid growth in expansion and refined medium.

The comparison of proliferative behavior differences between canine intestinal organoids grown in expansion versus refined medium by EdU incorporation assays revealed similar proliferation levels for all organoid types irrespective of the medium used. Yet, viability data of duodenal and jejunal organoids indicate that expansion medium does not support small intestinal organoid cultivation as effective as refined medium. The colonic epithelium is highly populated with various bacteria and has less digestive and absorptive function than small intestinal epithelium possibly resulting in more robustness with respect to cultivation. Therefore, colonic organoids can be expanded in both expansion and refined medium efficiently.

Importantly, generation of organoids from duodenal biopsies was more successful in refined than expansion medium. Not only the number of organoids per well was enhanced, but also their projected area. This feature has an important impact on canine intestinal disease modelling, especially when donor tissue stems from GI enteropathies with severely affected epithelium. The high suitability of refined medium for canine organoid establishment also matches the higher plating efficacy shown for human single-cell dissociated organoids grown in niche-inspired media [**25**].

5. CONCISE SUMMARY

We highly recommend using a refined medium for the creation and long-term culture of canine intestine organoids. We demonstrated that this medium supports the proliferation of stem cells and also encourages the differentiation of stem cells/immature cells into enterocytes, enteroendocrine, and goblet cells. Canine intestine organoids grown on a specialized medium offer a convenient, consistent, and reliable culture method, making them a more advanced in vitro model for disease research, drug testing, toxicity assessments, and customized therapy. The improved medium described here enables a more precise evaluation of genetic and epigenetic effects on canine intestinal cell differentiation compared to traditional expansion and differentiation media, advancing organoid research closer to in vivo conditions.

6. AT A GLANCE

Functional gastrointestinal diseases are significant health issues that have the potential to be life-threatening in humans. Research is focused on understanding the fundamental pathobiological mechanisms and developing treatment approaches. intestine organoids are a powerful in vitro model in this situation because they accurately replicate the structure and function of the specific intestine segment they mimic. Human-like intestinal illnesses can also impact dogs, making canine intestinal organoids a valuable resource for canine and comparative studies. We created organoids from different parts of a dog's digestive system and concentrated on both long-term growth and cell specialization to enhance their potential uses. Canine intestine organoids were cultured under varied circumstances and examined for cell viability, apoptosis, and differentiation using transcription profiling, proliferation assay, cell staining, and transmission electron microscopy. The standard expansion medium facilitated prolonged expansion of organoids regardless of their source, but hindered cell differentiation. On the other hand, moving organoids to a differentiation medium stimulated the growth of goblet cells and enteroendocrine cells, while also triggering apoptosis. Organoids were cultured with tyrosine kinase ligands to promote stem cell renewal and differentiation without hindrance. The distinct cellular variety of the canine duodenum, jejunum, and colon is clearly emphasized in our research, which is essential for creating precise in vitro models.

REFERENCES

1. Kim, H.P.; Crockett, S.; Shaheen, N.J. The Burden of Gastrointestinal and Liver Disease around the World. In GI Epidemiology; Wiley: Oxford, UK, 2014; pp. 1–13. [Google Scholar]
2. Bray, F.; Ferlay, J.; Soerjomataram, I.; Siegel, R.L.; Torre, L.A.; Jemal, A. Global cancer statistics 2018: GLOBOCAN estimates of incidence and mortality worldwide for 36 cancers in 185 countries. CA Cancer J. Clin. 2018, 68, 394–424. [Google Scholar] [CrossRef] [PubMed] [Green Version]
3. Rubin, S.I. Infectious Diseases of the GI Tract. Available online: https://www.msdvetmanual.com/digestive-system/digestive-system-introduction/infectious-diseases-of-the-gi-tract (accessed on 19 September 2019).
4. Albani, S.; Colomb, J.; Prakken, B. Translational Medicine 2.0: From Clinical Diagnosis–Based to Molecular-Targeted Therapies in the Era of Globalization. Clin. Pharmacol. Ther. 2010, 87, 642–645. [Google Scholar] [CrossRef]
5. Albani, S.; Prakken, B. The advancement of translational medicine—From regional challenges to global solutions. Nat. Med. 2009, 15, 1006–1009. [Google Scholar] [CrossRef]
6. Scherzer, M.; Kramer, N.; Unger, C.; Walzl, A.; Walter, S.; Stadler, M.; Hengstschläger, M.; Dolznig, H. Preclinical Cancer Models with the Potential to Predict Clinical Response. In Drug Discovery in Cancer Epigenetics; Elsevier BV: Oxford, UK, 2016; pp. 97–122. [Google Scholar]

7. Browning, T.H.; Trier, J.S. Organ culture of mucosal biopsies of human small intestine. J. Clin. Investig. 1969, 48, 1423–1432. [Google Scholar] [CrossRef] [PubMed] [Green Version]
8. Kedinger, M.; Haffen, K.; Simon-Assmann, P. Intestinal tissue and cell cultures. Differentiation 1987, 36, 71–85. [Google Scholar] [CrossRef] [PubMed]
9. Evans, G.S.; Flint, N.; Somers, A.S.; Eyden, B.; Potten, C.S. The development of a method for the preparation of rat intestinal epithelial cell primary cultures. J. Cell Sci. 1992, 101. [Google Scholar]
10. Ootani, A.; Li, X.; Sangiorgi, E.; Ho, Q.T.; Ueno, H.; Toda, S.; Sugihara, H.; Fujimoto, K.; Weissman, I.L.; Capecchi, M.R.; et al. Sustained in vitro intestinal epithelial culture within a Wnt-dependent stem cell niche. Nat. Med. 2009, 15, 701–706. [Google Scholar] [CrossRef] [Green Version]
11. Wang, X.; Yamamoto, Y.; Wilson, L.H.; Zhang, T.; Howitt, B.; Farrow, M.A.; Kern, F.; Ning, G.; Hong, Y.; Khor, C.C.; et al. Cloning and variation of ground state intestinal stem cells. Nature 2015, 522, 173–178. [Google Scholar] [CrossRef] [Green Version]
12. Sato, T.; Vries, R.G.; Snippert, H.J.; Van De Wetering, M.; Barker, N.; Stange, D.; Van Es, J.H.; Abo, A.; Kujala, P.; Peters, P.J.; et al. Single Lgr5 stem cells build crypt-villus structures in vitro without a mesenchymal niche. Nature 2009, 459, 262–265. [Google Scholar] [CrossRef]
13. Date, S.; Sato, T. Mini-Gut Organoids: Reconstitution of the Stem Cell Niche. Annu. Rev. Cell Dev. Boil. 2015, 31, 269–289. [Google Scholar] [CrossRef]
14. Sato, T.; Stange, D.; Ferrante, M.; Vries, R.G.; Van Es, J.H.; Brink, S.V.D.; Van Houdt, W.J.; Pronk, A.; Van Gorp, J.M.; Siersema, P.D.; et al. Long-term Expansion of Epithelial Organoids From Human Colon, Adenoma, Adenocarcinoma, and Barrett's Epithelium. Gastroenterology 2011, 141, 1762–1772. [Google Scholar] [CrossRef] [PubMed]
15. Wang, Y.; Kim, R.; Gunasekara, D.B.; Reed, M.I.; Disalvo, M.; Nguyen, D.L.; Bultman, S.J.; Sims, C.E.; Magness, S.T.; Allbritton, N.L. Formation of Human Colonic Crypt Array by Application of Chemical Gradients Across a Shaped Epithelial Monolayer. Cell. Mol. Gastroenterol. Hepatol. 2017, 5, 113–130. [Google Scholar] [CrossRef] [PubMed] [Green Version]
16. Powell, R.H.; Behnke, M. WRN conditioned media is sufficient for in vitro propagation of intestinal organoids from large farm and small companion animals. Boil. Open 2017, 6, 698–705. [Google Scholar] [CrossRef] [PubMed] [Green Version]

17. 2017 ACVIM Forum Research Abstract Program. J. Veter- Intern. Med. 2017, 31, 1225–1361. [CrossRef] [Green Version]

18. Nantasanti, S.; Spee, B.; Kruitwagen, H.S.; Chen, C.; Geijsen, N.; Oosterhoff, L.A.; Van Wolferen, M.E.; Peláez, N.; Fieten, H.; Wubbolts, R.W.; et al. Disease Modeling and Gene Therapy of Copper Storage Disease in Canine Hepatic Organoids. Stem Cell Rep. 2015, 5, 895–907. [Google Scholar] [CrossRef] [Green Version]

19. Kruitwagen, H.S.; Oosterhoff, L.A.; Vernooij, I.G.; Schrall, I.M.; Van Wolferen, M.E.; Bannink, F.; Roesch, C.; Van Uden, L.; Molenaar, M.; Helms, J.B.; et al. Long-Term Adult Feline Liver Organoid Cultures for Disease Modeling of Hepatic Steatosis. Stem Cell Rep. 2017, 8, 822–830. [Google Scholar] [CrossRef] [Green Version]

20. Derricott, H.; Luu, L.; Fong, W.Y.; Hartley, C.S.; Johnston, L.; Armstrong, S.D.; Randle, N.; Duckworth, C.A.; Campbell, B.J.; Wastling, J.M.; et al. Developing a 3D intestinal epithelium model for livestock species. Cell Tissue Res. 2018, 375, 409–424. [Google Scholar] [CrossRef] [Green Version]

21. Hamilton, C.A.; Young, R.; Jayaraman, S.; Sehgal, A.; Paxton, E.; Thomson, S.; Katzer, F.; Hope, J.; Innes, E.A.; Morrison, L.; et al. Development of in vitro enteroids derived from bovine small intestinal crypts. Veter- Res. 2018, 49, 54. [Google Scholar] [CrossRef] [Green Version]

22. Pierzchalska, M.; Grabacka, M.; Michalik, M.; Zyla, K.; Pierzchalski, P. Prostaglandin E2 supports growth of chicken embryo intestinal organoids in Matrigel matrix. Biotechniques 2012, 52, 307–315. [Google Scholar] [CrossRef] [Green Version]

23. Cerquetella, M.; Spaterna, A.; Laus, F.; Tesei, B.; Rossi, G.; Antonelli, E.; Villanacci, V.; Bassotti, G. Inflammatory bowel disease in the dog: Differences and similarities with humans. World J. Gastroenterol. 2010, 16, 1050–1056. [Google Scholar] [CrossRef] [PubMed]

24. Shearin, A.L.; Ostrander, E.A. Leading the way: Canine models of genomics and disease. Dis. Model. Mech. 2010, 3, 27–34. [Google Scholar] [CrossRef] [PubMed] [Green Version]

25. Fujii, M.; Matano, M.; Toshimitsu, K.; Takano, A.; Mikami, Y.; Nishikori, S.; Sugimoto, S.; Sato, T. Human Intestinal Organoids Maintain Self-Renewal Capacity and Cellular Diversity in Niche-Inspired Culture Condition. Cell Stem Cell 2018, 23, 787–793.e6. [Google Scholar] [CrossRef] [PubMed] [Green Version]

26. Pfaffl, M.W. A new mathematical model for relative quantification in real-time RT-PCR. Nucleic Acids Res. 2001, 29, 45. [Google Scholar] [CrossRef] [PubMed]

27. Grün, D.; Muraro, M.J.; Boisset, J.-C.; Wiebrands, K.; Lyubimova, A.; Dharmadhikari, G.; Born, M.V.D.; Van Es, J.; Jansen, E.; Clevers, H.; et al. De Novo Prediction of Stem Cell Identity using Single-Cell Transcriptome Data. Cell Stem Cell 2016, 19, 266–277. [Google Scholar] [CrossRef] [Green Version]

28. Audie, J.P.; Janin, A.; Porchet, N.; Copin, M.C.; Gosselin, B.; Aubert, J.P. Expression of human mucin genes in respiratory, digestive, and reproductive tracts ascertained by in situ hybridization. J. Histochem. Cytochem. 1993, 41, 1479–1485. [Google Scholar] [CrossRef]

29. Kim, Y.S.; Ho, S.B. Intestinal Goblet Cells and Mucins in Health and Disease: Recent Insights and Progress. Curr. Gastroenterol. Rep. 2010, 12, 319–330. [Google Scholar] [CrossRef] [Green Version]

30. Barker, N.; Van Es, J.H.; Kuipers, J.; Kujala, P.; Born, M.V.D.; Cozijnsen, M.; Haegebarth, A.; Korving, J.; Begthel, H.; Peters, P.J.; et al. Identification of stem cells in small intestine and colon by marker gene Lgr5. Nature 2007, 449, 1003–1007. [Google Scholar] [CrossRef]

31. Munoz, J.; Stange, D.; Schepers, A.G.; Van De Wetering, M.; Koo, B.-K.; Itzkovitz, S.; Volckmann, R.; Kung, K.S.; Koster, J.; Radulescu, S.; et al. The Lgr5 intestinal stem cell signature: Robust expression of proposed quiescent '+4' cell markers. EMBO J. 2012, 31, 3079–3091. [Google Scholar] [CrossRef] [Green Version]

32. Jenny, M.; Uhl, C.; Roche, C.; Duluc, I.; Guillermin, V.; Guillemot, F.; Jensen, J.; Kedinger, M.; Gradwohl, G. Neurogenin3 is differentially required for endocrine cell fate specification in the intestinal and gastric epithelium. EMBO J. 2002, 21, 6338–6347. [Google Scholar] [CrossRef] [Green Version]

33. Lopez-Diaz, L.; Jain, R.N.; Keeley, T.M.; VanDussen, K.L.; Brunkan, C.S.; Gumucio, D.L.; Samuelson, L.C. Intestinal Neurogenin 3 directs differentiation of a bipotential secretory progenitor to endocrine cell rather than goblet cell fate. Dev. Boil. 2007, 309, 298–305. [Google Scholar] [CrossRef] [Green Version]

34. Kingsbury, D.; Sun, L.; Qi, Y.; Fredericks, J.; Wang, Q.; Wannemuehler, M.; Jergens, A.; Allenspach, K. DDW Abstract: Optimizing the Development and Characterization of Canine Small Intestinal Crypt Organoids as a Research Model. Gastroenterology 2017, 152 (Suppl. 1). [Google Scholar] [CrossRef]

35. Chandra, L.; Borcherding, D.C.; Kingsbury, D.; Atherly, T.; Ambrosini, Y.M.; Bourgois-Mochel, A.; Yuan, W.; Kimber, M.; Qi, Y.; Wang, Q.; et al. Derivation of adult canine intestinal organoids for translational research in gastroenterology. BMC Boil. 2019, 17, 33. [Google Scholar] [CrossRef] [PubMed]

36. Kozuka, K.; He, Y.; Koo-McCoy, S.; Kumaraswamy, P.; Nie, B.; Shaw, K.; Chan, P.; Leadbetter, M.; He, L.; Lewis, J.G.; et al. Development and Characterization of a Human and Mouse Intestinal Epithelial Cell Monolayer Platform. Stem Cell Rep. 2017, 9, 1976–1990. [Google Scholar] [CrossRef] [PubMed] [Green Version]

37. Wallach, T.E.; Bayrer, J.R. Intestinal Organoids. J. Pediatr. Gastroenterol. Nutr. 2017, 64, 180–185. [Google Scholar] [CrossRef] [Green Version]

38. Meng, Y.; Ren, Z.; Xu, F.; Zhou, X.; Song, C.; Wang, V.Y.-F.; Liu, W.; Lu, L.; Thomson, J.A.; Chen, G. Nicotinamide Promotes Cell Survival and Differentiation as Kinase Inhibitor in Human Pluripotent Stem Cells. Stem Cell Rep. 2018, 11, 1347–1356. [Google Scholar] [CrossRef] [Green Version]

39. Uchida, R.; Saito, Y.; Nogami, K.; Kajiyama, Y.; Suzuki, Y.; Kawase, Y.; Nakaoka, T.; Muramatsu, T.; Kimura, M.; Saito, H. Epigenetic silencing of Lgr5 induces senescence of intestinal epithelial organoids during the process of aging. NPJ Aging Mech. Dis. 2018, 4, 1. [Google Scholar] [CrossRef]

40. Heikal, A.A. Intracellular coenzymes as natural biomarkers for metabolic activities and mitochondrial anomalies. Biomark. Med. 2010, 4, 241–263. [Google Scholar] [CrossRef] [Green Version]

08 PP2A DEFICIENCY ENHANCES CARCINOGENESIS OF LGR5⁺ INTESTINAL STEM CELLS BOTH IN ORGANOIDS AND IN VIVO

1. INTRODUCTION: AN OVERVIEW

The specific cells from which most malignancies originate have not been identified. Creating mice models of chemical carcinogenesis that mimic most human malignancies caused by exposure to environmental carcinogens is challenging to accomplish in a cell-specific way[1]. Current methodologies for studying the cellular origins of cancers involve the use of genetically modified mouse models (GEMMs) that utilize transgenic or conditionally targeted gene technologies to create tumors in various cellular environments [2]. Additionally, the development of cancer in both models is a time-consuming process, which hinders advancements in cancer research.

The most applied animal model for studying intestinal tumorigenesis is based on activating mutations in the Wnt pathway, which relies on adenomatous polyposis coli (Apc) depletion [3] and beta-catenin (CTNNB1) activation [4], leading to beta-catenin stabilization and constitutive transcription of its down-stream genes. Recent progress in the understanding of the cell of origin of intestinal tumor was made using this model, although several inconsistencies were observed. After in vivo Apc depletion in leucine-rich-repeat containing G-protein-coupled receptor 5 $(Lgr5)^+$ crypt stem cells, tumor formation occurred within 3–5 weeks [3]. However, Apc depletion or being combined with $Kras^{G12D}$ mutation in progenitor and differentiated cells did not induce tumor formation [5,6]. However, tumor-initiating mutations can occur in $Lgr5^+$ crypt stem cells and in differentiated $Lgr5^-$ cells [4], indicating that the two hypotheses are not mutually exclusive. Ablation of $Lgr5^+$ cells in orthotopically transplanted tumors, generated by genetic modification in differentiated villus cells, suppressed tumor growth [**7**]. Interestingly, $Lgr5^+$ cells reappeared and tumors recurred when ablation was terminated 4 days later. The generation of $Lgr5^+$ cells from $Lgr5^-$ cells after $Lgr5^+$ ablation was also observed in the xenograft mouse model of human colon cancer stem cells (CSCs) [**8**]. However, the specific mechanism of $Lgr5^+$ cell generation from remaining $Lgr5^-$ cells remains unclear.

Irregular activation of a signal transduction pathway, a process that alternates between being active and inactive, can change a healthy cell into a cancerous one or give cancer cells the ability to withstand therapy. Activating mutations in genes encoding kinases or signaling molecules, such as RAS and PI3K, switch on the signaling, continuously activating a survival and/or proliferation pathway, while activations of phosphatases, such as the serine/threonine phosphatase PP2A family, switch off the signaling [**9**]. Previous efforts through high-throughput screens of tyrosine kinome and tyrosine phosphatome have identified several driver or passenger mutations in a spectrum of malignancies, including intestinal tumor [**10,11,12**]. However, there are few if any studies focusing on the altered signalings driven by serine/threonine kinase mutations [**13**]. Human intestinal tumors contain active mutations in genes encoding proteins involved in the WNT, MAPK, TGF-beta, and PI3K pathways [**14**]. Ingenuity pathway analysis (IPA) of TCGA-COAD revealed PP2A complex and its subunits, such as PPP2R1A and PPP2CA, are intercalated among several driver mutation pathways. Moreover, endogenous PP2A inhibitors, SET and CIP2A [**15**], are highly expressed in intestinal tumors in comparison to their matched normal tissue samples. We showed that PP2A was suppressed in intestinal tumor stem cells (CSCs), thereby activating its substrate kinases to enhance survival under hypoxia and serum depletion [**16**], thereby increasing resistance to anti-angiogenesis therapy [**17**]. Our recent studies also demonstrated that reduced PP2A activity in colorectal and lung CSCs enhances suspension survival and induces tumor initiation [**18**], revealing the tumor suppressive role of PP2A [**19**]. Although higher numbers of Apc, p53, $Kras^{G12D}$, and Smad4 driver mutations may be required for human colorectal tumorigenesis, there are some intestinal tumors carry only one or no alteration in these driver mutations [**20**]. For example, gene fusions involving R-spondin 1 occurring in 10% of intestinal tumor are mutually exclusive with active Wnt signaling caused by APC or CTNNB1 mutations [**20**]. The new intestinal tumorigenesis animal models will help in understanding the molecular mechanisms of these tumors.

Considering that cancer arises from intricate interactions between genetic and environmental factors, utilizing chemical carcinogens that activate kinases along with GEMM containing phosphatase deficiency is a rational method to study the intricate relationship between genetic vulnerability and environmental influences. [**21**]. To investigate the cell origin of intestinal tumor, we first combined treatment with carcinogen 7,12-dimethylbenzanthracene (DMBA) that has previously been known to induce rodent s in the presence of 1,2-dimethyl-hydrazine [22] and PP2A inhibition via okadaic acid (OA) treatment or genetic deficiency. DMBA not only activates multiple mutations in different codons of ras [23] but also induces activation in other pathways, such as Notch [24], providing a screening approach for identifying key kinases or molecules. Besides DMBA, we also investigated the effects of N-methyl-N-nitrosourea (MNU) and 2-amino-1-methyl-6-phenylimidazo-[4,5-b]pyridine (PhIP) on intestinal carcinogenesis. MNU is one of the direct alkylating agents, which does not require metabolic activation for initiating carcinogenesis [25]. PhIP has received considerable attention because it has multi-organ targets and it was developed upon broiling of fish and meat [26]. Moreover, we established primary intestinal organoid models that recapitulate the rodent intestinal tumorigenesis paradigm [27]. These models of carcinogenesis in rodent intestines are valuable for developing innovative approaches to target mouse intestinal cancer stem cells and cure intestinal tumors.

2. MATERIALS AND METHODS

2.1. Mouse Colonies

Ppp2r1aflox/flox mice, carrying conditional alleles with loxP sites flanking exon 5–6 of Ppp2r1a, were purchased from the Jackson Laboratory and crossed to Lgr5-EGFP-CreERT2 or Villin-Cre mice to generate Lgr5-EGFP-CreERT2; Ppp2r1aflox/flox or Villin-Cre; Ppp2r1a flox/flox mice. NOD/SCID mice were purchased from Lasco Co., Ltd. (Taiwan). All animal studies and care of live animals were approved and performed following the guidelines made by the China Medical University Institutional Animal Care and Use Committee 2016-398-1; 2017-239.

2.2. Mouse Intestinal Organoid Cell Isolation, Culture, and Passage

Organoid culture was preformed according to a protocol modified from previously described methods [28]. In brief, the intestines were dissected, opened longitudinally and cut into small (2 mm) pieces. The tissues were rocked in dissociation reagent and incubated at room temperature (15–25 °C) for 15 min. The tissues were then mixed and filtered through a 70 μm sterile cell strainer. The crypts were collected by centrifugation at 140× g for 5 min at 4 °C. Approximately 500 crypts were suspended in 50 μL growth factor reduced phenol-free Matrigel (BD Biosciences, San Jose, CA, USA). Next, a 50 μL droplet of Matrigel/crypt mix was placed and polymerized in the center well of a 48-well plate. The basic culture medium (Dulbecco's modified Eagle's medium/F12 supplemented with penicillin/streptomycin), was supplemented with 50 ng/mL murine recombinant epidermal growth factor (EGF; Peprotech, Hamburg, Germany), Noggin (5% final volume) and R-spondin 1 (5% final volume) called "ENR" medium. Medium change was performed every 3–4 days. Each condition was examined in triplicate with multiple (>15) organoids in each sample. Each experiment was repeated twice.

2.3. Dysplasia Index

Histologic changes were scored blindly on the levels of four histological characteristics as previously described [27]: nuclear grade (enlarged nuclei with diffuse membrane irregularities and prominent nucleoli); stratification; mitoses and invasion (>2 foci). The dysplasia index was evaluated by all microscopic fields containing viable organoids with 5 fields per sample (n).

2.4. Primary Organoid Transplantation

For transplantation, cells from passage 7; day 50 organoid cultures were collected. Dissociated cells were pelleted by centrifugation and resuspended with Matrigel (50% Matrigel (BD), in a total volume of 100 μL containing indicated cell numbers and injected s.c. into NOD-SCID mice.

2.5. Immunofluorescence and Immunohistochemistry

Freshly isolated intestines were prepared according to a protocol modified from previously described methods [27]. The intestines were then applied for immunostaining. For immunostaining, the organoid cells were rinsed three times in ice-cold PBS. The organoid cells were spun down at 900 rpm for 10 min at 4 °C. Sections were deparaffinized and stained with H&E for the initial histology analysis. The immunofluorescence was performed on paraffin-embedded sections (5 μm). The permeabilized organoid cell samples were incubated with primary antibodies overnight at 4 °C. The samples were incubated with anti-PPP2R1A (GTX102206; GeneTex, Hsinchu City, Taiwan), anti-CK20 (GTX110600 Genetex), anti-Lgr5 (GTX50839 Genetex), anti-SMA (Abcam, ab5694, Cambridge, MA, USA), anti-beta-catenin (BD Transduction Labs, San Jose, CA, USA; 610154); the secondary antibodies used were DyLight® 650 Conjugated goat anti-rabbit (cat no. A120-101D5; Bethyl Laboratories Inc., Montgomery, TX, USA) and Goat anti-Rabbit IgG Antibody-FITC (Bethyl cat no. A120-101F) and DAPI (Molecular Probes) for 1 h at room temperature. The slides were mounted with SlowFade (SlowFade® AntiFade Kit, Molecular Probes, Waltham, MA, USA) followed by covering with a coverslip, and the edges were sealed to prevent drying. The specimens were examined with a Zeiss 710 Laser Scanning confocal microscope (Zeiss, Oberkochen, Germany).

The intestinal tissue was preserved and prepared into paraffin blocks using established protocols. Immunohistochemistry for beta-catenin was conducted following established protocols. [3]. Immunohistochemistry protocol hold as following: freshly isolated intestines were flushed with 10% formalin in PBS and fixed by incubation in a 10-fold excess of formalin overnight at room temperature. The formalin was removed and the intestines washed twice in PBS at room temperature. The intestines were then transferred to a tissue cassette and dehydrated by serial immersion in 20-fold volumes of 70, 96 and 100% EtOH for 2 h each at 4 °C. Excess ethanol was removed by incubation in xylene for 1.5 h room temperature and the cassettes then immersed in liquid paraffin (56 °C) overnight. Paraffin blocks were prepared using standard methods and 4μm tissue sections generated. These sections were de-waxed by immersion in xylene (2 × 5 min) and hydrated by serial immersion in 100% EtOH (2 × 1 min), 96% EtOH (2 × 1 min), 70% EtOH (2 × 1 min) and distilled water (2 × 1 min). Endogenous peroxidase activity was blocked by immersing the slides in peroxidase blocking buffer (0.040 M citric acid, 0.121 M disodium hydrogen phosphate, 0.030 M sodium azide, 1.5% hydrogen peroxide) for 15 min at room temperature. For beta-catenin, antigen retrieval involved 20 min boiling in Tris-EDTA pH 9.0, and blocking buffer (1% BSA in PBS) added to the slides for 30 min at room temperature. For beta-catenin (BD Transduction Labs, 610154), staining involved 1/100 dilution in blocking buffer (0.05% BSA in PBS) for 2 h at room temperature.

The slides were then rinsed in PBS and secondary antibody added (polymer HRP-labeled anti-mouse/rabbit, Envision) for 30 min at room temperature (Dako, Trappes, France). Slides were again washed in PBS and bound peroxidase detected by adding DAB substrate for 10 min at room temperature. Slides were then washed 2× in PBS and nuclei counterstained with Mayer's hematoxylin for 2 min, followed by two rinses in distilled water. Sections were dehydrated by serial immersion for 1 min each in 50 and 60% EtOH, followed by 2 min each in 70, 96, and 100% EtOH and xylene. Slides were mounted in mounting medium and a coverslip placed over the tissue section.

For immunohistochemistry (IHC) analysis, nuclei expressing beta-catenin after IHC staining were counted under 200× magnification. The Histological score (H-score) was determined based on the intensity and percentage of nucleus staining at each intensity [29], and calculated as follows: H-score = (nucleus showing highly beta-catenin expression) × 3 + (nucleus showing beta-catenin expression) × 2 + (nucleus showing weak beta-catenin expression) × 1.

2.6. Viral Infection of Organoids

For in vitro deficiency of the Ppp2r1a, organoid cultures containing floxed Ppp2r1a alleles were infected with adenovirus-encoding Cre recombinase (Ad-Cre) (Vector Biolabs, Philadelphia, PA, USA) at a titer of 100 multiplicity of infection (MOI) [27].

2.7. Tamoxifen Induction

Mice aged 6–8 weeks were injected intraperitoneally with a single 200 μL dose of tamoxifen in sunflower oil at 10 mg/mL.

2.8. Organoid Disaggregation, FACS, and Immunoblotting

Organoid cultures were recovered and dissociated from collagen gel by collagenase IV incubation, followed by incubation with 0.05% trypsin and EDTA. After extensive washing with 10% FBS, cells were filtered with 40-μm cell strainers (BD Falcon) Pellets were resuspended with FACS staining solution (5% FCS in PBS). Stringent wash was applied using ice-cold PBS, followed by isolation of $Lgr5^{-}EGFP^{+}$ cells using an FACSAria II (BD) [**30**]. For immunoblotting, the organoid cells were lysed in lysis buffer (1% Triton X-100, 150 mmol/L NaCl, 10 mmol/L Tris pH 7.4, 1 mmol/L EDTA pH 8.0, protease inhibitor cocktail) and then sonicated. The protein concentration was then measured. Next, equal amounts of protein (20 μg/well) were separated by SDS-polyacrylamide gel electrophoresis, transferred to nitrocellulose, and immunoblotted with primary antibodies. The membranes were blocked with CISblock buffer purchased from Cis-biotechnology, Taiwan. The following antibodies were used: anti-phospho-AKT (Ser-473), anti-AKT; anti-phospho-ERK1/2 (Thr-202/Tyr-204), anti-ERK, and anti-PP2A from Cell Signaling; anti-Lgr5 and anti-alkaline phosphate intestinal (Alpi) (Genetex, epitope C-terminus), beta-catenin (BD Transduction Labs, 610154), anti-Villin (Santa Cruz, Dallas, TX, USA), and anti-beta-actin and GAPDH (Sigma-Aldrich, St. Louis, MO, USA). Following the primary antibody incubation, the nitrocellulose membranes were incubated with secondary antibodies and visualized by ECL.

2.9. Antibody Arrays of Mouse AKT Pathway Phosphorylation

The RayBio™ Mouse AKT Pathway Phosphorylation Array Kit (cat. no. AAH-AKT1-2) was purchased and preformed according to a protocol modified from RayBiotech Inc. (Norcross, GA, USA). Briefly, the array membranes were blocked with blocking buffer for 30 min at room temperature. The membranes were then incubated with 2 mL of lysate prepared from organoid cultures with different treatments after normalization with equal amounts of protein. After extensive washing with wash buffer I (3 washings of 5 min each), and wash buffer II (3 washings of 5 min each) to remove unbound materials, the membranes were incubated with the Detection Antibody Cocktail for 1.5 to 2 h at room temperature, followed by wash with wash buffer I and II. Then the membranes were incubated with HRP-Anti-Rabbit IgG for 2 h at room temperature. The unbound HRP antibody was washed out with wash buffer I and II. Finally, each array membrane was exposed to X-ray film using a chemiluminescence detection system (Perkin Elmer, Wellesley, MA, USA).

2.10. Transcriptome Analysis

RNA was extracted from organoid culture using an RNeasy Kit (Qiagen, Hilden, Germany). RNA integrity was assessed using the RNA Nano6000 assay kit (Agilent Technologies, Santa Clara, CA, USA). For RNA-seq, library preparation and sequencing were performed by Novogene Technology. The output data (FASTQ files) were mapped to the target genome (TopHat v2.0.12), which can generate a database of splice junctions based on the gene model annotation file. HTSeq v0.6.1 was used to count the reads numbers mapped to each gene. Then the FPKM of each gene was calculated based on the length of the gene and reads count mapped to this gene. Differential expression heatmap results and biological variability were analyzed by ClustVis free web server [**31**] and gene set enrichment analysis (GSEA) [**32**], respectively. Data were submitted and approved by Gene Expression Omnibus (GEO; accession number GSE120241).

2.11. Whole-Exome Sequencing, Alignment, and Annotation

Exome sequences were captured with SureSelect^{XT} Mouse All Exon Kit (G7550E-001, Agilent, CA, USA) following the standard protocols. The products of exome capture should pass criteria: the length of fragments: 300 ± 30 bp and total amount: >600 ng. After exome capturing, the index-tagged samples were pooled and sequenced on Illumina HiSeq 2000. Burrows-Wheeler Alignment (v0.7.12) was employed to align reads to the reference genome (mm10) with default parameters. Aligned reads were sorted by picard-tools (v1.8). The duplicated reads were marked by picard-tools. Indel Realignment were performed with GenomeAnalysisTK (v3.5) using mm10 dbsnp database as known sites. Base quality score recalibration was also performed with GenomeAnalysisTK (v3.5) using mm10 dbsnp database. SNPs and indels were called by GenomeAnalysisTK HaplotypeCaller (v3.5), which used default parameters. Whole exome sequencing raw data was submitted to SRA database (SRA; **http://trace.ncbi.nlm.nih.gov/Traces/sra/**, accession number SRP162613)

2.12. Statistics

The p-values were determined using two-tailed Student's t-test (t groups) and One-way ANOVA (>2 groups). A p-value less than 0.05 was considered significant.

3. RESULTS

3.1. DMBA and OA treatment combination leads to dysplasia and oncogenic transformation in organoid culture

We utilized an organoid culture system supplemented with epidermal growth factor (EGF), Noggin, and R-spondin 1 (ENR) media to study the potential neoplastic transformation induced by DMBA and/or OA. As mentioned earlier [**27**], small intestine or colon organoids predominantly exhibited a well-organized, stereotyped epithelial single-layer organization at 7 days of culture, and maintained the similar morphology over a 50-day period of culture (**Figure 1**). At day 7, DMBA did not affect colony (organoid)-forming efficiency. OA induced a slight increase in both colony-forming efficiency, while a combination of DMBA and OA induced a large and significant increase in colony-forming efficiency (**Figure 1**A). At day 50, DMBA did not affect organoid morphology, OA induced mild enlargement in part of the epithelial layer with crowded nuclei, while a combination of DMBA and OA induced a very large malformation involving the entire epithelium with a confluent sheet of nuclear pleomorphism (**Figure 1**B), similar to that observed only when combining Apc, p53, KrasG12D, and Smad4 mutations in differentiated villus cells [**27**].

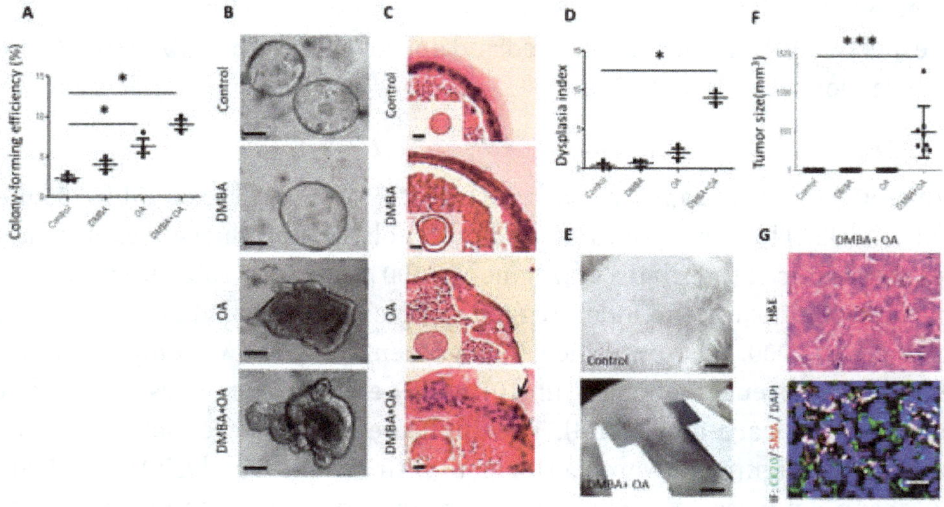

Figure 1. Combination of DMBA and okadaic acid (OA) induces dysplasia and oncogenic transformation in wild-type intestinal organoid culture. In vitro culture of wild type intestinal organoids without (control) or with DMBA or/and tamoxifen (TAM) in the presence of EGF, Noggin, and R-spondin 1 (500 single cells/well). (A) Colony (organoid)-forming efficiency was calculated at day 7. Experiment has been carried out in triplicate and each time 100 organoids were counted in each group. (B) Bright-field of organoid culture at day 50. Scale bar, 100 μm. (C) H&E staining and histologic characterization of cystic stratified epithelium with nuclear pleomorphism (arrow). Scale bar, 50 μm. (D) Dysplasia index at day 50 (experiment were repeated twice with n = 3 microscopic fields containing viable organoids). (E) Dissociated cells in Matrigel (500,000 cells/100 μL) were injected s.c. into NOD-SCID mice. In vivo tumor formation 45 days later (For those without tumor formation, observation was extended for up to 3 months, experiment were repeated twice with n = 3). (F) Tumor size 45 days after s.c. implantation (n = 8). (G) H&E staining and immunofluorescence of CK20 and SMA for tumor sections. Scale bar, 100 μm. *, $p < 0.05$; ***, $p < 0.0001$ as determined with one-way ANOVA.

Histological analysis revealed that organoids treated with DMBA alone had a single-layer epithelium, similar to the control. OA-treated organoids showed multi-cell-layer-changes in only a small part of the epithelium, while those treated with DMBA in combination with OA showed multi-cell-layer-changes with loss of the cell border in nearly the entire epithelium (**Figure 1**C), similar to the histology achieved only by quadruple mutants, Apc/KrasG12D/p53/Smad4 [**27**]. A dysplasia index quantification of proliferation, nuclear atypia, invasion, and cellular stratification in organoids indicated that DMBA did not induce dysplasia compared to the control, OA induced a marginal increase in dysplasia, while the combination of DMBA and OA induced a large and significant increase in dysplasia (**Figure 1**D). Furthermore, the combination of DMBA and OA, but not DMBA or OA alone, endowed organoids with robust in vivo tumorigenicity, forming alpha-smooth muscle actin (SMA)$^+$ and CK20$^+$ intestinal tumor after subcutaneous transplantation (**Figure 1**E–G).

3.2. Combination of DMBA Treatment and PP2A Deficiency Induces Dysplasia and Oncogenic Transformation in Organoid Culture

We further characterized the transformation effect of DMBA or/and adenovirus carrying recombinase (Ad-Cre-GFP)-mediated-PP2A deficiency in Ppp2r1aflox/flox mice-derived organoids.

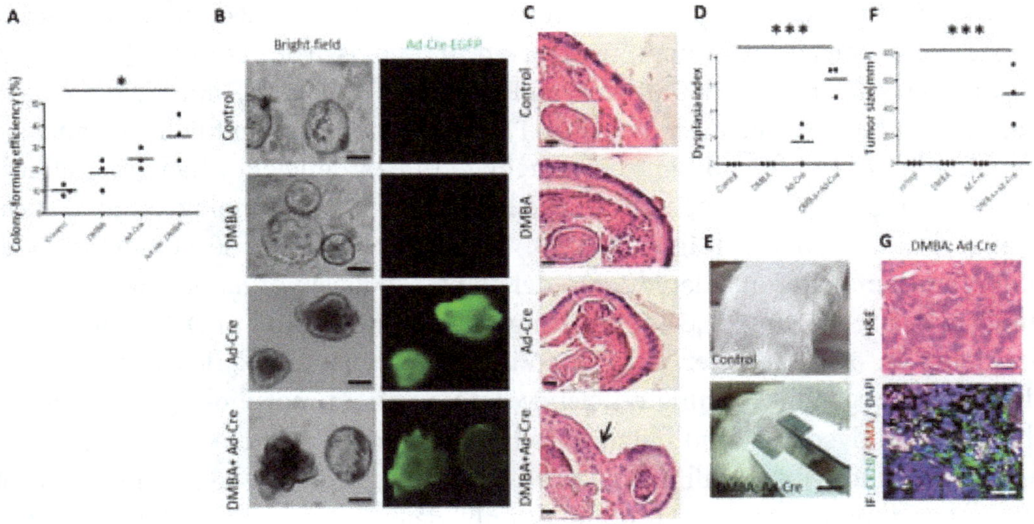

Figure 2. Combination of DMBA and Ad-Cre induces dysplasia and oncogenic transformation in Ppp2r1aflox/flox intestinal organoid culture. In vitro culture of Ppp2r1aflox/flox intestinal organoids without (control) or with DMBA or/and Ad-Cre-GFP (Ad-Cre) infection in the presence of EGF, Noggin and R-spondin 1 (500 single cells/well). (A) Colony (organoid)-forming efficiency was calculated at day 7. At least 100 organoids were counted in each group. (B) Bright-field and fluorescence images of organoid culture at day 50. Scale bar, 100 µm. (C) H&E staining and histologic characterization of cystic stratified epithelium with nuclear pleomorphism (arrow indicated). Scale bar, 50 µm. (D) Dysplasia index at day 50 (experiments were repeated twice with n = 3 microscopic fields containing viable organoids). (E) Dissociated cells in Matrigel (500,000 cells/100 µL) were injected s.c. into NOD-SCID mice. In vivo tumor formation 45 days later (for those without tumor formation, observation was extended for up to 3 months, experiments were repeated twice with n = 3). (F) Tumor size 45 days after s.c. implantation (n = 3). (G) H&E staining and immunofluorescence of CK20 and SMA for tumor sections. Scale bar, 100 µm. *, $p < 0.05$; ***, $p < 0.0001$ as determined with one-way ANOVA.

Similarly, DMBA had no significant effects, Ad-Cre-GFP mediated-PP2A deficiency had mild effects, and the combination of DMBA and Ad-Cre-GFP mediated-PP2A deficiency had large effects on early organoid forming efficiency, late organoid morphology, histological changes, and dysplasia (**Figure** 2A–D). Furthermore, only the combination of DMBA and Ad-Cre-GFP-mediated-PP2A deficiency fully endowed organoids with robust in vivo tumorigenicity (**Figure** 2E–G).

3.3. Combination of DMBA Treatment and PP2A Deficiency in Lgr5+ Rather than in Differentiated Villus Cells Induces Dysplasia and Oncogenic Transformation in Organoid Culture

To investigate whether Lgr5+ crypt stem cells or differentiated villus cells serve as the cell of origin of tumors, we treated organoids from Lgr5-EGFP-CreERT2; Ppp2r1aflox/flox mice with DMBA or/and tamoxifen. Similarly, DMBA did not have significant effects, tamoxifen mediated-PP2A deficiency had mild effects, and the combination of DMBA and tamoxifen-mediated-PP2A deficiency had great effects on early organoid forming efficiency, late organoid morphology, histological changes, and dysplasia (**Figure** 3A–E). Furthermore, only the combination of DMBA and tamoxifen-mediated-PP2A deficiency endowed organoids with in vivo tumorigenicity (**Figure** 3F,G). Interestingly, the combination of DMBA and PP2A deficiency in organoids derived from Villin-Cre; Ppp2r1aflox/flox mice did not affect early organoid forming efficiency, late organoid morphology, histological changes, and dysplasia, and failed to induce in vivo tumorigenicity. Of note, the recombinase activity in Villin-Cre mice is gradually reduced from villus to crypt [**33**], nevertheless, Ppp2r1a protein is only deleted in sorted villus cells but not in sorted Lgr5+ cells. These data suggest that Lgr5+ crypt stem cells but not differentiated villus cells serve as the cell of origin of intestinal tumor.

3.4. Combination of DMBA Treatment and PP2A Deficiency in Lgr5+ Cells Induces Upregulation in Stem Cell and EMT Markers, Downregulation in Differentiated Markers, and Tumorigenicity in Organoid Culture

Flow cytometric analysis (**Figure** 4A) revealed that DMBA did not increase the Lgr5+ cell ratio (as assayed by Lgr5-EGFP). PP2A deficiency induced a marginal increase, while the combination of DMBA and PP2A deficiency induced a significant increase in the Lgr5+ cell ratio. Comparative gene expression analysis of RNA samples isolated from organoid culture of Lgr5-EGFP-CreERT2; Ppp2r1aflox/flox mice 50 days after DMBA and tamoxifen administration revealed marked upregulation of stem cell genes, such as Lgr5, CD44, Ephb3, Egr2, Notch1, and Sox4; as well as EMT markers, such as Snail1, Snail2, Twist1, fibronectin, and vimentin;

and a marked downregulation of genes associated with differentiated cells, such as Paneth, enterocyte, goblet, and secretory cells compared to other treatment groups (**Figure 4**B). Furthermore, a small number (10^3) of $Lgr5^+$ but not $Lgr5^-$ cells isolated from organoid culture treated with DMBA and tamoxifen possessed in vivo tumorigenicity (**Figure 4**C). Collectively, these data suggest that the combination of DMBA and PP2A deficiency converted $Lgr5^+$ crypt stem cells into CSCs.

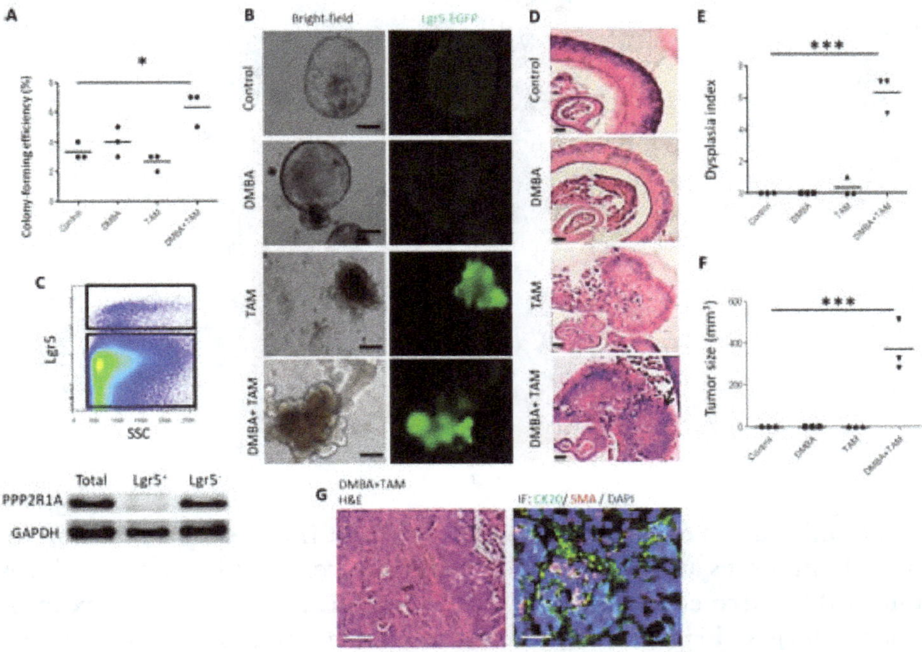

Figure 3. Combination of DMBA and TAM induces dysplasia and oncogenic transformation in Lgr5-EGFP-CreERT2; Ppp2r1aflox/flox intestinal organoid culture. In vitro culture of Lgr5-EGFP-CreERT2; Ppp2r1aflox/flox intestinal organoids without (control) or with DMBA or/and tamoxifen (TAM) in the presence of EGF, Noggin and R-spondin 1 (500 single cells/well). (A) Colony (organoid)-forming efficiency was calculated at day 7. At least 100 organoids were counted in each group. (B) Bright-field and fluorescence images of organoid culture at day 50. Scale bar, 100 μm. (C) Fluorescence-activated cell sorting (FACS) isolation of $Lgr5^+$ and $Lgr5^-$ populations. After FACS, PPP2R1A protein levels were detected by western blot. (D) H&E staining and histologic characterization of cystic stratified epithelium with nuclear pleomorphism (arrow). Scale bar, 50 μm. (E) Dysplasia index at day 50 (experiments were repeated twice with n = 3 microscopic fields containing viable organoids). (F) Dissociated cells in Matrigel (500,000 cells/100 μL) were injected s.c. into NOD-SCID mice. In vivo tumor formed 45 days later (for those without tumor formation, observation was extended for up to 3 months, experiments were repeated twice with n = 3). (G) H&E staining and immunofluorescence of CK20 and SMA for tumor sections. Scale bar, 100 μm. *, $p < 0.05$; ***, $p < 0.0001$ as determined with one-way ANOVA.

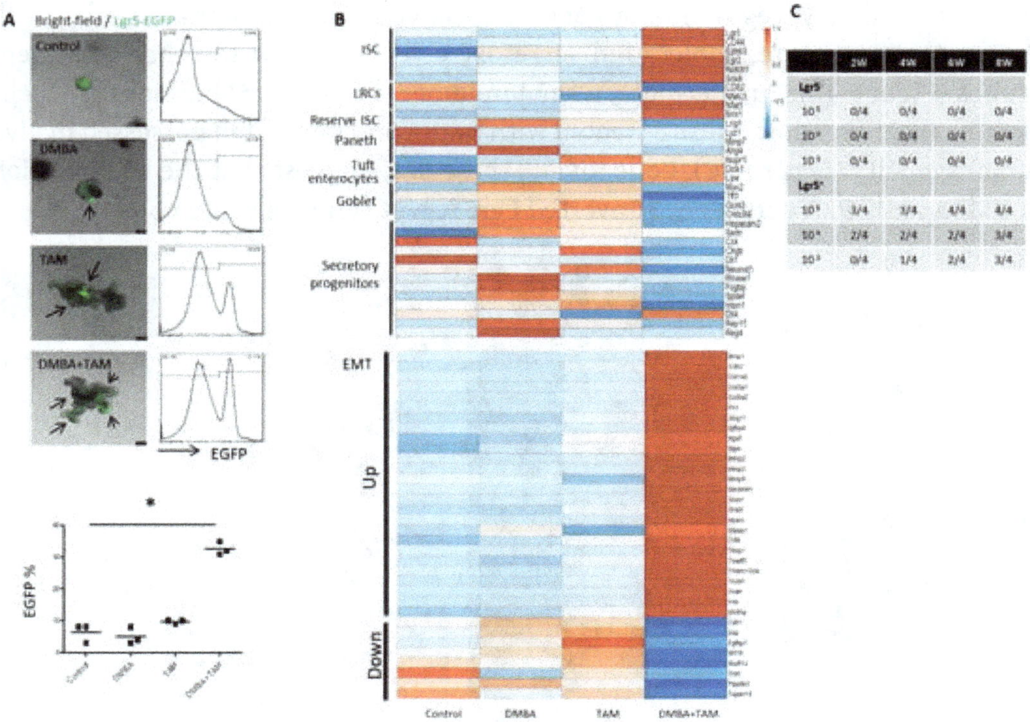

Figure 4. Combination of DMBA and PP2A deficient induces upregulation in stem cell and EMT markers and downregulation in differentiated markers in intestinal organoid. (A) In vitro culture of Lgr5-EGFP-CreERT2; Ppp2r1aflox/flox intestinal organoids. Merged bright-field and fluorescence images of organoid culture treated without (control) or with DMBA or/and tamoxifen (TAM) for 50 days in the presence of EGF, Noggin and R-spondin 1. Lgr5-EGFP were denoted as arrows. Scale bar, 100 μm. Flow cytometric analysis and quantification of GFP expression (bottom panel). No fluorescence organoid culture was serve as negative control to decide the threshold. *, $p < 0.05$ as determined with one-way ANOVA. (B) RNA-sequencing (seq) analysis of transcriptomes for 50-day organoids. The upper heat map shows clustering to previously reported RNA-seq data of sorted ISC (Intestinal Stem Cell); reserve ISC; paneth cell; LRCs (label retaining cells); tuft; enterocytes; goblet and secretory progenitor cells. The lower heat map shows clustering to EMT (epithelial-mesenchymal transition). (C) Tumor incidence in limiting dilution assay. Tumorigenic potential characterization of indicated numbers of $Lgr5^+$ and $Lgr5^-$ cells from the 50-day organoid culture. Dissociated cells in Matrigel (100 μL) were injected s.c. into NOD-SCID mice. Incidence of tumor formation was calculated more than 2 months.

3.5. Combination of DMBA Treatment and PP2A Deficiency Generates CSCs through PI3K, ERK, and Wnt Activation

To understand the molecular characteristics of the genes and pathways involved in organoid culture of Lgr5-EGFP-CreERT2; Ppp2r1aflox/flox mice after DMBA and tamoxifen administration, RNA-seq and gene set enrichment analysis (GSEA) were performed. Similar to previous findings that intestinal tumor begins with specific molecular alterations in Wnt-beta-catenin pathway [**13,23**], Wnt signaling was upregulated upon oncogenic transformation of organoid culture (**Figure 5**A). Western blotting of nuclear proteins (**Figure 5**B) and immunofluorescence (**Figure 5**C) revealed that nuclear accumulation of beta-catenin was predominantly observed in organoids with both of DMBA treatment and PP2A deficiency. Screening with a serine/threonine phosphorylation protein array followed by confirmation with western blotting further revealed that PI3K/AKT/GSK-3beta and Raf/ERK were activated in organoids with both DMBA treatment and PP2A depletion compared to other treatment groups (**Figure 5**D,E). Interestingly, treatment with the PI3K inhibitor LY294002, MEK inhibitor PD98059, and Wnt inhibitor DKK1 reduced the formation of malformed organoids, inhibited dysplasia (**Figure 5**F,G), and completely blocked in vivo tumorigenicity (**Figure 5**H). Notably, not only the WNT signaling was the most, but also the PI3K and RAS-MAPK (ERK) signalings were common altered pathways in human intestinal tumor, as revealed by The Cancer Genome Atlas (TCGA) Project [**14**]. These data suggest that CSC generation by DMBA treatment and PP2A deficiency depends on the activation of PI3K, ERK, and Wnt signals.

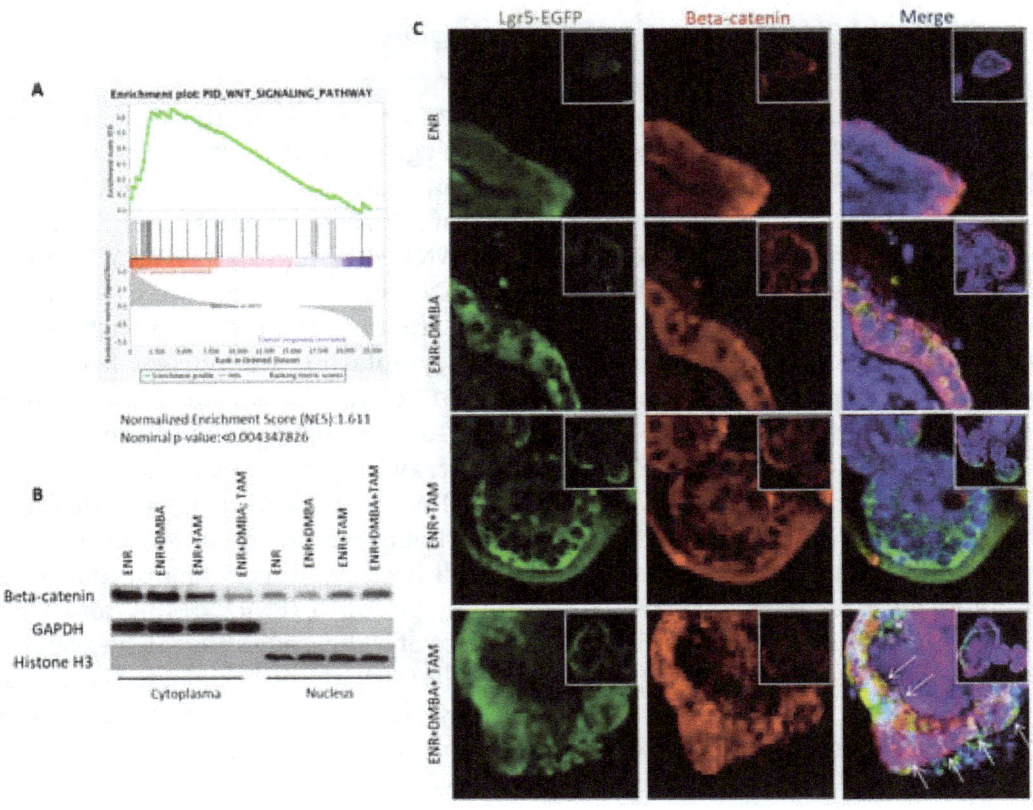

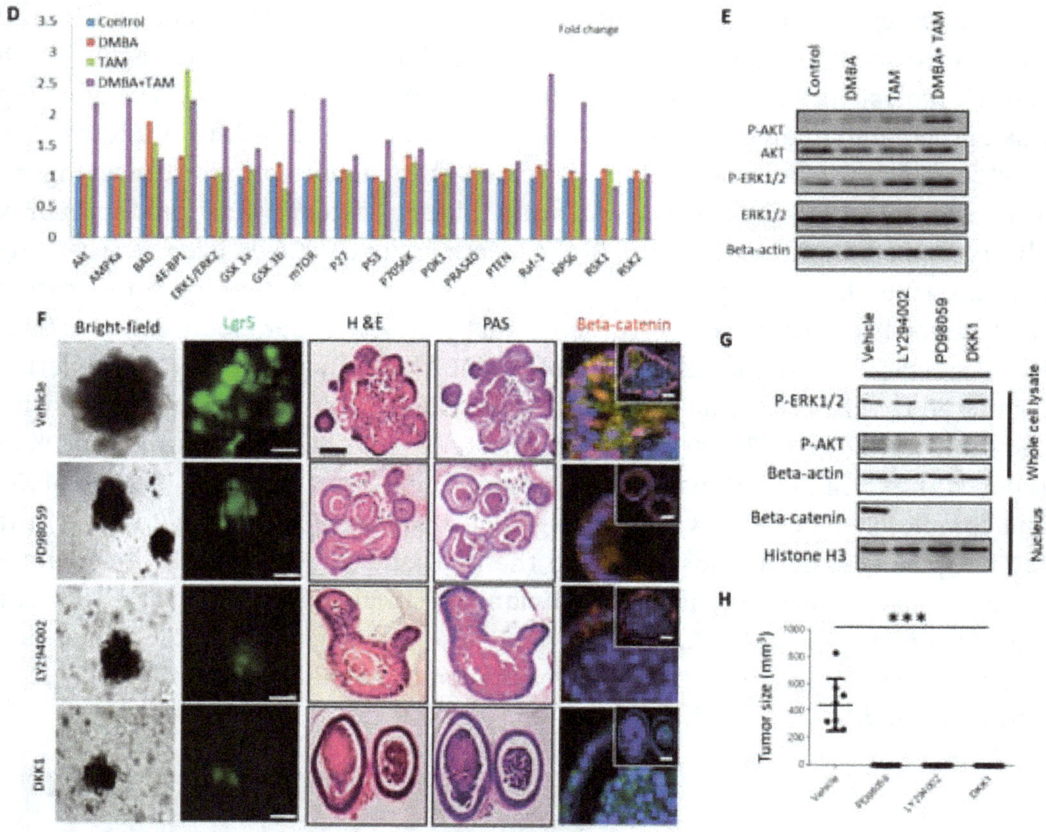

Figure 5. Beta-catenin activation caused by PI3K and ERK mediates dysplasia and oncogenic transformation in organoid culture. Lgr5-EGFP-CreERT2; Ppp2r1aflox/flox intestinal organoids were treated without (control) or with DMBA or/and tamoxifen (TAM) for 50 days in the presence of EGF, Noggin and R-spondin 1. (A) Gene set enrichment analysis (GSEA) shows "WNT SIGNALING PATHWAY" for the organoids treated with DMBA and TAM group versus control group, $p < 0.05$. (B) Western blotting of nuclear and cytoplasmic fractions. GAPDH and Histone H3 were used as protein loading controls for the cytoplasmic and nuclear fractions, respectively. (C) Immunofluorescence of Lgr5-EGFP and beta-catenin expression in organoid (denoted by arrows). Scale bar, 100 μm. (D) Graphs of mouse AKT pathway phosphorylation protein expression array (original data in Extended Data Figure 3) and densitometric analyses, n = 1. (E) Western blotting. (F) Bright-field, fluorescence images, H&E, PAS staining and beta-catenin immunofluorescence images. (G) Western blot analysis of whole cell lysate and nuclear fraction from organoid cultures treated with EGF, Noggin, R-spondin 1 (ENR), DMBA, and TAM for 50 days in the absence (Vehicle) or presence of indicated inhibitor treatment. (H) Dissociated cells in Matrigel (500,000 cells/100 μL) were injected s.c. into NOD-SCID mice. In vivo tumor formed 45 days later (For those without tumor formation, observation was extended for up to 3 months, n = 8). ***, $p < 0.0001$ as determined with one-way ANOVA.

3.6. Lgr5⁺ CSCs Are R-Spondin 1-Dependent

CSCs isolated from human intestinal tumor specimens express the Lgr5 crypt marker [**34**]. R-spondin is expressed by the intestinal stroma and is differentially upregulated during Citrobacter rodentium- and dextran sulfate sodium (DSS)-induced colitis in mice, which reflects human ulcerative colitis, a precancerous stage [**35**].

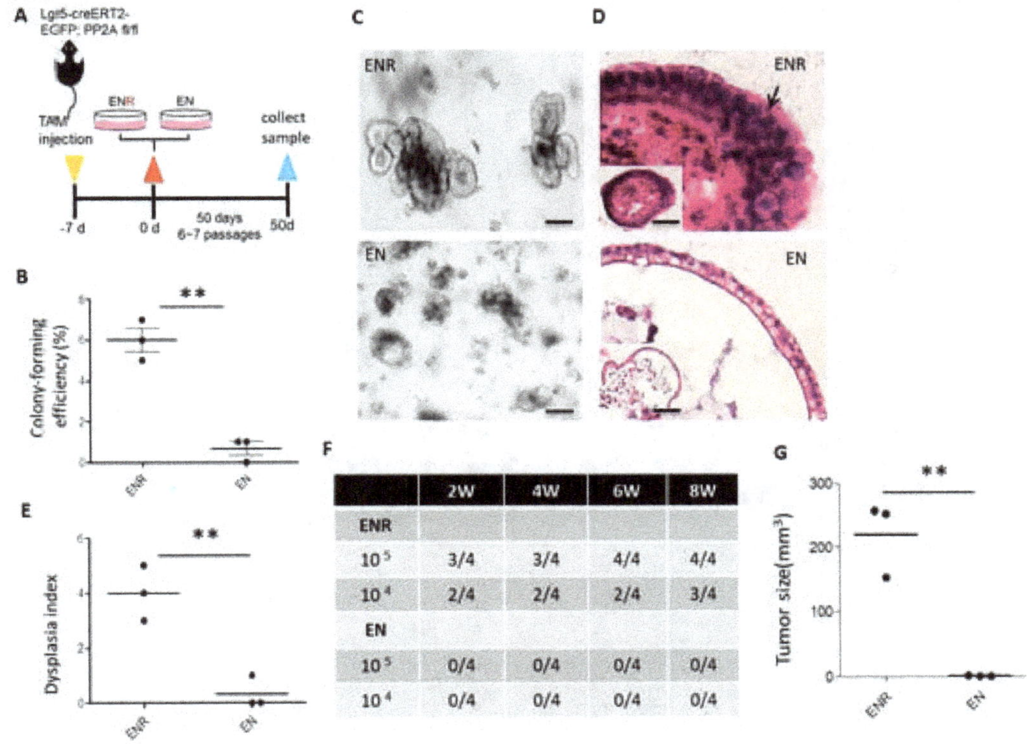

	2W	4W	6W	8W
ENR				
10^5	3/4	3/4	4/4	4/4
10^4	2/4	2/4	2/4	3/4
EN				
10^5	0/4	0/4	0/4	0/4
10^4	0/4	0/4	0/4	0/4

Figure 6. R-spondin 1 drives Wnt-dependent dysplasia and oncogenic transformation in the intestinal organoid culture. In vitro culture of Lgr5-EGFP-CreERT2; Ppp2r1aflox/flox intestinal organoids (500 single cells/well) treated with DMBA and tamoxifen (TAM) in the presence of EGF, Noggin, and with (ENR) or without R-spondin-1 (EN). (A) Schematic illustration of the experimental design. (B) Colony (organoid)-forming efficiency at day 7. At least 100 organoids were counted in each group. (C) Bright-field images at day 50. Scale bar, 100 μm. (D) H&E staining and histologic characterization of cystic stratified epithelium with nuclear pleomorphism (arrow). Scale bar, 50 μm. (E) Dysplasia index at day 50 (experiment was repeated twice with n = 3 microscopic fields containing viable organoids). (F) Incidence of tumor formation at indicated time periods, and (G) tumor size in NOD-SCID mice after s.c. injection 45 days later of indicated cell numbers from 50-day organoid. **, $p < 0.01$ as determined with Student's t-test.

These data suggest a role for R-spondin 1 and its receptor Lgr5 in the maintenance of undifferentiated status and tumorigenesis of human colorectal CSCs. In contrast to tumorigenesis initiated by dedifferentiation (tumor generated from intestinal epithelial cell of villin-creERT2/APC lox/lox/K-rasG12D/+ mice) [**4**], where tumor cells were $Lgr5^-$ and generated independently of R-spondin 1, tumor cells in the current study were $Lgr5^+$ and generated dependently on R-spondin 1 (**Figure 6**), suggesting that tumor cells generated by DMBA treatment and PP2A deficiency in mouse $Lgr5^+$ cells were indeed intestinal CSCs and could serve as surrogates of human colorectal CSCs [**34**].

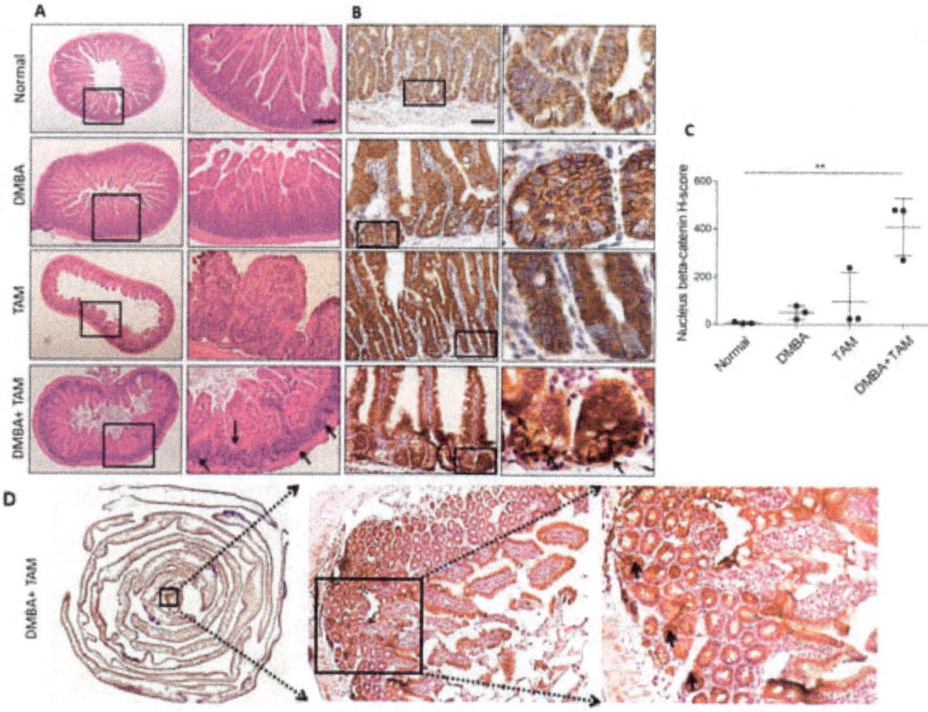

Figure 7. Combination of DMBA treatment with PP2A deficient in $Lgr5^+$ drives intestinal neoplasia in both the small intestine and colon. (A) H&E staining and (B) Beta-catenin IHC were performed on the serial sections. Multiple beta-$catenin^{high}$ adenomas were observed throughout the colon 36 days after induction. (C) Quantitative analysis of nucleus beta-catenin H-score from (B). (D) High level expression of beta-catenin was apparent in the transformed stem cell compartment (Peyer's patches are stained blue). Multiple beta-$catenin^{high}$ transformed cells were observed throughout the intestinal 36 day after induction (magnified at right panel, denoted by arrows). Original magnifications: (A) left, 4×; (A) right, 10×; (B) left, 20×; (B) right, 40×; (D) center, 20×; (D) right, 40×; Scale bar, 100 µm. **, $p < 0.01$ as determined with one-way ANOVA.

Earlier studies utilizing tumorigenesis models created through genetic modification in differentiated villus cells, albeit having modest tumorigenesis efficiency [27], have shown significant involvement of Lgr5+ cells in carcinogenesis/ metastasis. [7,**8**].

3.7. Combination of DMBA Treatment with PP2A Deficiency in Lgr5⁺ Also Induces Tumor Formation In Vivo

We investigated whether tumorigenesis generated by DMBA treatment and PP2A deficiency in mouse Lgr5⁺ cells reflects tumor formation in vivo. Lgr5-EGFP-CreERT2; Ppp2r1aflox/flox mice treated with DMBA and tamoxifen formed adenocarcinoma in the small intestine and colorectal regions 36 days later. Histological analysis revealed that mice receiving DMBA and tamoxifen increased the incidence of multiple foci adenoma compared to other groups (**Figure** 7A). IHC analysis revealed that beta-catenin accumulated in the nuclei of tumor cells mainly in the crypt area (**Figure** 7B) and quantitative evaluation of nucleus beta-catenin accumulation [**29**] further showed that nucleus beta-catenin H-score was significantly greater in mice receiving DMBA and tamoxifen compared to other groups (**Figure** 7C,D). The efficiency and rapidity were much greater than tumorigenesis generated by Apc deficiency in either Lgr5⁺ crypt stem cell- [**3**] or differentiated villus cell-based models [**4**].

3.8. Not Only DMBA but Also Other Carcinogens Induce Tumors from Lgr5⁺ Intestinal Stem Cells of PP2A Deficient Mice

To demonstrate carcinogen-induced tumor from Lgr5⁺ intestinal stem cells of PP2A deficient mice was not limited to DMBA, N-methyl-N-nitrosourea (MNU) and 2-amino-1-methyl-6-phenylimidazo-[4,5-b]pyridine (PhIP) were also administered in combination with tamoxifen treatment in organoid cultures derived from Lgr5-EGFP-CreERT2; Ppp2r1aflox/flox mice and from Villin-Cre; Ppp2r1aflox/flox mice. Interestingly, increased early organoid forming efficiency, late organoid with irregular nuclei and prominent nucleoli morphology and dysplasia, and in vivo tumorigenicity were only observed in organoid cultures derived from Lgr5-EGFP-CreERT2; Ppp2r1aflox/flox mice but not from Villin-Cre; Ppp2r1aflox/flox mice. More importantly, we found that tumorigenicity induced by combination of MUN or PhIP with PP2A deficiency also depended on the activation of PI3K, ERK, and Wnt signals. Similarly, combination of MUN or PhIP treatment with PP2A deficiency in Lgr5⁺ cells also induced tumor formation in vivo.

3.9. Mutational Landscapes of Intestinal Tumors Derived from Lgr5⁺ Cells Treated with Carcinogen and PP2A Deficiency

To gain insight of the genetic alterations that drove these pathways in the models, we performed whole-exome sequencing (WES) . Somatic variants in each chemical induced tumor organoid sample were identified with a tumor-control paired strategy by removing the variants in their paired control samples and the variants affecting protein coding sequence were further filtrated. The numbers of somatic mutations, including synonymous and nonsynonymous mutations, for organoid cultures with combined DMBA, MUN, or PhIP treatment with PP2A deficiency in Lgr5⁺ cells.

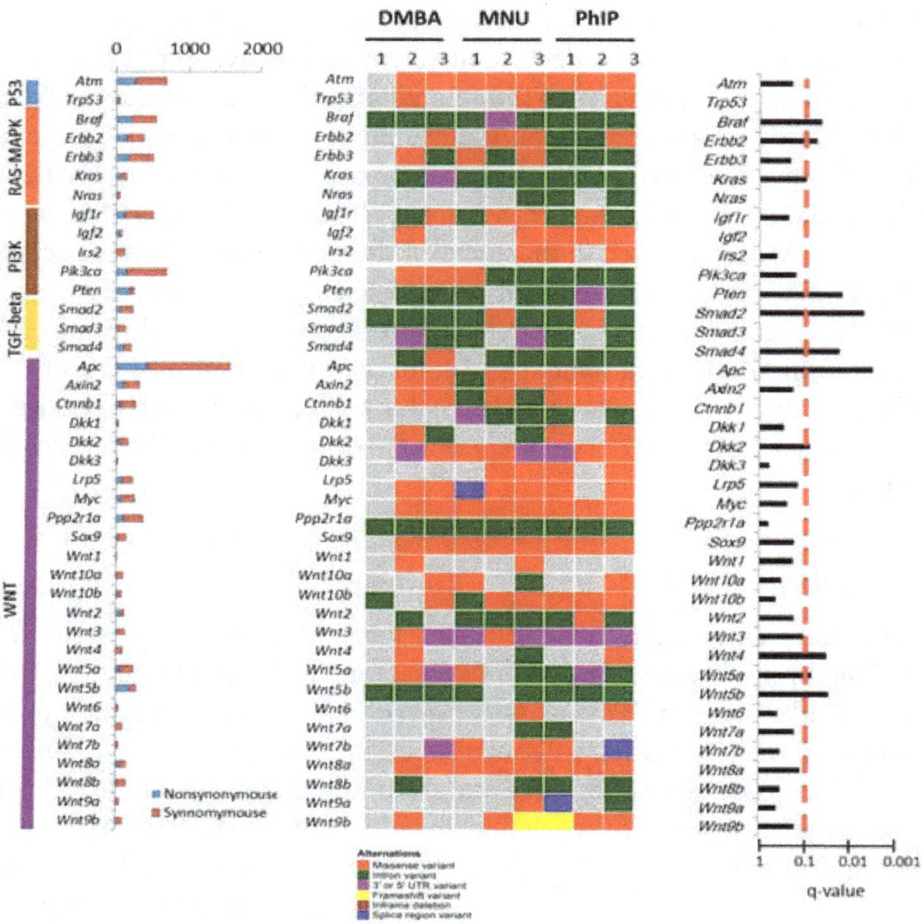

Figure 8. Landscape of somatic mutant genes in three carcinogen treated organoid cultures. Data matrix shows number of somatic mutant genes in each carcinogen treated organoid cultures and were classified according to their pathway. Somatic mutations are presented according to the type of mutation (missense variant, intron variant, 3′ or 5′ prime UTR variant, frameshift variant, inframe deletion, or splice region variant) On the left, the total number of mutations of each gene within all three groups is shown with a bar plot, while the q-value of each significantly mutated gene is shown on the right.

IPA analysis of 270 mutated genes shared by DMBA, MUN, and PhIP treatment with PP2A deficiency in Lgr5⁺ cells revealed 10 top significantly enriched pathways, including the intestinal tumor metastasis signaling (p-value = 2.12×10^{-57}) and Wnt/beta-catenin signaling (p-value = 1.40×10^{-55}). Furthermore, beta-catenin (CTNNB1) seemed to be a common downstream hub as identified by the Path Explorer function in IPA. There were five core pathways related with human intestinal tumor found by TCGA, including p53, RAS-MAPK, PI3K, TGF-beta, and WNT pathways (**Figure 8**) [**14**]. We identified several recurrent mutations with FDR < 0.1, including Braf, erbb2, kras, pten, Smad2, Smad4, Apc, DKK2, Wnt4, Wnt5a, and Wnt5b (**Figure 8**). Based on these analyses, the mouse intestinal tumor organoid models based on combined use of chemical carcinogen and genetic modification can recapitulate the human colorectal cancer development process in response to complex interactions between the genotype and environmental factor.

4. DISCUSSION

Enhancing carcinogenesis in GEMMs requires numerous gene alterations for increased effectiveness. GEMMs provide a simplified representation of the frequency and types of mutations in human malignancies, with mutation rates ranging from less than 0.1 to over 50 mutations per megabase. [36-**37**]. The use of GEMMs in combination with carcinogenesis increased the tumor spectrum or speeded the tumor formation observed in some GEMMs, such as the $p53^{-/-}$ mouse model in combination with exposure to carcinogens or radiation [**21,38**]. In the current study, Ppp2r1a-/- mouse model in combination with exposure to different carcinogens induced tumorigenesis through similar signaling pathways, while GEMM or carcinogen exposure alone did not induce tumorigenesis. These data suggest that the combination of GEMMs with exposure to carcinogen or other environmental agents is a logical approach in studying tumorigenesis and cancer progression.

PP2A is a tumor suppressor that regulates many oncogenic pathways. In fact, decreased PP2A activity has been reported as a common event in colorectal cancer [**39**]. DMBA and MNU are important environmental carcinogens. PhIP, a food-borne carcinogen produced while cooking meat and fish, models human colon cancer in rodents [**40**]. Here, we demonstrated that DMBA, MNU, or PhIP each induced intestinal organoid transformation when combined with PP2A deficiency in $Lgr5^{+}$ intestinal stem cells but not in differentiated villus cells, suggesting that PP2A plays a role in suppressing colorectal tumorigenesis induced by chemical carcinogen exposure. Our results provide further experimental evidence to demonstrate that the cell of origin of intestinal tumor is crypt stem cells instead of differentiated villus cells. We did not focus on the molecular mechanism underlying the differential tumorigenicity pathways between stem cells and differentiated cells, which requires further investigation.

A recent study shows that unless the R-spondin and Wnt ligands are both present, the default fate of $Lgr5^{+}$ crypt stem cells is differentiation [**41**]. However, gain-of-function studies reveal that R-spondin and Wnt ligands have qualitatively distinct, non-interchangeable roles in crypt stem cells. Wnt proteins confer a basal competency unto the $Lgr5^{+}$ crypt stem cell by inducing R-spondin receptor expression that enables R-spondin-driven $Lgr5^+$ crypt stem cell self-renewal. In the current study, using a combination of carcinogen treatment and PP2A deficiency, intestinal organoids derived from Lgr5-cre; Ppp2r1aflox/flox, but not Villin-Cre; Ppp2r1aflox/flox, underwent oncogenic transformation and exhibited CSC phenotypes that were dependent on the presence of R-spondin 1 in the culture media. These studies together suggest the important roles of R-spondin signaling in stem cell self-renewal and preventing differentiation. The discrepancy of R-spondin 1 dependence between tumorigenicity induced by the current method and previous GEMM relied on Apc depletion or CTNNB1 activation [**4**] is supported by the mutual exclusion of R-spondin fusion and Apc or CTNNB1 mutation identified in human intestinal tumors [**20**]. The Lgr5/R-spondin 1 complex degrades Rnf43 and Znrf3, two transmembrane E3 ligases that remove Wnt receptors from the stem cell surface. Consistently, simultaneous deficient of these two E3 ligases in the intestinal epithelium induced the formation of unusual adenomas consisting entirely of $Lgr5^+$ stem cells and their niche [**42**].

Concurrent exposure to a carcinogen and targeted removal of PP2A in villus cells did not lead to the development of tumors, enhanced cell growth, or abnormal tissue growth in gut organoids. The current study did not investigate the mechanism that distinguishes Lgr5+ crypt stem cells from mature villus cells regarding susceptibility to carcinogenesis. Our current findings indicate that the Wnt and Rspondin/Lgr5 signaling pathways are crucial for the localization of nuclear-beta catenin, a process essential for stem cell self-renewal and potentially triggering cancer if disrupted.

5. CONCISE SUMMARY

In summary, we demonstrated that carcinogen-induced cancer arises from $Lgr5^+$ crypt stem cells in $Ppp2r1a^{-/-}$ mice. In addition, combing carcinogenesis with GEMM recapitulated the developmental process of environmentally induced human tumor, while increasing the rate and percentage of tumorigenesis. Interestingly, exposure to different carcinogens, such as DMBA, MNU, or PhIP, when combined with PP2A deficiency in $Lgr5^+$ intestinal stem cells induced tumorigenesis that was dependent on the activation of pathways including Wnt, PI3K, and RAS-MAPK signalings, the common altered pathways revealed by TCGA human intestinal tumor project [**14**]. These data indicate that PP2A acts as a tumor suppressor in the development of intestinal cancer. This organoid platform offers experimental proof of its effectiveness in detecting crucial oncogenes and suppressor genes as early molecular epidemiological biomarkers of carcinogenesis. It is also beneficial in human cancer prevention efforts.

6. AT A GLANCE

The cellular origin and the impact of intrinsic and extrinsic variables on transformation are not well understood in most malignancies. There are no existing models for carcinogenesis unique to cells. We created a tumorigenesis model by combining carcinogenesis and genetically altered mice models to study the cellular origin in carcinogenesis. In organoids, the absence of protein phosphatase 2A (PP2A) triggered cancer in Lgr5+ intestinal lineage when treated with any of three carcinogens: DMBA, MNU, or PhIP, but not in differentiated cells. The altered cells exhibited an increase in stem cell characteristics, upregulation of EMT markers, and gained tumorigenic properties. Tumorigenesis was shown to rely on the activation of Wnt, PI3K, and RAS-MAPK pathways using a mechanistic approach. Tumor growth occurred when a carcinogen was combined with PP2A deficiency in vivo. We show that these intestinal cancers exhibit a mutation landscape and core driving pathways similar to those found in human intestinal tumors in The Cancer Genome Atlas (TCGA) using whole-exome sequencing. The data offer insight into how external carcinogens and internal genetic changes interact, indicating that PP2A acts as a tumor suppressor in intestinal cancer development.

REFERENCES

1. Poirier, M.C. Chemical-induced DNA damage and human cancer risk. Nat. Rev. Cancer 2004, 4, 630–637. [Google Scholar] [CrossRef]
2. Visvader, J.E. Cells of origin in cancer. Nature 2011, 469, 314–322. [Google Scholar] [CrossRef] [PubMed]
3. Barker, N.; Ridgway, R.A.; van Es, J.H.; van de Wetering, M.; Begthel, H.; van den Born, M.; Danenberg, E.; Clarke, A.R.; Sansom, O.J.; Clevers, H. Crypt stem cells as the cells-of-origin of intestinal cancer. Nature 2009, 457, 608–611. [Google Scholar] [CrossRef] [PubMed]
4. Schwitalla, S.; Fingerle, A.A.; Cammareri, P.; Nebelsiek, T.; Goktuna, S.I.; Ziegler, P.K.; Canli, O.; Heijmans, J.; Huels, D.J.; Moreaux, G.; et al. Intestinal tumorigenesis initiated by dedifferentiation and acquisition of stem-cell-like properties. Cell 2013, 152, 25–38. [Google Scholar] [CrossRef] [PubMed] [Green Version]
5. Tetteh, P.W.; Basak, O.; Farin, H.F.; Wiebrands, K.; Kretzschmar, K.; Begthel, H.; van den Born, M.; Korving, J.; de Sauvage, F.; van Es, J.H.; et al. Replacement of lost Lgr5-positive stem cells through plasticity of their enterocyte-lineage daughters. Cell Stem Cell 2016, 18, 203–213. [Google Scholar] [CrossRef]
6. Westphalen, C.B.; Asfaha, S.; Hayakawa, Y.; Takemoto, Y.; Lukin, D.J.; Nuber, A.H.; Brandtner, A.; Setlik, W.; Remotti, H.; Muley, A.; et al. Long-lived intestinal tuft cells serve as colon cancer-initiating cells. J. Clin. Investig. 2014, 124, 1283–1295. [Google Scholar] [CrossRef] [Green Version]
7. De Sousa e Melo, F.; Kurtova, A.V.; Harnoss, J.M.; Kljavin, N.; Hoeck, J.D.; Hung,

J.; Anderson, J.E.; Storm, E.E.; Modrusan, Z.; Koeppen, H.; et al. A distinct role for Lgr5+ stem cells in primary and metastatic colon cancer. Nature 2017, 543, 676–680. [Google Scholar] [CrossRef]

8. Shimokawa, M.; Ohta, Y.; Nishikori, S.; Matano, M.; Takano, A.; Fujii, M.; Date, S.; Sugimoto, S.; Kanai, T.; Sato, T. Visualization and targeting of LGR5(+) human colon cancer stem cells. Nature 2017, 545, 187–192. [Google Scholar] [CrossRef]
9. Ruvolo, P.P. The broken "Off" switch in cancer signaling: PP2A as a regulator of tumorigenesis, drug resistance, and immune surveillance. BBA Clin. 2016, 6, 87–99. [Google Scholar] [CrossRef] [Green Version]
10. Bardelli, A.; Parsons, D.W.; Silliman, N.; Ptak, J.; Szabo, S.; Saha, S.; Markowitz, S.; Willson, J.K.; Parmigiani, G.; Kinzler, K.W.; et al. Mutational analysis of the tyrosine kinome in colorectal cancers. Science 2003, 300, 949. [Google Scholar] [CrossRef]
11. Wang, Z.; Shen, D.; Parsons, D.W.; Bardelli, A.; Sager, J.; Szabo, S.; Ptak, J.; Silliman, N.; Peters, B.A.; van der Heijden, M.S.; et al. Mutational analysis of the tyrosine phosphatome in colorectal cancers. Science 2004, 304, 1164–1166. [Google Scholar] [CrossRef]
12. Samuels, Y.; Wang, Z.; Bardelli, A.; Silliman, N.; Ptak, J.; Szabo, S.; Yan, H.; Gazdar, A.; Powell, S.M.; Riggins, G.J.; et al. High frequency of mutations of the PIK3CA gene in human cancers. Science 2004, 304, 554. [Google Scholar] [CrossRef] [PubMed] [Green Version]
13. Parsons, D.W.; Wang, T.L.; Samuels, Y.; Bardelli, A.; Cummins, J.M.; DeLong, L.; Silliman, N.; Ptak, J.; Szabo, S.; Willson, J.K.; et al. Colorectal cancer: Mutations in a signalling pathway. Nature 2005, 436, 792. [Google Scholar] [CrossRef] [PubMed]
14. Cancer Genome Atlas, N. Comprehensive molecular characterization of human colon and rectal cancer. Nature 2012, 487, 330–337. [Google Scholar] [CrossRef] [PubMed] [Green Version]
15. Westermarck, J.; Hahn, W.C. Multiple pathways regulated by the tumor suppressor PP2A in transformation. Trends Mol. Med. 2008, 14, 152–160. [Google Scholar] [CrossRef] [PubMed]
16. Lin, S.P.; Lee, Y.T.; Wang, J.Y.; Miller, S.A.; Chiou, S.H.; Hung, M.C.; Hung, S.C. Survival of cancer stem cells under hypoxia and serum depletion via decrease in PP2A activity and activation of p38-MAPKAPK2-Hsp27. PLoS ONE 2012, 7, e49605. [Google Scholar] [CrossRef] [PubMed] [Green Version]
17. Lin, S.P.; Lee, Y.T.; Yang, S.H.; Miller, S.A.; Chiou, S.H.; Hung, M.C.; Hung, S.C.

Colon cancer stem cells resist antiangiogenesis therapy-induced apoptosis. Cancer Lett. 2013, 328, 226–234. [Google Scholar] [CrossRef] [PubMed]

18. Liu, C.C.; Lin, S.P.; Hsu, H.S.; Yang, S.H.; Lin, C.H.; Yang, M.H.; Hung, M.C.; Hung, S.C. Suspension survival mediated by PP2A-STAT3-Col XVII determines tumour initiation and metastasis in cancer stem cells. Nat. Commun. 2016, 7, 11798. [Google Scholar] [CrossRef] [PubMed] [Green Version]
19. Cheng, Y.; Ren, X.; Yuan, Y.; Shan, Y.; Li, L.; Chen, X.; Zhang, L.; Takahashi, Y.; Yang, J.W.; Han, B.; et al. eEF-2 kinase is a critical regulator of Warburg effect through controlling PP2A-A synthesis. Oncogene 2016, 35, 6293–6308. [Google Scholar] [CrossRef]
20. Seshagiri, S.; Stawiski, E.W.; Durinck, S.; Modrusan, Z.; Storm, E.E.; Conboy, C.B.; Chaudhuri, S.; Guan, Y.; Janakiraman, V.; Jaiswal, B.S.; et al. Recurrent R-spondin fusions in colon cancer. Nature 2012, 488, 660–664. [Google Scholar] [CrossRef]
21. Donehower, L.A.; Harvey, M.; Slagle, B.L.; McArthur, M.J.; Montgomery, C.A., Jr.; Butel, J.S.; Bradley, A. Mice deficient for p53 are developmentally normal but susceptible to spontaneous tumours. Nature 1992, 356, 215–221. [Google Scholar] [CrossRef] [PubMed]
22. Cheng, J.L.; Futakuchi, M.; Ogawa, K.; Iwata, T.; Kasai, M.; Tokudome, S.; Hirose, M.; Shirai, T. Dose response study of conjugated fatty acid derived from safflower oil on mammary and colon carcinogenesis pretreated with 7,12-dimethylbenz[a]anthracene (DMBA) and 1,2-dimethylhydrazine (DMH) in female Sprague-Dawley rats. Cancer Lett. 2003, 196, 161–168. [Google Scholar] [CrossRef]
23. Brown, K.; Buchmann, A.; Balmain, A. Carcinogen-induced mutations in the mouse c-Ha-ras gene provide evidence of multiple pathways for tumor progression. Proc. Natl. Acad. Sci. USA 1990, 87, 538–542. [Google Scholar] [CrossRef] [PubMed] [Green Version]
24. Kimura, K.; Satoh, K.; Kanno, A.; Hamada, S.; Hirota, M.; Endoh, M.; Masamune, A.; Shimosegawa, T. Activation of Notch signaling in tumorigenesis of experimental pancreatic cancer induced by dimethylbenzanthracene in mice. Cancer Sci. 2007, 98, 155–162. [Google Scholar] [CrossRef] [PubMed] [Green Version]
25. Reddy, B.S.; Narisawa, T.; Maronpot, R.; Weisburger, J.H.; Wynder, E.L. Animal models for the study of dietary factors and cancer of the large bowel. Cancer Res. 1975, 35, 3421–3426. [Google Scholar] [PubMed]
26. Wakabayashi, K.; Nagao, M.; Esumi, H.; Sugimura, T. Food-derived mutagens

and carcinogens. Cancer Res. 1992, 52, 2092s–2098s. [Google Scholar]

27. Li, X.; Nadauld, L.; Ootani, A.; Corney, D.C.; Pai, R.K.; Gevaert, O.; Cantrell, M.A.; Rack, P.G.; Neal, J.T.; Chan, C.W.; et al. Oncogenic transformation of diverse gastrointestinal tissues in primary organoid culture. Nat. Med. 2014, 20, 769–777. [Google Scholar] [CrossRef] [Green Version]
28. Sato, T.; Vries, R.G.; Snippert, H.J.; van de Wetering, M.; Barker, N.; Stange, D.E.; van Es, J.H.; Abo, A.; Kujala, P.; Peters, P.J.; et al. Single Lgr5 stem cells build crypt-villus structures in vitro without a mesenchymal niche. Nature 2009, 459, 262–265. [Google Scholar] [CrossRef]
29. Bilalovic, N.; Sandstad, B.; Golouh, R.; Nesland, J.M.; Selak, I.; Torlakovic, E.E. CD10 protein expression in tumor and stromal cells of malignant melanoma is associated with tumor progression. Mod. Pathol. 2004, 17, 1251–1258. [Google Scholar] [CrossRef]
30. Mahe, M.M.; Aihara, E.; Schumacher, M.A.; Zavros, Y.; Montrose, M.H.; Helmrath, M.A.; Sato, T.; Shroyer, N.F. Establishment of gastrointestinal epithelial organoids. Curr. Protoc. Mouse Biol. 2013, 3, 217–240. [Google Scholar] [CrossRef] [Green Version]
31. Metsalu, T.; Vilo, J. ClustVis: A web tool for visualizing clustering of multivariate data using Principal Component Analysis and heatmap. Nucleic Acids Res. 2015, 43, W566–W570. [Google Scholar] [CrossRef] [PubMed]
32. Subramanian, A.; Tamayo, P.; Mootha, V.K.; Mukherjee, S.; Ebert, B.L.; Gillette, M.A.; Paulovich, A.; Pomeroy, S.L.; Golub, T.R.; Lander, E.S.; et al. Gene set enrichment analysis: A knowledge-based approach for interpreting genome-wide expression profiles. Proc. Natl. Acad. Sci. USA 2005, 102, 15545–15550. [Google Scholar] [CrossRef] [PubMed] [Green Version]
33. Madison, B.B.; Dunbar, L.; Qiao, X.T.; Braunstein, K.; Braunstein, E.; Gumucio, D.L. Cis elements of the villin gene control expression in restricted domains of the vertical (crypt) and horizontal (duodenum, cecum) axes of the intestine. J. Biol. Chem. 2002, 277, 33275–33283. [Google Scholar] [CrossRef] [PubMed] [Green Version]
34. Kemper, K.; Prasetyanti, P.R.; De Lau, W.; Rodermond, H.; Clevers, H.; Medema, J.P. Monoclonal antibodies against Lgr5 identify human colorectal cancer stem cells. Stem Cells 2012, 30, 2378–2386. [Google Scholar] [CrossRef]
35. Kang, E.; Yousefi, M.; Gruenheid, S. R-spondins are expressed by the intestinal stroma and are differentially regulated during citrobacter rodentium- and DSS-induced colitis in mice. PLoS ONE 2016, 11, e0152859. [Google Scholar] [CrossRef] [Green Version]
36. Vogelstein, B.; Papadopoulos, N.; Velculescu, V.E.; Zhou, S.; Diaz, L.A., Jr.;

Kinzler, K.W. Cancer genome landscapes. Science 2013, 339, 1546–1558. [Google Scholar] [CrossRef]

37. Westcott, P.M.; Halliwill, K.D.; To, M.D.; Rashid, M.; Rust, A.G.; Keane, T.M.; Delrosario, R.; Jen, K.Y.; Gurley, K.E.; Kemp, C.J.; et al. The mutational landscapes of genetic and chemical models of Kras-driven lung cancer. Nature 2015, 517, 489–492. [Google Scholar] [CrossRef] [Green Version]
38. Lee, C.L.; Mowery, Y.M.; Daniel, A.R.; Zhang, D.; Sibley, A.B.; Delaney, J.R.; Wisdom, A.J.; Qin, X.; Wang, X.; Caraballo, I.; et al. Mutational landscape in genetically engineered, carcinogen-induced, and radiation-induced mouse sarcoma. JCI Insight 2019, 4. [Google Scholar] [CrossRef] [Green Version]
39. Cristobal, I.; Manso, R.; Rincon, R.; Carames, C.; Senin, C.; Borrero, A.; Martinez-Useros, J.; Rodriguez, M.; Zazo, S.; Aguilera, O.; et al. PP2A inhibition is a common event in colorectal cancer and its restoration using FTY720 shows promising therapeutic potential. Mol. Cancer Ther. 2014, 13, 938–947. [Google Scholar] [CrossRef] [Green Version]
40. Kakiuchi, H.; Watanabe, M.; Ushijima, T.; Toyota, M.; Imai, K.; Weisburger, J.H.; Sugimura, T.; Nagao, M. Specific 5'-GGGA-3'-->5'-GGA-3' mutation of the Apc gene in rat colon tumors induced by 2-amino-1-methyl-6-phenylimidazo [4,5-b] pyridine. Proc. Natl. Acad. Sci. USA 1995, 92, 910–914. [Google Scholar] [CrossRef] [Green Version]
41. Yan, K.S.; Janda, C.Y.; Chang, J.; Zheng, G.X.Y.; Larkin, K.A.; Luca, V.C.; Chia, L.A.; Mah, A.T.; Han, A.; Terry, J.M.; et al. Non-equivalence of Wnt and R-spondin ligands during Lgr5(+) intestinal stem-cell self-renewal. Nature 2017, 545, 238–242. [Google Scholar] [CrossRef] [PubMed]
42. Koo, B.K.; Spit, M.; Jordens, I.; Low, T.Y.; Stange, D.E.; van de Wetering, M.; van Es, J.H.; Mohammed, S.; Heck, A.J.; Maurice, M.M.; et al. Tumour suppressor RNF43 is a stem-cell E3 ligase that induces endocytosis of Wnt receptors. Nature 2012, 488, 665–669. [Google Scholar] [CrossRef] [PubMed]

09 MOUSE EMBRYONIC STEM CELL-DERIVED URETERIC BUD PROGENITORS STIMULATE NEPHROGENESIS

1. INTRODUCTION: AN OVERVIEW

Pluripotent stem cells (PSCs) have the ability to differentiate into several cell types, making them valuable for research in developmental biology and regenerative medicine[**1**]. Kidney organoids created from pluripotent stem cells have demonstrated the ability to replicate the formation and function of kidney structure in a laboratory setting[**2,3,4**]. Renal organoids in a four-dimensional (4D) culture system, which includes three dimensions plus time, autonomously form intricate tissue-specific structures that can accurately represent tissue growth, diseases, and damage[**5,6,7,8**. Utilizing genome editing and stem cell technologies enables the creation of individualized kidney organoids, serving as effective tools for treating kidney diseases, assessing drug toxicity, and regenerating tissues[**9,10**].

Several procedures have been reported recently that allow for the creation of renal cell types from mouse and human pluripotent stem cells. We and multiple other studies observed the activation of nephron progenitors, which can potentially mature into epithelial nephron-like structures. [**2,3,4,8,11,12,13,14,15,16,17,18**]. Other groups have shown the derivation of ureteric bud (UB) progenitors [**19**]. However, they did not show nephron progenitor induction and also lacked the connection between collecting ducts and nephrons [**2,19**]. A newly published study has shown generation of UB structures from PSCs, which possessed UB-like branching morphogenesis when aggregated with the primary metanephric mesenchyme (pMM) to form chimeric kidney organoids [**8**]. However, the protocol is technically complex, which limits its application. Analysis of these reports suggests that we still need further studies to develop simple, reproducible, and stable protocols for UB progenitor generation. Here, we report a simple protocol to direct differentiation of mouse embryonic stem cells (mESCs) into

UB progenitor cells. The newly generated UB progenitor cells have a potential to develop into ureteric bud structures and have a capacity to induce nephrogenesis when co-cultured with dissociated pMM. Within reconstructed kidney organoids, the primitive metanephric mesenchyme (pMM) transformed into nephron structures, while ureteric bud (UB) progenitor cells gave rise to collecting ducts that interconnected with the nephron tubules. The chimeric kidney organoids also exhibit the existence of endothelial cells that create a vascular network. Our study developed a simple and repeatable strategy for creating UB progenitors from PSCs, which can be utilized to induce tubulogenesis.

2. MATERIALS AND METHODS

The animal care and experimental procedures in this work complied with Finnish national laws for the use of laboratory animals and the European Convention for the protection of vertebrate animals used for scientific purposes. (ETS 123), and the EU Directive 86/609/EEC. Animal experimentation was also authorized by the Finnish National Animal Experiment Board (ELLA) as being compliant with the EU guidelines for animal research and welfare.

2.1. Mouse ES Cell Line Generation and Maintenance

mESC line Sv129S6 was obtained from the Biocenter Oulu Transgenic core facility. The Sv129S6 mESC line was derived from Taconic's W4/129S6 inbred mouse strain and has been tested to have a normal karyotype [**19**]. The mESC and mESC-GFP (Green Fluorescent Protein, pcDNA3.1 transfected) line was described previously [**20**]. It was maintained on mitotically inactivated mouse embryonic fibroblasts (MEFs) in mESC medium: Dulbecco's Modified Eagle's Medium (DMEM; Life Technologies, Waltham, MA, USA) supplemented with 10% fetal bovine serum (FBS, Gibco, Waltham, MA, USA), 1% (v/v) nonessential amino acids (Life Technologies), 100 mM 2-mercaptoethanol (Nacalai Tesque, Kyoto, Japan), and 1000 U/mL leukemia inhibitory factor (LIF, Millipore, Espoo, Finland).

2.2. Directed Differentiation of mESCs to UB Progenitors

Mouse ESCs were cultured as described above in MEF-coated 6-well plates in mESCs medium up to 70%–90% confluency. The cells were passaged on 1% geltrex-coated 24-well plates at 30,000 cells/cm^2 in 500 μL 50% ReproFF2 (ReproCELL, Glasgow, UK)—50% CM (conditioned MEF medium) supplied with 10 ng/mL fibroblast growth factor (FGF) 2 (PeproTech Nordic, Stockholm, Sweden) and 10 ng/mL Activin A (Cell Guidance Systems, Cambridge, UK). After 2 days, the cells reached 60–80% of confluency, and the medium was changed to differentiation medium: Advanced RPMI (Thermo Fisher Scientific, Waltham, MA, USA) supplemented with 8 μM CHIR99021 (Reagents Direct, Encinitas, CA, USA) and 4–8 ng/mL Noggin (R&D systems, Minneapolis, MN, USA) for 2 days, followed by treatment of the cells with

Activin A (10 ng/mL) for 2 days and then 3 days with FGF9 (40 ng/mL) (PeproTech Nordic, Stockholm, Sweeden) in Advanced RPMI medium (ThermoFisher Scientific).

2.3. Gene Expression Analysis

Total RNA was extracted using an RNeasy kit from Qiagen, Germantown, MD, USA, following the manufacturer's instructions. cDNA was synthesized using the First Strand cDNA Synthesis Kit from ThermoFisher Scientific in Waltham, MA, USA, following normal techniques. A quantitative polymerase chain reaction (qPCR) was conducted using a CFX96 BioRad thermocycler. Brilliant III SYBR® Green QPCR Master Mix (Agilent Technologies, Santa Clara, CA, USA) was used according to the manufacturer's instructions. GAPDH probe served as a control to normalize the data. The data was analyzed using the $2^{-\Delta\Delta CT}$ method. Gene expression measurements were performed in triplicates on three independent experiments.

2.4. Chimera 3D Kidney Organoids Formation

On day 9 of mESCs differentiation, when the cells were at the UB progenitor cells stage, they were separated into individual cells using TrypLE select (Life Technologies). Cells were washed three times in phosphate buffer saline (PBS) and then resuspended in organ culture media consisting of DMEM supplemented with 10% fetal bovine serum and 1% penicillin-streptomycin. For generation of kidney organoids, we mixed dissected and dissociated pMM cells (from CD-1 pregnant females, at E11.5), as described before **[21]**, with differentiated UB progenitors at a ratio of 3:1, respectively. Briefly, kidney rudiments were dissected out of E11.5 embryos and treated with trypsin/pancreatin solution for 30–40 s to separate the UB from the pMM **[22]**. The MM cells were dissociated using 2.0 mg/mL Collagenase IV solution (Wortington, Lakewood, NJ, USA) in 0.1% bovine serum albumin (BSA) in 1×PBS. 10 min incubation was interrupted by pipetting and continued until cells were separated. The reaction was stopped by washing three times in complete organ culture medium **[22]**. The pMM- and mESC-derived UB cells were mixed in a 3:1 ratio and centrifuged for 4 min at 1380× g to form a pellet (5×10^4 cells) in Lo-Binding Eppendorf tubes. Following centrifugation, we carefully transferred the differentiated UB and pMM pellets to filter into Trowel culture to aggregate as an organoid. The organ culture medium was changed every 3–4 days.

For generation of whole kidney organoids, we dissected mouse kidney rudiments at E11.5 from CD-1 pregnant females. Kidney rudiments were dissociated into single cell suspension as described previously **[19]**. After dissociation, the embryonic kidney cells (7×10^4) were mixed with undifferentiated mESC or differentiated mESCs-derived UB progenitors (1×10^4) to make the pellet. We then continued the procedure as described above.

2.5. Whole-Mount Immunohistochemistry

Kidney organoids were washed 2 times with PBS and fixed with 100% cold methanol (–20 °C) for 30 min at room temperature (RT) or with 4% paraformaldehyde in PBS (organoid with GFP or dye) for 30 min at RT in the dark. After fixation, the organoids were washed at least three times in PBS and blocked in 0.1% Triton-X100 (Sigma, Lyon, France), 1% BSA, and 10% goat serum/0.02M glycine-PBS for 1–3 h at room temperature. Incubation of the organoids with primary antibodies was performed in a blocking buffer overnight at 4 °C. The samples were washed 6 times with PBS and incubated with secondary antibodies Alexa Fluor 405, 488, 568, 546, or 647 (1:1000, Life technologies) and fluorescein anti-LTL (Lotus Tetragonolobus Lectin, 1:350, #FL-1321, Vector Laboratories, Burlingame, CA, USA) overnight at 4 °C and counter-stained with Hoechst (Thermo Fisher Scientific). The primary antibodies used in stainings were: Wt1 (1:100, #05-753, Millipore), Pax2 (1:200, #PRB-276P, Covance, Cambridge, MA, USA), Troma1 (1:200, DSHB, Iowa City, IA, USA), Gata3 (1:20, #AF2605-SP, R&D Systems), E-cad (1:300, #610181, BD Biosciences, Franklin Lakes, NJ, USA), Synaptopodin (SYNPO) (1:4, #ABIN112223, antibody on line.com, Aachen, Germany), Umod (1:25, #LS-C150268, LSBio, Seattle, WA, USA), CD31 (1:100, #550274 BD Biosciences), Laminin (1:200, #L9393, Sigma), and Cleaved Caspase-3 (1:200, #9661s, Cell Signaling Technology, Leiden, Netherlands). Stained organoids were mounted with Shandon™ Immu-Mount™ (Thermo Scientific™). A Zeiss LSM780 microscope and Zeiss Axiolab (Zeiss, Oberkochen, Germany) were used for image capture and analysis.

2.6. Nephrotoxicity Assay

3D kidney organoids were cultured in organ culture medium supplemented with gentamicin at 5 mg/mL (#G1264, Sigma) for 48 h, or with cisplatin at 5, 20, or 50 μM (#P4394 Sigma) for 24 h after day 8 of organ culture. Organoids were then fixed with 100% cold methanol for 30 min for whole-mount immunohistochemistry. The Notch inhibitor, N-S-phenyl-glycine-t-butyl ester (DAPT, #D5942, Sigma), was used (10μM) to investigate toxicity towards proximal tubule development.

2.7. Statistical Evaluation

Data is displayed as mean ± standard deviation (SD) and is based on at least three independent experiments. A two-tailed t-test was utilized for statistical analysis by the student. A p-value less than 0.05 was deemed significant.

3. RESULTS

3.1. Direct Differentiation of mESCs into UB Progenitor Cells

Both the nephron and ureteric bud progenitor cells originate from the intermediate mesoderm (IM) throughout development. We initially developed mouse embryonic stem cells (mESCs) into the intermediate mesoderm (IM) to build a technique for directing development into the UB lineage. (**Figure 1**A). We treated the mESCs with FGF2 and activin A to differentiate mESCs into epiblast in monolayer culture. The differentiated cells showed expression of epiblast markers such as Fgf5 and T (Brachyury) .

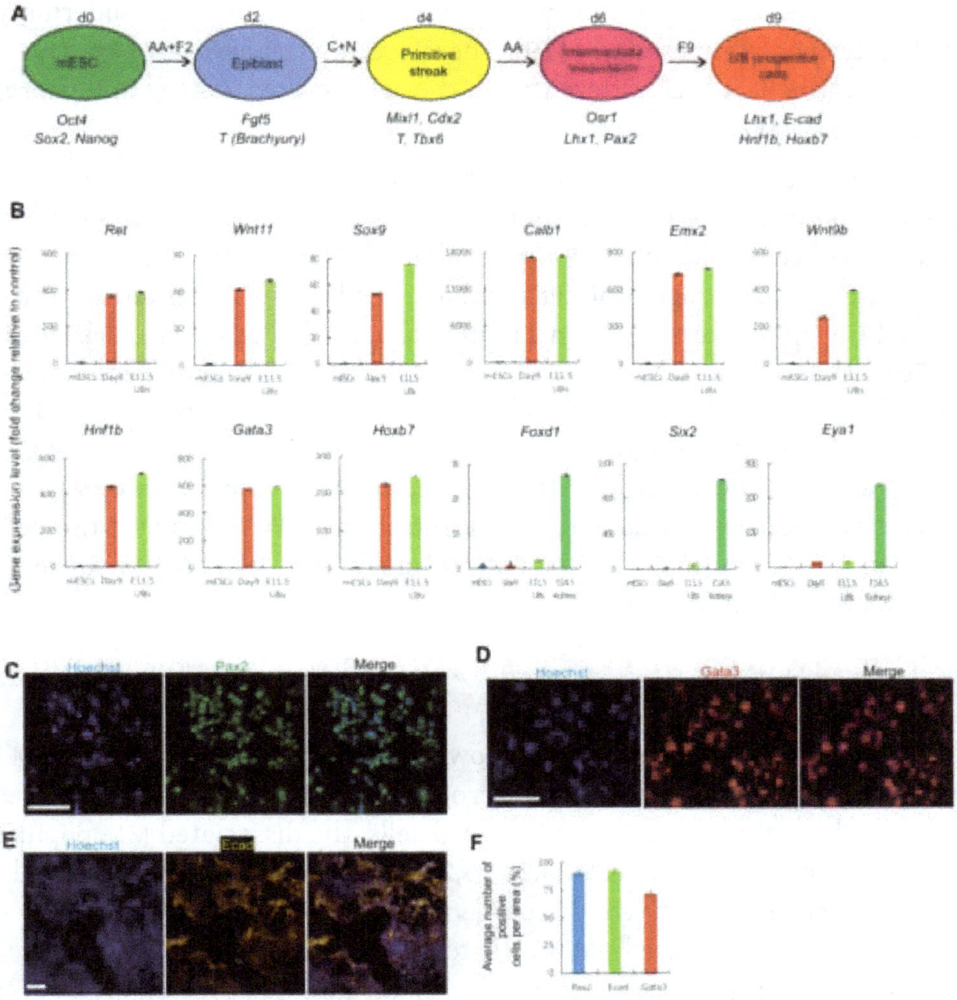

Figure 1. Differentiation of mouse embryonic stem cells (mESCs) to ureteric bud (UB) progenitor cells. (A) Schematic of the differentiation protocol of mESCs into UB progenitor cells. AA: Activin A; F2: FGF2; C: CHIR99021; N: Noggin; F9: FGF9. (B) Graphs of qPCR results showing the gene expression (fold change) of ureteric bud markers relative to mESC. No expression of stroma (Foxd1) and nephron progenitor cell markers (Six2 and Eya1) was observed at day 9 of differentiation. (n = 3). (C–E) Immunocytochemistry of Pax2, Ecad, and Gata3 in mESCs on day 9 of differentiation. Scale bars, 50 μm. (F) Quantification of the number of cells expressing Pax2, Ecad, and Gata3 at day 9 of differentiation. n = 3 samples per marker (3 randomly chosen areas in 3 independent experiments).

We then used glycogen synthase kinase-3β (GSK-3β) inhibitor, CHIR99021 (CHIR), together with a low concentration of bone morphogenetic protein (BMP) signaling inhibitor, Noggin (suppresses number of cells differentiated to lateral plate mesoderm) [**2**], to activate differentiation of mouse epiblast cells into primitive streak (PS). The Noggin-treated cells expressed PS markers Cdx2, T, Tbx6, and Mixl1. Activin A has been previously used for specification of the mesodermal cells towards intermediate mesoderm [**19**]. Therefore, we followed for two days with activin A treatment, which differentiated the cells to the IM stage and expressed Osr1, Lhx1, and Pax2.

Previous studies have demonstrated that FGF9 is able to induce renal lineage differentiation from the IM population [**2**]. Therefore, we treated these cells with a moderate concentration of FGF9 for an additional three days, directing them to differentiate into UB progenitor cells with expression of UB markers. These cells expressed UB tip markers: Ret, Wnt11, and Sox9, as well as other markers of UB: Lhx1, Ecad, Hnf1b, Wnt7b, Wnt9b, Calb1, Emx2, Gata3, Hoxb7, and Tacstd2 (**Figure 1**B). In addition, expression of stromal cell marker Foxd1 nephron progenitor cell markers, Six2 and Eya1 (**Figure 1**B), or other epithelial segment markers, were observed at day nine of differentiation. Immunofluorescence staining further revealed that the use of a moderate concentration of FGF9 induced the cells to express Pax2, E-cadherin (Ecad), and Gata3 (**Figure 1**C–F), which may suggest that these differentiated cells represent putative UB progenitor cells.

3.2. Creating Kidney Organoids using UB Progenitor Cells derived from mESCs and dissociated Primary MM Population

Previous studies, including ours, have shown that breaking apart mouse pMM into individual cells preserves the nephron progenitor stemness. When stimulated by an inducer like embryonic UB or spinal cord cells, the dissociated MM population transforms into nephrons. [**8,21,23,24,25,26,27**]. To establish the potential and function of the mESC-derived UB progenitor cells, we aggregated these cells with mouse E11.5-dissociated pMM cells to generate a kidney organoid. The cell aggregates were cultured for up to 11 days in a traditional Trowell organ culture system, during which they spontaneously formed kidney organoids with complex structures (**Figure 2**A,B). On day three, we observed Troma1+ UB structures and the formation of renal vesicles adjacent to the UB (**Figure 2**C–D).

Whole-mount immunostaining of day eight chimeric organoids showed development of nephrons with positive staining of glomerular markers Wilms tumor 1 (Wt1+) and Synaptopodin (Synpo+), proximal tubule marker Lotus Tetragonolobus Lectin (LTL+), and distal tubules markers Pax2+LTL– and Ecad+ .

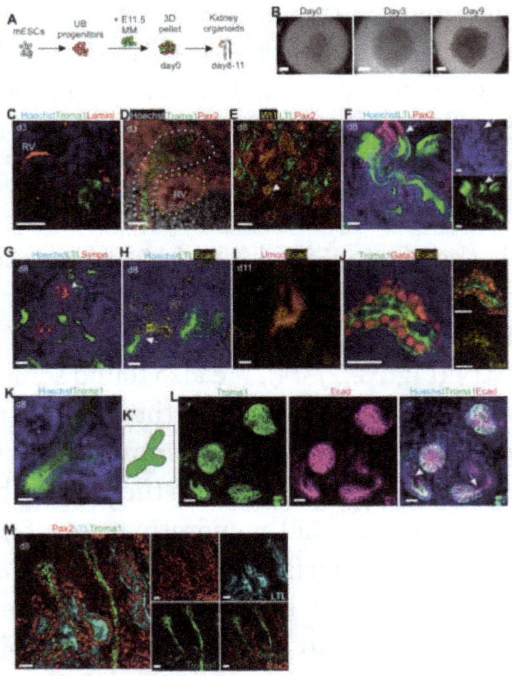

Figure 2. Generation of renal organoids by mESC-derived UB progenitors and primary metanephric mesenchyme (pMM) cells. (A) Schematic of generation of kidney organoids from mESC-derived UB progenitors with mouse E11.5-dissociated pMM. (B) Global bright field images of self-organizing kidney organoids in a Trowel organ culture system. Scale bars, 500 μm. (C) Immunofluorescence of kidney organoids at day 3 show formation of a renal vesicle next to the Troma1+ structure generated by mESC-derived UB progenitor cells. (D) Confocal image at day 3 showing Pax2+ renal vesicle (yellow dotted line) surrounded by Troma+Pax2+ ureteric epithelium (white dotted line). (E–M) Immunofluorescence of kidney organoids at day 8 or 11. (E) Glomeruli are marked with Wt1, proximal tubules are marked with LTL, and distal tubules are marked with Pax2+LTL–. The arrowhead shows the connection location of glomeruli with proximal tubule. (F) Immunostaining of distal tubule marked with Pax2 and proximal tubule marked with LTL, with all nuclei stained with DAPI. The arrow shows the proximal tubules (Pax2+LTL+) connected with distal tubules (Pax2+LTL–). (G) Glomeruli (Synpo+) adjacent to proximal tubules (LTL+) (the arrowhead marks the place of connection). (H) Immunostaining of proximal tubule with LTL and distal tubule with Ecad. Confocal image shows proximal tubules (LTL+) connected with distal tubules (Ecad+LTL–) (marked with an arrow). (I) Confocal image of Loops of Henle marked by Umod and Ecad on day 11. (J) Confocal images of Troma1+Gata3+Ecad+ collecting duct structure. (K-K') A "T" shaped UB structure in the kidney organoid. (L) mESC-derived UB progenitor cells-generated collecting ducts (Troma1+Ecad+) connecting with nephron's distal tubules (Troma1–Ecad+) (marked with an arrow). (M) Kidney organoids developed collecting duct trunk structures. Scale bars, (B) 500 μm, (E) 50 μm, (C–D, F–M) 20 μm.

Moreover, we found numerous Synpo+ and Wt1+ glomeruli adjacent to LTL+ proximal tubules, which connected with Pax2+LTL–/Ecad+ distal tubules (**Figure 2**E–H marked with arrowheads and arrows), indicating a proper nephron structure with glomerulus/proximal tubule/distal tubule organization. On day 11, the organoids also displayed Henle's loop with the expression of uromodulin (Umod+) and Ecad+ (**Figure 2**I).

We also tested whether the mESC-derived UB progenitor cells have in vivo UB capacity to form the collecting duct system. On day eight, we observed Troma1+Gata3+Ecad+Pax2+LTL– collecting duct structures in the kidney organoids by immunocytochemistry (**Figure 2**J–M). We also found some Troma1+ "T" shaped UB structures (**Figure 2**K, K'), indicating that the mESC-derived UB progenitors behave in a manner similar to UB cells in vivo. Importantly, we observed that the collecting ducts (Troma1+Ecad+) connected with the distal tubules (Ecad+Troma1–) of the nephron structure (**Figure 2**L), generating an interconnection between collecting ducts and nephrons, which is essential for urine drainage. The collecting ducts displayed the morphology of branches and long collecting duct trunks (**Figure 2**M). Altogether, the in vitro reconstructed organoids developed kidney structures that are similar to in vivo kidney, although it is unclear if the generated UB structures form a proper network.

We have also tried to stimulate the formation of blood vessels in the growing glomeruli within these kidney organoids. Prior research has shown that rho-associated protein kinases (ROCK) serve as downstream effectors of vascular endothelial growth factor (VEGF) and inhibit the process of angiogenesis. [**28**]. We utilized the ROCK inhibitor to boost angiogenesis in the renal organoids. The therapy did not result in an increase in the endothelial network area, and CD31+ cells were not present in the growing glomerular tuft.

3.3. Characterization of Kidney Organoids

To rule out the possibility that the differentiated cells (mESC-derived UB progenitors) could give rise to nephrons when induced by the embryonic UB, we aggregated day nine differentiated cells with E11.5-dissociated UB cells and grew them in organ culture. Since UB survival and development depend on the presence of metanephric mesenchyme, in the organ cultures, the purified UB failed to branch in the presence of UB-differentiated cells. Next, we wanted to verify that nephron structures in the organoids were generated via the MM population induced by the mESC-derived UB progenitors, and not by contamination of the MM with the primary UB cells. To assess this possibility, we cultured E11.5 MM tissue in isolation. The tissue already underwent apoptosis at the second day of culture and died at day three. This result also confirmed that without a suitable inducer, the MM cells will not undergo nephrogenesis and cannot survive for a long time under the organ culture conditions in vitro. These data suggest that we did differentiate mESC towards UB progenitors, and that they can further develop into collecting ducts when co-cultured with pMM.

We confirmed that the nephron structures and collecting ducts originated from pMM- and mESC-derived UB progenitors by aggregating pMM population obtained from mTmG mice (td-tomato+) with differentiated mESCs (unlabeled). (**Figure** 3A). The aggregates formed well-developed nephron structures (WT1+ glomeruli, LTL+ proximal tubules, Ecad+Troma1– distal tubules), which originated from MM cells (mTmG+) (**Figure** 3B) and Troma1-labeled collecting duct, which was mTmG– and therefore originated from the mESC-derived UB progenitors (**Figure** 3C–E). We also generated an mESC line with stable expression of the GFP. We differentiated these cells into UB progenitors and used them to induce pMM cells. Immunofluorescence analysis confirmed that the Troma1+Ecad+ collecting ducts were derived from GFP+ mESCs (**Figure** 3F). Altogether, these data demonstrate that the nephrogenesis occurring in generated kidney organoids is specifically derived from an interaction between the pMM and mESC-derived UB progenitors.

3.4. mESC-Derived UB Progenitor Cells Integrated into the 3D Ureteric Bud Structures

In order to identify the mESC-derived UB progenitors from wild-type UB cells in chimeric organoids, and to ensure that they will only generate UB cells, we generated an organoid with an mESC-GFP line. We dissociated a whole E11.5 embryonic kidney rudiment (MM and UB) and mixed it with undifferentiated mESC or mESC-derived UB progenitors generating chimeric kidney organoids [**19,21,27**] (**Figure** 4A).

The undifferentiated mESCs aggregated with dissociated embryonic kidney rudiments randomly localized within the organoids and had a negative effect on nephrogenesis. The undifferentiated mESC had formed groups within the renal structures; however, there were only a few structures, and very few Troma1+ ureteric buds could be observed (**Figure** 4B). When we aggregated the mESCs-derived UB progenitors with the dissociated embryonic kidney, we noticed much more robust tubulogenesis and numerous chimeric ureteric bud structures (**Figure** 4C). The UB progenitor cells did not interfere with renal development, but efficiently and specifically integrated into the mouse ureteric buds, as indicated by Troma1 and GFP+ staining (**Figure** 4C and D). Moreover, the immunostaining of day three organoids with nephron progenitor's marker, Six2, presented integration of mESC-derived UB progenitors (GFP+) into the UB structure (**Figure** 4D). The data show that mESC-derived UB progenitors integrate effectively into ureteric bud structures in chimeric renal organoids. They can make UB de novo and create chimeric structures.

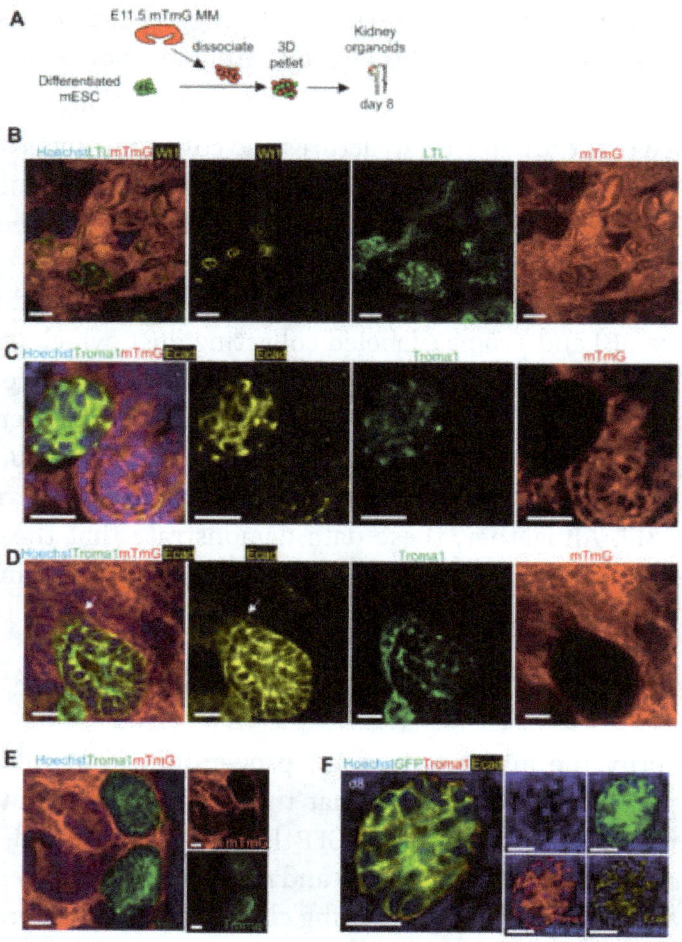

Figure 3. UB structures in kidney organoids are specifically derived from differentiated mESCs. (A) Schematic of generation of kidney organoids from mESC-derived UB progenitors with mouse E11.5-dissociated mTmG (td-tomato+) pMM. (B) Confocal images of three-dimensional (3D) kidney organoids derived from E11.5 mTmG+ pMM and mESC-derived UB progenitors. Nephron structures such as WT1+ glomeruli and LTL+ proximal tubules were derived from mTmG+ pMM. Scale bars, 50 μm. (C) Confocal images of kidney organoids showing ureteric bud structures (Ecad+Troma1+) being generated by mESC-derived UB progenitor cells. Scale bars, 20 μm. (D) Confocal images showed Troma1+Ecad+ collecting duct derived from mTmg– cells (mESC-derived UB progenitors) and connected with Troma1–Ecad+ renal tubules (connection marked with an arrow). Scare bars, 20 μm. (E) The Troma1+ UB structures derived from mTmG– cells (mESC-derived UB progenitors). Scale bar: 20 μm. (F) Troma1+Ecad+ collecting ducts are derived from GFP+ mESCs-derived UB progenitors. Scale bar: 20 μm.

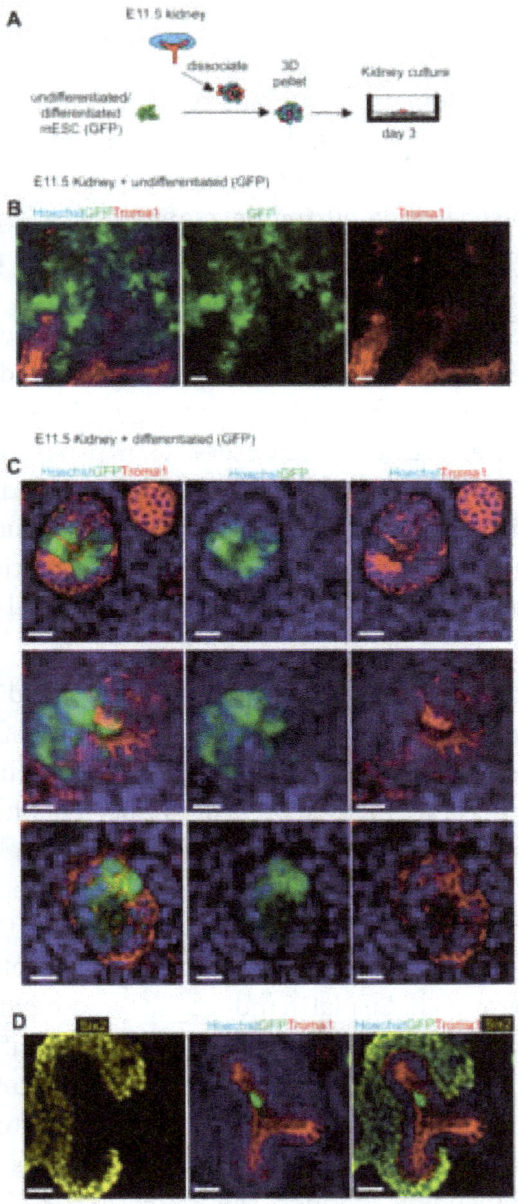

Figure 4. Mouse ESC-derived UB progenitor cells form anembryonic UB in 3D organ culture in vitro. (A) Schematic of kidney organoid generation from mESC-derived UB progenitors with mouse E11.5-dissociated kidney rudiments. (B) Immunofluorescence analysis demonstrating random localization of undifferentiated mESCs in organ co-cultures. Scale bars, 20 μm. (C) Immunofluorescence analysis demonstrating mESC-derived UB progenitors integrated into the UB structures and enhanced chimeric ureteric bud formation. Scale bars, 20 μm. (D) Confocal image showing localization of mESC-derived UB progenitor cells (GFP+) in Troma1+ UB structures of the chimeric organoid and not in the Six2+ nephron progenitor's region. Scale bars: 20 μm.

3.5. Using kidney organoids as models to research kidney development and drug toxicity

After transfer of the 3D chimeric organoids to organ culture, they self-organized and generated a well-structured kidney organoid with proper nephron and collecting duct structures. As patterning of the nephron into its different segments begins at the renal vesicle stage during development [**29,30**], we postulated that developmental patterning could be changed by chemical modulation of these endogenous signals. A previous report revealed that Notch signaling is required for proximal tubule fate acquisition in a mammalian nephron [**31**]. We therefore treated the organoids (pMM cells mixed with mESC-derived UB progenitor cells in a ratio of 3:1, **Figure 2**A) with a Notch signaling inhibitor, N-S-phenyl-glycine-t-butyl ester (DAPT). DAPT leads to suppression of proximal tubules' formation in the human nephron organoid culture [**4,31,32**]. We added DAPT to the culture medium from day 3 to 11 of 3D organoid culture. Immunofluorescence analysis of the cells demonstrated that with the DAPT treatment, formation of glomerulus and ureteric bud ducts was normal, but development of proximal tubules was severely suppressed.

In order to use stem cell-derived kidney organoids for disease modelling and drug screening, they need to present functional maturation of the nephrons within the organoids. To test whether these organoids could be used to study kidney injury and toxicity in vitro, we focused on drug-induced nephrotoxicity, which has been shown as an important cause of acute kidney injury in hospitalized patients [**33**]. We treated the chimeric kidney organoids with gentamicin, a commonly used antibiotic with well-established proximal tubular toxicity, after nine days of organ culture for 48 h [**34**]. We also treated organoids with another nephrotoxicant, cisplatin, from day 10 for 24 h. Cisplatin induces caspase-mediated acute apoptosis of proximal tubular cells in the kidney [**35**]. Whole-mount immunostaining of control organoids with caspase 3 showed random apoptotic interstitial cells; however, both gentamicin and cisplatin induced acute apoptosis in LTL+ proximal tubules. The percentage of apoptotic proximal tubular cells induced by cisplatin increased in a dose-dependent manner: the 5 and 20 μM cisplatin doses mainly affected the proximal tubule compartment, 32% and 62% respectively, while 50 μM cisplatin led to apoptosis of almost all of the proximal tubule cells (≈96%), but was also toxic to other cell types presenting a global type of nephrotoxicity at this concentration. In summary, our research demonstrates that mouse embryonic stem cell-derived ureteric bud progenitors stimulate kidney development in mouse metanephric mesenchyme cells. Additionally, chimeric kidney organoids created from these progenitors exhibit the anticipated reaction to harmful substances and medications. We showed that the kidney organoid system is capable of assessing the nephrotoxic effects of medicines and substances in a laboratory setting.

4. DISCUSSION

Kidney development initiates by the interplay of two precursor tissues of the kidney, UB and MM. The MM cell population consists mainly of nephron progenitor cells (NPCs) that will develop into nephrons, while the ureteric bud will give rise to the collecting duct tree. Protocols for differentiation of mouse and human pluripotent stem cells to renal progenitor cells, and further to self-organized kidney organoids containing nephrons, have been well established [**2,3,4,13,36**], but current methods of differentiation of pluripotent stem cells, specifically to ureteric bud progenitor cells, need further development [**8,19**]. Previous studies on generation of ESC-derived UB have shown derivation of a UB-like population by selective induction with metanephric mesenchyme cells [**19**] or through CHIR99021 treatment for nephron differentiation of both ureteric bud and nephron structures [**2**]. However, the ESC-derived UB-like cells did not show nephron progenitor induction [**19**], and therefore, an inter-nephron connection with collecting ducts was lacking [**2**]. Another group recently published a protocol for derivation of UB structures from PSCs, and generation of kidney organoid composed of mESCs-derived UB aggregated with pMM, or mESCs-derived UB combined with mESC-derived NPC and primary stromal progenitor cells (SPs). Although successful, their protocol requires a knock-in of markers in the PSCs, which later involves sorting of cells for the specific marker [**8**]. More recently, Mae and colleagues reported a protocol for generation of branching ureteric bud tissues from human pluripotent stem cells (hPSC) with a series of growth factors, but there was no evidence of nephrogenesis [**37**] . While these published protocols produce functional kidney organoids, they are technically complex. Here, we reported an establishment of a simple (directed with growth factors), efficient (>90% of Pax2+, Ecad+ and >70% Gata3+ cells), and reproducible differentiation protocol of mESC to ureteric bud progenitor cells. These mESC-derived UB progenitor cells induced pMM cells to undergo nephrogenesis leading to development of well-structured nephrons. The nephrons were composed of glomeruli, proximal tubules, loops of Henle, and distal tubules, and were linked to collecting duct structures formed by mESC-derived UB cells. Furthermore, the mESC-derived UB progenitor cells created a UB from scratch when mixed with pMM cells, and they produced chimeric structures when joined with kidney rudiment cells (pUB and pMM).

Although our current culturing conditions yielded functional kidney organoids, additional research is required to optimize these conditions. Prior research indicated that ROCK kinases act as downstream effectors of VEGF, exerting a negative regulatory influence on angiogenesis. [**28**]. We added ROCK inhibitor (Y27) to culture expecting an increase in angiogenesis. However, we failed to see a difference between control and Y27-treated samples. Better results could be obtained by supplementing the medium with VEGF, which was already published by Freedman and co-workers, although they still did not observe endothelial cells entering the glomerular tuft in their system [**9**]. Similarly, development of a vascular glomeruli in organotypic kidney cultures and renal organoids was reported earlier by our research team [**38**]. It seems that in the absence of the blood flow, the endothelial cells are not able to properly interact with developing nephrons [**39**] and formation of glomerular vasculature does not proceed further than migration of endothelial cells into the vascular cleft region of an S-shaped stage nephron. Sufficient vascularization of the organoids may be achieved by treatment with angiogenic factors, co-culture with blood vessel organoids [**40**], by providing flow to the system [**15**], or with a combination of the aforementioned treatments.Even though organoids generated by mESC-derived UB progenitor cells did not have a proper vascular network, the developed nephrons did respond to toxicological tests as expected. Research conducted by us and others[**4**], has demonstrated that the administration of gentamicin plus cisplatin triggers apoptosis in proximal tubular cells. Therefore, these organoids provide a practical method to evaluate drug-induced kidney damage.

We have created a simple and replicable procedure for producing UB progenitors from mESCs. This work establishes a solid basis for in vitro kidney research, such as disease modeling and drug discovery methods, which can be challenging to conduct using animal models or primary cells that may not fully replicate all aspects of developmental or disease processes. In the near future, researchers want to create fully functional nephrons in kidney organoids using UB and MM pieces obtained from PSC. Utilizing these cells will allow for the creation of both well-organized nephrons and the collecting duct tree. This is the initial stage in creating high-throughput gene discovery models and developing tissue engineering for organ transplantation. Nevertheless, these organoids must be effectively vascularized and developed to the required size. The research described here offer fresh perspectives on renal pathophysiology and create opportunities for creating novel treatment approaches.

5. AT A GLANCE

Kidney organoids can be created from pluripotent stem cells (PSCs) and are considered a promising method for researching kidney development, diseases, and regeneration. Research on guiding PSCs to develop into renal cell types is well-documented, with a focus on producing nephron progenitor cells from PSCs. So far, the process of differentiating PSCs into ureteric bud (UB) progenitor cells has been largely unsuccessful. We outline a straightforward, effective, and replicable procedure for inducing the differentiation of mouse embryonic stem cells (mESCs) into UB progenitor cells. When the mESC-derived UB cells were co-cultured with primary metanephric mesenchyme (pMM), they were capable of initiating nephrogenesis. The embryonic pMM in kidney organoids established nephron structures, while the mESC-derived UB cells created many collecting ducts connecting to the nephron tubules. Our study successfully created a simple and consistent method to produce ureteric bud progenitors from mouse embryonic stem cells.

REFERENCES

1. Robinton, D.A.; Daley, G.Q. The promise of induced pluripotent stem cells in research and therapy. Nature 2012, 481, 295–305. [Google Scholar] [CrossRef]

2. Takasato, M.; Er, P.X.; Chiu, H.S.; Maier, B.; Baillie, G.J.; Ferguson, C.; Parton, R.G.; Wolvetang, E.J.; Roost, M.S.; Chuva de Sousa Lopes, S.M.; et al. Kidney organoids from human iPS cells contain multiple lineages and model human nephrogenesis. Nature 2015, 526, 564–568. [Google Scholar] [CrossRef]

3. Freedman, B.S.; Brooks, C.R.; Lam, A.Q.; Fu, H.; Morizane, R.; Agrawal, V.; Saad, A.F.; Li, M.K.; Hughes, M.R.; Werff, R.V.; et al. Modelling kidney disease with CRISPR-mutant kidney organoids derived from human pluripotent epiblast spheroids. Nat. Commun. 2015, 6, 8715. [Google Scholar] [CrossRef] [Green Version]

4. Morizane, R.; Lam, A.Q.; Freedman, B.S.; Kishi, S.; Valerius, M.T.; Bonventre, J.V. Nephron organoids derived from human pluripotent stem cells model kidney development and injury. Nat. Biotechnol. 2015, 33, 1193–1200. [Google Scholar] [CrossRef] [Green Version]

5. Boreström, C.; Jonebring, A.; Guo, J.; Palmgren, H.; Cederblad, L.; Forslöw, A.; Svensson, A.; Söderberg, M.; Reznichenko, A.; Nyström, J.; et al. A CRISP(e)R view on kidney organoids allows generation of an induced pluripotent stem cell–derived kidney model for drug discovery. Kidney Int. 2018, 94, 1099–1110. [Google Scholar] [CrossRef] [PubMed] [Green Version]

6. Kim, Y.K.; Nam, S.A.; Yang, C.W. Applications of kidney organoids derived from human pluripotent stem cells. Korean J. Intern. Med. 2018, 33, 649–659. [Google Scholar] [CrossRef] [PubMed]

7. Hale, L.J.; Howden, S.E.; Phipson, B.; Lonsdale, A.; Er, P.X.; Ghobrial, I.; Hosawi, S.; Wilson, S.; Lawlor, K.T.; Khan, S.; et al. 3D organoid-derived human glomeruli for personalised podocyte disease modelling and drug screening. Nat. Commun. 2018, 9, 1–17. [Google Scholar] [CrossRef] [Green Version]

8. Taguchi, A.; Nishinakamura, R. Higher-Order Kidney Organogenesis from Pluripotent Stem Cells. Cell Stem Cell 2017, 21, 730–746. [Google Scholar] [CrossRef] [PubMed] [Green Version]

9. Czerniecki, S.M.; Cruz, N.M.; Harder, J.L.; Menon, R.; Annis, J.; Otto, E.A.; Gulieva, R.E.; Islas, L.V.; Kim, Y.K.; Tran, L.M.; et al. High-Throughput Screening Enhances Kidney Organoid Differentiation from Human Pluripotent Stem Cells and Enables Automated Multidimensional Phenotyping. Cell Stem Cell 2018, 22, 929–940. [Google Scholar] [CrossRef] [PubMed] [Green Version]

10. Cruz, N.M.; Song, X.; Czerniecki, S.M.; Gulieva, R.E.; Churchill, A.J.; Kim, Y.K.; Winston, K.; Tran, L.M.; Diaz, M.A.; Fu, H.; et al. Organoid cystogenesis reveals a critical role of microenvironment in human polycystic kidney disease. Nat. Mater. 2017, 16, 1112–1119. [Google Scholar] [CrossRef] [Green Version]

11. Araoka, T.; Mae, S.; Kurose, Y.; Uesugi, M.; Ohta, A.; Yamanaka, S.; Osafune, K. Efficient and Rapid Induction of Human iPSCs/ESCs into Nephrogenic Intermediate Mesoderm Using Small Molecule-Based Differentiation Methods. PLoS ONE 2014, 9, e84881. [Google Scholar] [CrossRef] [Green Version]

12. Takasato, M.; Er, P.X.; Becroft, M.; Vanslambrouck, J.M.; Stanley, E.G.; Elefanty, A.G.; Little, M.H. Directing human embryonic stem cell differentiation towards a renal lineage generates a self-organizing kidney. Nat. Cell Biol. 2014, 16, 118–126. [Google Scholar] [CrossRef] [PubMed]

13. Taguchi, A.; Kaku, Y.; Ohmori, T.; Sharmin, S.; Ogawa, M.; Sasaki, H.; Nishinakamura, R. Redefining the in vivo origin of metanephric nephron progenitors enables generation of complex kidney structures from pluripotent stem cells. Cell Stem Cell 2014, 14, 53–67. [Google Scholar] [CrossRef] [PubMed] [Green Version]

14. Garreta, E.; Prado, P.; Tarantino, C.; Oria, R.; Fanlo, L.; Martí, E.; Zalvidea, D.; Trepat, X.; Roca-Cusachs, P.; Gavaldà-Navarro, A.; et al. Fine tuning the extracellular environment accelerates the derivation of kidney organoids from human pluripotent stem cells. Nat. Mater. 2019, 18, 397–405. [Google Scholar] [CrossRef] [PubMed]

15. Homan, K.A.; Gupta, N.; Kroll, K.T.; Kolesky, D.B.; Skylar-Scott, M.; Miyoshi, T.; Mau, D.; Valerius, M.T.; Ferrante, T.; Bonventre, J.V.; et al. Flow-enhanced vascularization and maturation of kidney organoids in vitro. Nat. Methods 2019, 16, 255–262. [Google Scholar] [CrossRef]

16. Allison, S.J. Fluid flow enhances vascularization and maturation of kidney organoids. Nat. Reviews. Nephrol. 2019, 15, 254. [Google Scholar] [CrossRef] [PubMed]

17. Low, J.H.; Li, P.; Chew, E.G.Y.; Zhou, B.; Suzuki, K.; Zhang, T.; Lian, M.M.; Liu, M.; Aizawa, E.; Rodriguez Esteban, C.; et al. Generation of Human PSC-Derived Kidney Organoids with Patterned Nephron Segments and a De Novo Vascular Network. Cell Stem Cell 2019, 25, 373–387. [Google Scholar] [CrossRef]

[PubMed]

18. Przepiorski, A.; Sander, V.; Tran, T.; Hollywood, J.A.; Sorrenson, B.; Shih, J.; Wolvetang, E.J.; McMahon, A.P.; Holm, T.M.; Davidson, A.J. A Simple Bioreactor-Based Method to Generate Kidney Organoids from Pluripotent Stem Cells. Stem Cell Rep. 2018, 11, 470–484. [Google Scholar] [CrossRef] [PubMed] [Green Version]

19. Xia, Y.; Nivet, E.; Sancho-Martinez, I.; Gallegos, T.; Suzuki, K.; Okamura, D.; Wu, M.; Dubova, I.; Esteban, C.R.; Montserrat, N.; et al. Directed differentiation of human pluripotent cells to ureteric bud kidney progenitor-like cells. Nat. Cell Biol. 2013, 15, 1507–1515. [Google Scholar] [CrossRef]

20. Aro, E.; Salo, A.M.; Khatri, R.; Finnilä, M.; Miinalainen, I.; Sormunen, R.; Pakkanen, O.; Holster, T.; Soininen, R.; Prein, C.; et al. Severe Extracellular Matrix Abnormalities and Chondrodysplasia in Mice Lacking Collagen Prolyl 4-Hydroxylase Isoenzyme II in Combination with a Reduced Amount of Isoenzyme I. J. Biol. Chem. 2015, 290, 16964–16978. [Google Scholar] [CrossRef] [Green Version]

21. Junttila, S.; Saarela, U.; Halt, K.; Manninen, A.; Pärssinen, H.; Lecca, M.R.; Brändli, A.W.; Sims-Lucas, S.; Skovorodkin, I.; Vainio, S.J. Functional genetic targeting of embryonic kidney progenitor cells ex vivo. J. Am. Soc. Nephrol. 2015, 26, 1126–1137. [Google Scholar] [CrossRef] [Green Version]

22. Rak-Raszewska, A. Experimental Tubulogenesis Induction Model in the Mouse. In Kidney Organogenesis; Methods in Molecular Biology; Vainio, S., Ed.; Humana Press: New York, NY, USA, 2019; Volume 1926, pp. 39–51. [Google Scholar]

23. Ganeva, V.; Unbekandt, M.; Davies, J.A. An improved kidney dissociation and reaggregation culture system results in nephrons arranged organotypically around a single collecting duct system. Organogenesis 2011, 7, 83–87. [Google Scholar] [CrossRef] [PubMed] [Green Version]

24. Hendry, C.E.; Vanslambrouck, J.M.; Ineson, J.; Suhaimi, N.; Takasato, M.; Rae, F.; Little, M.H. Direct Transcriptional Reprogramming of Adult Cells to Embryonic Nephron Progenitors. J. Am. Soc. Nephrol. Jasn. 2013, 24, 1424–1434. [Google Scholar] [CrossRef] [Green Version]

25. Lusis, M.; Li, J.; Ineson, J.; Christensen, M.E.; Rice, A.; Little, M.H. Isolation of clonogenic, long-term self renewing embryonic renal stem cells. Stem Cell Res. 2010, 5, 23–39. [Google Scholar] [CrossRef] [PubMed] [Green Version]

26. Saxén, L.; Sariola, H. Early organogenesis of the kidney. Pediatr. Nephrol. 1987, 1, 385–392. [Google Scholar] [CrossRef] [PubMed]

27. Unbekandt, M.; Davies, J.A. Dissociation of embryonic kidneys followed by

reaggregation allows the formation of renal tissues. Kidney Int. 2010, 77, 407–416. [Google Scholar] [CrossRef] [PubMed] [Green Version]

28. Kroll, J.; Epting, D.; Kern, K.; Dietz, C.T.; Feng, Y.; Hammes, H.P.; Augustin, H.G. Inhibition of Rho-dependent kinases ROCK I/II activates VEGF-driven retinal neovascularization and sprouting angiogenesis. Am. J. Physiol.—Heart Circ. Physiol. 2009, 296, H893–H899. [Google Scholar] [CrossRef] [Green Version]

29. Georgas, K.; Rumballe, B.; Valerius, M.T.; Chiu, H.S.; Thiagarajan, R.D.; Lesieur, E.; Aronow, B.J.; Brunskill, E.W.; Combes, A.N.; Tang, D.; et al. Analysis of early nephron patterning reveals a role for distal RV proliferation in fusion to the ureteric tip via a cap mesenchyme-derived connecting segment. Dev. Biol. 2009, 332, 273–286. [Google Scholar] [CrossRef] [Green Version]

30. Little, M.; Georgas, K.; Pennisi, D.; Wilkinson, L. Kidney development: Two tales of tubulogenesis. Curr. Top. Dev. Biol. 2010, 90, 193. [Google Scholar]

31. Cheng, H.T.; Kim, M.; Valerius, M.T.; Surendran, K.; Schuster-Gossler, K.; Gossler, A.; McMahon, A.P.; Kopan, R. Notch2, but not Notch1, is required for proximal fate acquisition in the mammalian nephron. Development 2007, 134, 801–811. [Google Scholar] [CrossRef] [Green Version]

32. Cheng, H.; Miner, J.H.; Lin, M.; Tansey, M.G.; Roth, K.; Kopan, R. Gamma-secretase activity is dispensable for mesenchyme-to-epithelium transition but required for podocyte and proximal tubule formation in developing mouse kidney. Development 2003, 130, 5031–5042. [Google Scholar] [CrossRef] [Green Version]

33. Uchino, S.; Kellum, J.A.; Bellomo, R.; Doig, G.S.; Morimatsu, H.; Morgera, S.; Schetz, M.; Tan, I.; Bouman, C.; Macedo, E.; et al. Beginning and Ending Supportive Therapy for the Kidney (BEST Kidney) Investigators, for the Acute Renal Failure in Critically Ill Patients: A Multinational, Multicenter Study. JAMA 2005, 294, 813–818. [Google Scholar] [CrossRef] [Green Version]

34. Whiting, P.H.; Brown, P.A.J. The Relationship Between Enzymuria and Kidney Enzyme Activities in Experimental Gentamicin Nephrotoxicity. Ren. Fail. 1996, 18, 899–909. [Google Scholar] [CrossRef] [PubMed]

35. Mese, H.; Sasaki, A.; Nakayama, S.; Alcalde, R.E.; Matsumura, T. The role of caspase family protease, caspase-3 on cisplatin-induced apoptosis in cisplatin-resistant A431 cell line. Cancer Chemother. Pharm. 2000, 46, 241–245. [Google Scholar] [CrossRef] [PubMed]

36. Takasato, M.; Little, M.H. A strategy for generating kidney organoids: Recapitulating the development in human pluripotent stem cells. Dev. Biol. 2016, 420, 210–220. [Google Scholar] [CrossRef] [PubMed]

37. Mae, S.; Ryosaka, M.; Toyoda, T.; Matsuse, K.; Oshima, Y.; Tsujimoto, H.; Okumura, S.; Shibasaki, A.; Osafune, K. Generation of branching ureteric bud tissues from human pluripotent stem cells. Biochem. Biophys. Res. Commun. 2018, 495, 954–961. [Google Scholar] [CrossRef]

38. Halt, K.J.; Pärssinen, H.E.; Junttila, S.M.; Saarela, U.; Sims-Lucas, S.; Koivunen, P.; Myllyharju, J.; Quaggin, S.; Skovorodkin, I.N.; Vainio, S.J. CD146+ cells are essential for kidney vasculature development. Kidney Int. 2016, 90, 311–324. [Google Scholar] [CrossRef] [PubMed] [Green Version]

39. Serluca, F.C.; Drummond, I.A.; Fishman, M.C. Endothelial Signaling in Kidney Morphogenesis: A Role for Hemodynamic Forces. Curr. Biol. 2002, 12, 492–497. [Google Scholar] [CrossRef] [Green Version]

40. Wimmer, R.A.; Leopoldi, A.; Aichinger, M.; Wick, N.; Hantusch, B.; Novatchkova, M.; Taubenschmid, J.; Hämmerle, M.; Esk, C.; Bagley, J.A.; et al. Human blood vessel organoids as a model of diabetic vasculopathy. Nature 2019, 565, 505–510. [Google Scholar] [CrossRef]

10 COMPARING TRADITIONAL AND ADVANCED CELL CULTURES IN HEMATOPOIETIC STEM CELL RESEARCH

1. INTRODUCTION:AN OVERVIEW

Blood is a connective tissue composed of around 34% cells and 66% plasma, responsible for delivering nutrients, gasses, and chemicals throughout the body. Hematopoiesis is the formation of blood cells that replenishes the blood system throughout an individual's life. Hematopoiesis is a complex process that relies heavily on the differentiation and proliferation of hematopoietic stem cells (HSCs). Every cell in the hematopoietic hierarchy can be identified by unique surface marks that have epitopes detected by antibodies [**1,2,3**]. **Figure 1** shows the main markers in human hematopoietic hierarchy. The hematopoietic process in humans starts in the yolk sac (mesoblastic phase). Then, it is transferred to the liver and spleen. Eventually, the bone marrow assumes the primary role in hematopoiesis. Hematopoietic stem cells (HSCs) in the bone marrow possess the ability of indefinite self-renewal, generating offspring that is identical to the parent cell. They are typically in the G0 phase of the cell cycle and possess the ability to develop into specialized cells.

2. HEMATOPOIETIC STEM CELLS

The medullary microenvironment has a role in the dormancy, regeneration, growth, development, and cell death of hematopoietic stem cells. It consists of several cell types such as mesenchymal stem cells, endothelial cells, fibroblasts, osteoblasts, reticular cells, and adipocytes. These cells produce cytokines, growth factors, glycoproteins, and glycosaminoglycans, along with other regulatory substances. Various combinations of these chemicals create distinct microenvironments in the medullary cavity, referred to as niches. [**4**]. Histologically defined microenvironments are subdivided into four regions: endosteal, subendosteal, central, and perisinusoidal. Granulocytes and monocytes are found in all regions of the bone marrow, whereas erythroblasts proliferate preferentially in the central region [**5**]. Concerning the dynamics of the lymphoid lineage, B lymphocyte precursors are found in the subendosteal region, gradually decreasing toward the central region, whereas mature B cells are found throughout the bone marrow [**6**]. HSCs are located in the endosteal region, also known as the osteoblastic niche, but studies suggest that HSCs may migrate to the perisinusoidal region or vascular niche and remain quiescent or differentiate depending on the needs of the organism [**2**,**5**,**7**,**8**,**9**]. In fact, studies with new markers for HSCs and niche cells, new image techniques, including labeling protocols, have shown that most HSCs reside adjacent to sinusoidal vessels, leading to the proposed existence of a perivascular niche for HSCs [**10**].

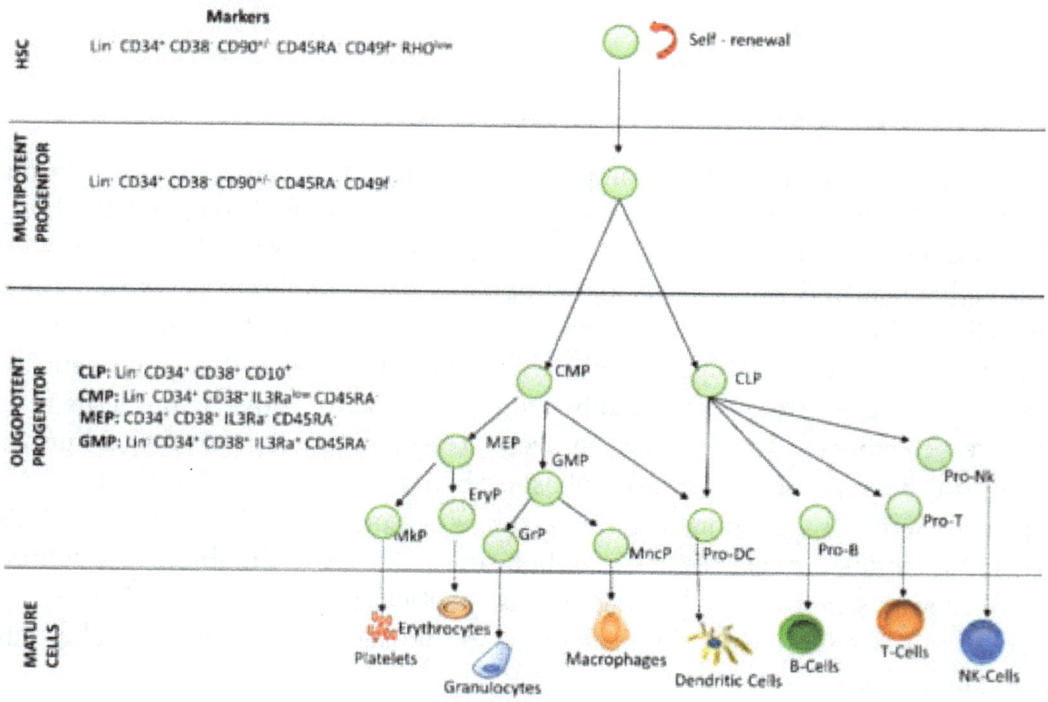

Figure 1. Hierarchy of human hematopoiesis. LT-HSC: Long Term-Hematopoietic Stem Cell; ST-HSC: Short Term-Hematopoietic Stem Cell; MPP: Multipotent Progenitor; OPP: Oligopotent Progenitor; LRP: Lineage Restricted Progenitor; MEC: Mature Effector Cell. The markers of the most important lineages are listed: Common Lymphoid Progenitor (CLP); Common Myeloid Progenitor (CMP); Megakaryocyte-Erythrocyte Progenitor (MEP); Granulocyte-Macrophage Progenitor (GMP). Restricted lineage progenitor cells: Megakaryocyte Progenitor (MkP); Erythrocytic Progenitor (EryP); Granulocytic Progenitor (GrP); Monocyte Progenitor (MncP); Dendritic Progenitor Cell (Pro DC); Progenitor Cell-T (Pro-T); Progenitor Cell-B (Pro-B); Progenitor Cell-Nk (Pro-Nk).

It is assumed that in the bone marrow, there are at least two different niches: the endosteal niche, which would harbor quiescent HSCs, and the perivascular niche, which would harbor cycling HSCs [**11**]. Although most studies have been done on non-humans, researchers suppose that the data reflect what happens in humans. It has previously been proposed that HSCs are maintained in the endosteal (osteoblastic) niche; however, the available evidence does not seem to support this model. Nevertheless, the endosteal niche seems to support the maintenance of a subset of lymphoid progenitors [**10**]. Approximately 80% of dividing and non-dividing HSCs have been described to be associated with sinusoidal vessels, with another 10% of HSCs being adjacent to arterioles, and almost another 10% in transition zone vessels [**10**]. A small percentage of HSCs are located in the endosteum. In fact, a quantitative model of cellular components that could define these microenvironments, and the preferential location of HSCs in the bone marrow are still lacking [**12**]. Obstacles to recognizing the HSCs in the bone marrow include the low frequencies at which HSCs are found in the bone marrow and the cellular complexity of the bone marrow microenvironment.

Cell signaling in the HSC niche is a complex process and passes through an extensive signaling network balancing self-renewal and differentiation [**13**]. This signaling involves several substances, such as growth factors and cytokines that are secreted by both the medullary stroma cells and hematopoietic stem cells and are important signaling factors for hematopoiesis, proliferation, and differentiation [**14**].

The Jak/STAT, Ras/Erk, and PI3K/Akt signaling pathways have been described as important inducers of erythropoiesis transduction by activation of the erythropoietin receptor, and these intracellular pathways are responsible for the survival, proliferation, and differentiation of normal erythropoietic progenitors [**15**].

Other intracellular signaling pathways that are important for the control of hematopoiesis have been described, such as the Notch, Wingless-type (Wnt), and Hedgehog pathways [**16**], which have been associated with self-renewal and maintenance of HSCs. Notch proteins are highly conserved receptors on the surface of the cell membrane that regulate the development of stem cells, and mutations in this receptor may cause leukemia [**17**] and breast cancer [**18**]. Activation of the Notch pathway is necessary to keep HSCs undifferentiated. This pathway is more active in HSCs and less active in differentiated cells. Inhibition of the Notch pathway potentiates the differentiation of HSCs and loss of the bone marrow reconstitution capacity of sub-lethally irradiated animals; thus, Notch has been used as a marker of undifferentiated HSCs [**19**]. Wnt protein regulates several phenomena during fetal development, and this protein has been related to the self-renewal of stem cells [**20**]. Hedgehog (Hh) protein has been described as regulating embryonic and adult stem cell activity. In mammals, three genes are known to be responsible for this protein—Sonic Hedgehog (SHh), Indian Hedgehog (IHh), and Desert Hedgehog (DHh) [**21,22**].

Soluble factors are also closely associated with the maintenance and regulation of the undifferentiated state of HSCs in the bone marrow of adults, in addition to regulating the proliferation and differentiation of this population. Stromal-cell-derived factor-1 (SDF-1/CXCL12) and its CXCR4 linker are activated to recruit endothelial progenitor cells (EPCs) and regulate HSCs [**2,13,23**]. Other soluble factors act to promote the maintenance of HSCs in their niche; for example, the stem cell factor (SCF/Kit-ligand) and its c-Kit receptor (CD117) are both required by HSCs for their maintenance. SCF is an important soluble cytokine for hematopoiesis, and THE c-Kit receptor is expressed on the HSCs surface; altered forms of this receptor have been associated with several types of cancer [**24,25**]. Thrombopoietin (TPO) and its MPL ligand are also important soluble factors necessary for the maintenance of HSCs in their niche. TPO is a primary physiological regulator responsible for the stimulation of platelet production, a primary dominant factor and megakaryocytopoiesis stimulator. In addition, recent in vitro studies have shown that TPO alone or in combination with growth factors, such as a c-Kit ligand, IL-3, or even Flt-3, stimulates the proliferation of hematopoietic progenitor cells [**26,27**]. Many other factors also modulate the function of HSCs but are not necessarily required, such as angiogenin, angiopoietin-1, G-CSF, IL-6, and TGFβ, among others [**25**].

3. STEM CELL CULTURE METHODS

Recreating the intricate milieu and cellular interactions in a laboratory setting is challenging. Enhanced methods can be used by researchers to replicate the bone marrow structure for studying hematopoiesis and producing cells in regenerative medicine.

Cell culture is the growth of cells from animal or plant in a favorable, artificial, and controlled environment. Today, cell culture is the basis of biology techniques and essential for regenerative medicine procedures [**28**]. These cells can originate directly from the tissue or after enzymatic or mechanically dissociated tissue or can be derived from an already established cell line.

Traditional cell culture, also known as 2D cell culture, is a very well-established method and easy-to-use culture model (**Figure** 2A,C). This technique depends on adherence to a flat surface, typically a culture flask, dish or polystyrene glass, to provide mechanical support for its growth in monolayers and access to nutrients and growth factors present in the culture media. Cells can also grow in suspension, as those derived from blood or bone marrow [29]. While this method offers benefits like cost-effectiveness and efficient functional assays, it also has drawbacks such as the inability to replicate natural tissue structures and effectively mimic cell-cell and cell-environment interactions. [29].

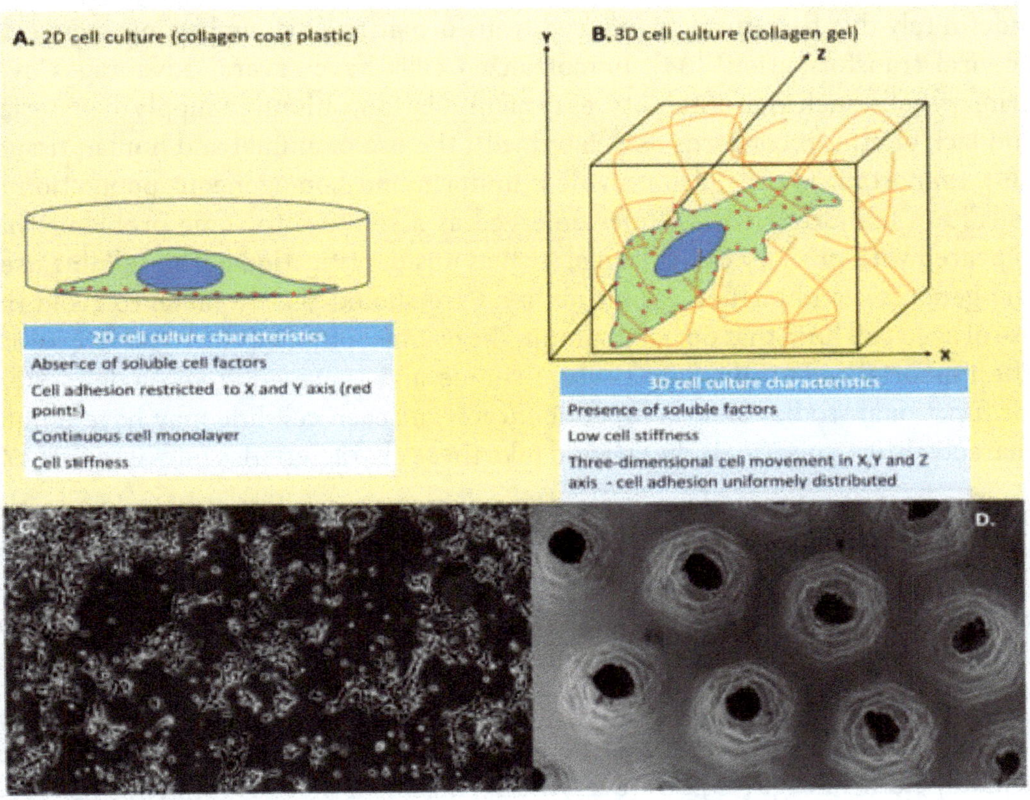

Figure 2. Two-dimensional (2D) and three-dimensional (3D) cell culture. (A) Schematic model of 2D cell culture. Standard model of 2D cell culture. Cells are cultured as a single layer in a culture flask. (B) Schematic model of 3D cell culture. 3D model of cell culture giving the notion of height, width and depth; cells are surrounded by the medium. (C) Example of 2D culture. HEK 293 cells in 2D cell culture; the adherence to a flat surface provides mechanical support for growth in monolayers. Scale bar 400 µm. (D) Example of 3D culture. HEK 293 cells 3D cell culture in agarose allowing the cells to grow or interact with their surroundings in all three dimensions. Scale bar 1000 µm.

Primary cell culture is a valuable tool in cellular biology for assessing many cellular characteristics such chemoresistance, karyotypes, cellular parameters, metabolism, and in vitro modeling of normal and pathological conditions. [30]. The isolated cells resemble their tissue of origin. Primary cell culture is complex and requires specific care, including storage, thawing-freezing procedures, or choice of enzymatic treatment, but the main problem is how to keep the primary cell in culture long enough to be established for experimental tests [31,32,33].

Primary culture can be representative of the cell types of the tissue from which they were isolated; although these cells are difficult to maintain, they best mimic a pathological condition or physiological function.

Immortalized cells or established cell lineages are cells that can grow in vitro indefinitely due to natural or induced transformation (e.g., embryonic stem cells or viral transformation) [**34**]. Immortalized cells have several advantages over primary cells, such as profitability, easy manipulation, unlimited supply of material, and lack of ethical concerns associated with the use of animal and human tissues [**35**]. Immortalized cells also provide a uniform and homogeneous population of cells [**36**]. Immortalized cell lines emerged as a solution to some problems that appeared with primary cell cultures, such as misidentification of the cell line used and genotypic and phenotypic instability. Care should also be taken to avoid the use of aged cell lines that do not maintain the original physiological characteristics. The immortalized strains constitute a simple and representative model system for functional studies and therapeutic targets. As each cell line may have unique characteristics, specific studies should take these characteristics into account [**37**].

The co-culture technique is used for numerous applications, including the study of natural or synthetic interactions between distinct populations of cells. Co-culture methods are of great importance in research, as they are used to observe cell–cell interactions, how cells are organized, how they participate in the development of diseases such as cancers, in which different types of cells are involved, including the microenvironment [**38**].

Both self-renewal and differentiation are required abilities in any cell of the hematopoietic lineage [**39**]. However, the expansion of these cells in vitro has been challenging for the scientific community, as regulation of these cells depends on several mechanisms of intercellular communication resulting from the secretion of local- and systemic-acting factors [**40**]. HSCs, which can also be obtained and expanded from umbilical cord blood, should respond to and integrate events in their microenvironment to ensure sustained production of all hematopoietic lineages [**41**].

Although HSCs have been extensively analyzed and characterized, their ex vivo expansion remains a problem [**42,43,44**]. It has been shown that the cell culture of HSCs is viable for at least 169 days but very much depends on the quality of the HSCs. There are currently several approaches to ex vivo expansion. Most first require the isolation of $CD34^+$ or $CD133^+$ cells from frozen or fresh hematopoietic tissue and incubation in culture medium supplemented with cytokines, granulocyte colony stimulating factor (G-CSF), stem cell factor (SCF), and thrombopoietin (TPO) [**45**].

Therefore, the cell culture of HSCs must take into account the microenvironment in which these cells are inserted so that it can reproduce the whole framework of the hematopoietic structure. The hematopoietic niche contains several types of cells, and mimicking this microenvironment in vitro requires a stromal layer, which controls multiple cellular parameters, including quiescence, self-renewal, differentiation, apoptosis and migration. Under the artificial culture conditions, HSCs undergo differentiation and apoptosis [**46**]. A support layer is required so HSCs can survive and proliferate.

Co-culture of HSCs is one of the most frequently used models for understanding how the highly specific bone marrow niche interacts ex vivo with hematopoietic cells, promoting their differentiation and expansion. The technique can focus on the importance of non-contact culture systems on the successful maintenance of hematopoietic cells [**47**] and on the use of the stroma as a cell layer to provide support for HSC culturing, as mentioned above. Several studies have shown that contact between HSCs and stromal cells is important for maintaining HSC function [**48,49**]. The stromal cells from bone marrow include osteoblasts, macrophages, endothelial cells, and mesenchymal cells [**50,51**]. Mesenchymal cells are multipotent progenitor cells that can differentiate into mesenchymal cells, such as osteoblasts, adipocytes, and chondrocytes, and also have the potential for differentiation into cells such as neurons and lung cells [**52**]. These multipotent cells have interactions with hematopoietic cells forming the framework of the HSC niche, supporting the development of hematopoiesis and acting as immunological regulators [**53,54**]. In addition, recent studies have indicated that other molecules, such as N6-methyladenosine (M6A), by modulating the expression of a group of YTHDF2 genes at the mRNA level, are important regulators of HSC self-renewal. Some authors have suggested that although extensive efforts have led to multiple methods for in vivo expansion of HSCs, it is not possible for some single molecules or pathways to be manipulated simultaneously due to a large number of essential targets for self-renewal of stem cells [**55**].

There are significant challenges to address, such as improving techniques for maintaining hematopoietic stem cells in a laboratory setting and expanding them outside the body for regenerative medicine purposes. This will lead to a deeper understanding of the hematopoietic niche and its regulators in both normal and diseased states. Enhancing the capacity to genetically reprogram hematopoietic stem cells (HSCs) for clinical therapeutic applications is still necessary[**56**].

4. 3D HEMATOPOIETIC STEM CELL CULTURE

Cell culture in 2D format is simple and provides excellent material for studying homogeneous populations [**57**]. However, it does not consider several other important parameters of cell physiology, such as cell–cell communication or communication between the cell and microenvironment or adjacent molecules [**58**]. Therefore, the major problem with 2D cell culture is its limits [**59**]. One of the main criticisms of this study format is that animal physiology cannot be mimicked using only one layer of cells, which certainly does not correspond to the original tissue considering the complexity of the cellular microenvironment in the tissue of origin [**60**].

As an alternative to the technical limitations of 2D cell culture, 3D cell culture allows a better simulation of the in vivo structural complexity, replicating several characteristics present in tissues (**Figure** 2B,D), not only the interaction of cells with their microenvironment, but also morphology, differentiation, polarity, proliferation rate, gene expression profiles, and cell heterogeneity [**61,62,63,64**]. In fact, 3D culture has proven to be a realer model for translating research results into in vivo applications.

Current 3D cell culture models and methods include spheroids, organoids, microcarrier cultures, organs-on-chips, and 3D bioprinting [**65,66**]. Organotypic explant culture methods are used mostly when a technical/specific requirement of the tissue is to be studied and mimicked [**67**]. However, although the complexity of the 3D system is evident, some criteria must be considered and cannot be disregarded, such as the choice of material for the scaffold and hydrogels and cell type and culture methods, which vary considerably according to the tissue studied [**66**].

Organoid culture is most commonly used to describe constructs derived from pluripotent stem cells (embryonic or induced cells) or adult stem cells from various organs, including the hematopoietic tissue [**68**]. Organoid culture is classified as either tissue organoids (i.e., organotypic) or stem cells depending on how the cell layers are formed [**69**]. Organotypic tissue refers to free stromal cells without parenchyma, and its application is mainly with epithelial cells because of their high intrinsic ability to self-organize. With this method, it is possible to study HSCs, and Christopher et al. [**70**] were able to produce mature T cells from stem cells and hematopoietic progenitors in a thymus organoid culture.

Spheroid culture models simulate the microenvironment conditions of a living cell. Compared to the classic 2D model, the spheroid culture model emphasizes the interactions between cells and their relationship to the extracellular matrix (ECM) [**71,72**]. Tissues are not composed of a homogeneous population of cells; they are complex structures formed by several different components, with an intricate relationship such as vessels, nerves, and stroma, which should be considered in any kind of tissue engineering. This complex interaction between cells and the extracellular compartment requires a 3D environment to best represent these interactions [**73,74**].

Spheroid cell culture can be used in scaffold and scaffold-free models. The scaffold methods comprise hydrogel support, decellularized extracellular matrix, and resistant polymeric material support. Hydrogel consists of polymeric groups with a water-swollen hydrophilic structure [75]. Depending on their nature, these compounds are classified into different categories, including ECM protein-containing hydrogels (ECMPs), natural hydrogels, or synthetic hydrogels, each one with its own properties [76,77]. Decellularization involves eliminating cells from the original tissue through chemical treatment while maintaining the extracellular matrix (ECM). The tissue can be regenerated with cultured cells and then transplanted in vivo or utilized for ex vivo cell differentiation. Decellularized scaffolds maintain the vascular organization, three-dimensional niches, and chemical composition of bone marrow, unlike artificial scaffolds. Extracellular matrix components have a crucial role in supporting cell viability by influencing cell behavior, signaling for survival, and proliferation. Resistant polymeric material supports are structures resembling fibers or sponges. Cells cultured in this support demonstrate a physiological activity similar to that of native tissue, like cartilaginous tissue. The most frequently utilized substance for the polymeric support is polystyrene, however biodegradable supports like polycaprolactone have also been utilized.

The development of a bioprinting system for the bone marrow microenvironment is important since it cannot be mimicked by methods such as organoids. Advanced 3D bone marrow models could serve for several different studies, including hematopoietic regulation, BM, MSCs, HSC interaction and expansion, interactions of hematological cancer cells, and evolution of several hematological diseases. In addition, these models could be used as a platform for expanding HSCs for transplantation. However, it is difficult to obtain a reliable BM model because of several critical technical challenges, from currently available 3D printing techniques to the possibility of precisely mimicking the different BM niches [**78**].

Relatively few studies have been done using hematopoietic stem cells in these methods. Decellularization of cartilaginous tissues has been tested for ex vivo culturing of hematopoietic cells [79]. A co-culture model of hematopoietic stem/progenitor cell (HSPC) spheroids using polydimethylsiloxane (PDMS) has shown that the effectiveness of three-dimensional culture for HSPC expansion for clinical use is still a strategy that needs further improvement [**80**].

A three-dimensional collagen-based culture using HSPC, bone-marrow-derived MSCs or the umbilical cord (UC) to mimic the main compartments of the bone marrow hematopoietic niche has been proposed [**81**]. Data analysis identified two compartments: (I) HSPC suspended above collagen and (II) migrating HSPC within the collagen fiber matrix. The various locations reflected the unique microenvironments within the bone marrow that greatly influence the destiny of hematopoietic stem and progenitor cells (HSPC). The authors proposed that the 3D culture system utilizing collagen and BM-MSC facilitated HSPC proliferation and offered a promising platform for in-depth research on niches, hematopoiesis, and their regulatory mechanisms.

A bone marrow composed of two compartments, solid and liquid, that act harmoniously, has been proposed [**82**]. A bone marrow structure was created using a macroporous PEG hydrogel that resembled the macroporous 3D architecture of the trabecular bone, site of the red bone marrow, and, therefore, where the HSPC niches are located. This bone marrow analog was found to be suitable for HSPC culture and for enhancing HSPC expansion compared to conventional 2D cell culture. The developed model of a perfused 3D bone marrow analogue mimicked the HSCs niche under steady-state or activated cell conditions that favor the maintenance or differentiation, respectively, of HSCs and allowed drug testing [**82**] It was concluded that the system reflected the behavior of HSPC in the niche under physiological conditions.

Some studies have shown that the interaction of bone marrow stromal cells with leukemic cells increases the resistance of these leukemic cells. Numerous scaffolds have been created to provide a minimal structure based on the 3D leukemic microenvironment [**73**]. As 3D culture could result in resistance to drugs, it can be a good screening tool for drug evaluation prior to the administration of chemotherapic drugs [**74,83**]. A classic example of scaffolds used to recreate the leukemic niche is polycaprolactone, which is an aliphatic and biodegradable polyester with good biocompatibility [**84,85**].

Recently, a scaffold of degradable zwitterionic hydrogel was tested for human HSPC expansion [**86**]. A 73-fold increase of long-term hematopoietic stem cells was observed (LT-HSC). The viscoelasticity and smoothness of the highly hydrated zwitterionic hydrogels seems to be important for the creation of cell niches, by their unique mechanical and antifouling properties.

The organs-on-chips technique was developed to study the mechanical and physiological response of a tissue, combining concepts of tissue engineering and microfluidics [**87**]. A bioelectronic device based on a conductive polymer scaffold was integrated with an electrochemical transistor configuration that allows 3D cell growth and the real-time monitoring of cell adhesion and growth.

This technique consists of manipulating small amounts (10^{-9} to 10^{-18} L) of fluids using small openings with micrometer dimensions. This methodology has been widely reported because it offers several advantages, such as using small amounts of samples and reagents, performing separations and detections with high resolution, and a short time for analysis [**61**]. Such techniques allow the precise control of fluids and particles in a given cell culture. This culture method enables the control of such nanoliter-scale fluids as described above and further enables and facilitates the simultaneous manipulation of cultured cells from a single cell [**62**]. Through precise manipulation of the components of the microfluidic culture medium, it is possible to transport nutrients, hormones, and oxygen growth factors to facilitate homeostasis and recreate mechanical signals that are absent in traditional culture [**88**].

This cell culture system offers several advantages for basic research applications, including the precision of micromanufacturing, which allows the presentation of a controllable and reproducible microenvironment [**64**]. Another advantage of this model is that it provides complete control over the conditions of the cell culture, including dynamic cell control, nutrient addition, removal of metabolites, stimulation with drugs and proteins, and simultaneous image and chip format [**62,89,90**].

The organs-on-chips method was utilized in cancer research, specifically in cancer-on-chip investigations, to recreate the microenvironment and produce consistent and dependable outcomes. [**91,92**]. However, up to now, it has been difficult to culture HSCs in an organs-on-chips model. A device with a central cavity that successfully mimics the bone and bone marrow has been described. This device is made from polydimethylsiloxane (PDMS) with bone inducers inserted. The central chamber of this device is composed of porous PDMS membranes, and cytokines are added in the microfluids [**93**]. Although several methods have been used, results using HSCs are generally poor [**94**].

5. CONCISE SUMMARY

Hematopoietic stem cells from bone marrow are the most commonly utilized stem cells in medicinal applications. Developing accurate methods to replicate bone marrow hematopoietic stem cells and their surroundings in a laboratory setting is difficult. Aside from hematopoietic stem cells (HSCs), many other cell types in the bone marrow, such as megakaryocytes, macrophages, monocytes, and endothelial cells, have a role in regulating HSCs and niche function. Two-dimensional cell cultures are commonly utilized because they are cost-effective and easy to work with. Nevertheless, 2D culture has various constraints. Consequently, 3D cell culture methods have been created. Despite the high current cost, the closer resemblance of a 3D culture to the tissue being examined is a significant advantage. Various techniques like spheroids, organoids, 3D bioprinting, and organs-on-chip are being used or developed to culture HSCs while preserving their characteristics. This accomplishment will enable the development of hematopoietic stem cells outside the body, opening up new possibilities for stem cell transplantation, pharmacological testing, and individualized therapy.

6. AT A GLANCE

Bone marrow's primary function is hematopoiesis. Human hematopoietic stem and progenitor cells are located in the bone marrow microenvironment, which is a key location for the emergence of hematopoietic disorders. Many changes related to the advancement of disease have been discovered in the bone marrow stem cell environment. The relationship between the bone marrow microenvironment and hematopoietic stem cells plays a crucial role in regulating the proliferation, differentiation, and balance of the stem cell population. Alterations in this highly controlled system can trigger the development of cancer. Our comprehension of human hematopoiesis and the related niche biology is restricted by the availability of human material and the constraints of in vitro culture models. Conventional culture systems used for studying human hematopoiesis do not include microenvironment niches, spatial marrow gradients, or high cell density, which limits their ability to accurately replicate bone marrow conditions outside the body. This review will explore the significance of 2D and 3D culture as a biologically relevant system for studying normal and pathological hematopoiesis.

REFERENCES

1. Ng, A.P.; Alexander, W.S. Haematopoietic stem cells: Past, present and future. *Cell Death Discov.* 2017, *3*, 17002. [Google Scholar] [CrossRef]
2. Chotinantakul, K.; Leeanansaksiri, W. Hematopoietic stem cell development, niches, and signaling pathways. *Bone Marrow Res.* 2012, *2012*, 270425. [Google Scholar] [CrossRef] [Green Version]
3. Wasnik, S.; Tiwari, A.; Kirkland, M.A.; Pande, G. Osteohematopoietic stem cell niches in bone marrow. *Int. Rev. Cell Mol. Biol.* 2012, *298*, 95–133. [Google Scholar]
4. Bianco, P.; Robey, P.G. Stem cells in tissue engineering. *Nature* 2001, *414*, 118–121. [Google Scholar] [CrossRef]
5. Calvi, L.M.; Link, D.C. Cellular complexity of the bone marrow hematopoietic stem cell niche. *Calcif. Tissue Int.* 2014, *94*, 112–124. [Google Scholar] [CrossRef]
6. Nilsson, S.K.; Johnston, H.M.; Coverdale, J.A. Spatial localization of transplanted hemopoietic stem cells: Inferences for the localization of stem cell niches. *Blood* 2001, *97*, 2293–2299. [Google Scholar] [CrossRef] [Green Version]
7. Kiel, M.J.; Morrison, S.J. Maintaining hematopoietic stem cells in the vascular niche. *Immunity* 2006, *25*, 862–864. [Google Scholar] [CrossRef] [Green Version]
8. Orkin, S.H.; Zon, L.I. Hematopoiesis: An evolving paradigm for stem cell biology. *Cell* 2008, *132*, 631–644. [Google Scholar] [CrossRef] [Green Version]

9. Calvi, L.M.; Adams, G.B.; Weibrecht, K.W.; Weber, J.M.; Olson, D.P.; Knight, M.C.; Martin, R.P.; Schipani, E.; Divieti, P.; Bringhurst, F.R.; et al. Osteoblastic cells regulate the haematopoietic stem cell niche. *Nature* 2003, *425*, 841–846. [Google Scholar] [CrossRef]

10. Oh, I.H.; Kwon, K.R. Concise review: Multiple niches for hematopoietic stem cell regulations. *Stem Cells* 2010, *28*, 1243–1249. [Google Scholar]

11. Crane, G.M.; Jeffery, E.; Morrison, S.J. Adult haematopoietic stem cell niches. *Nat. Rev. Immunol.* 2017, *17*, 573–590. [Google Scholar] [CrossRef]

12. Nies, C.; Gottwald, E. Advances in Tissue Engineering and Regenerative Medicine Artificial Hematopoietic Stem Cell Niches-Dimensionality Matters. *Adv. Tissue Eng. Regen. Med.* 2017, *2*, 42. [Google Scholar]

13. Gomariz, A.; Isringhausen, S.; Helbling, P.M.; Nombela-Arrieta, C. Imaging and spatial analysis of hematopoietic stem cell niches. *Ann. N. Y. Acad. Sci.* 2019. [Google Scholar] [CrossRef]

14. Blank, U.; Karlsson, G.; Karlsson, S. Signaling pathways governing stem-cell fate. *Blood* 2008, *111*, 492–503. [Google Scholar] [CrossRef]

15. Majka, M.; Janowska-Wieczorek, A.; Ratajczak, J.; Ehrenman, K.; Pietrzkowski, Z.; Kowalska, M.A.; Gewirtz, A.M.; Emerson, S.G.; Ratajczak, M.Z. Numerous growth factors, cytokines, and chemokines are secreted by human CD34(+) cells, myeloblasts, erythroblasts, and megakaryoblasts and regulate normal hematopoiesis in an autocrine/paracrine manner. *Blood* 2001, *97*, 3075–3085. [Google Scholar] [CrossRef] [Green Version]

16. Jafari, M.; Ghadami, E.; Dadkhah, T.; Akhavan-Niaki, H. PI3k/AKT signaling pathway: Erythropoiesis and beyond. *J. Cell. Physiol.* 2019, *234*, 2373–2385. [Google Scholar] [CrossRef]

17. Cerdan, C.; Bhatia, M. Novel roles for Notch, Wnt and Hedgehog in hematopoesis derived from human pluripotent stem cells. *Int. J. Dev. Biol.* 2010, *54*, 955–963. [Google Scholar] [CrossRef]

18. Aster, J.C.; Pear, W.S.; Blacklow, S.C. Notch signaling in leukemia. *Annu. Rev. Pathol.* 2008, *3*, 587–613. [Google Scholar] [CrossRef]

19. Tekmal, R.R.; Keshava, N. Role of MMTV integration locus cellular genes in breast cancer. *Front. Biosci.* 1997, *2*, 519–526. [Google Scholar]

20. Duncan, A.W.; Rattis, F.M.; DiMascio, L.N.; Congdon, K.L.; Pazianos, G.; Zhao, C.; Pazianos, G.; Zhao, C.; Yoon, K.; Cook, J.M.; et al. Integration of Notch and Wnt signaling in hematopoietic stem cell maintenance. *Nat Immunol.* 2005, *6*, 314–322. [Google Scholar] [CrossRef]

21. Gordon, M.D.; Nusse, R. Wnt signaling: Multiple pathways, multiple receptors, and multiple transcription factors. *J. Biol. Chem.* 2006, *281*, 22429–22433. [Google Scholar] [CrossRef] [PubMed] [Green Version]

22. Dyer, M.A.; Farrington, S.M.; Mohn, D.; Munday, J.R.; Baron, M.H. Indian hedgehog activates hematopoiesis and vasculogenesis and can respecify prospective neurectodermal cell fate in the mouse embryo. *Development* 2001, *128*, 1717–1730. [Google Scholar]

23. Shi, X.; Wei, S.; Simms, K.J.; Cumpston, D.N.; Ewing, T.J.; Zhang, P. Sonic Hedgehog Signaling Regulates Hematopoietic Stem/Progenitor Cell Activation during the Granulopoietic Response to Systemic Bacterial Infection. *Front. Immunol.* 2018, *9*, 349. [Google Scholar] [CrossRef] [PubMed]

24. Mendez-Ferrer, S.; Michurina, T.V.; Ferraro, F.; Mazloom, A.R.; Macarthur, B.D.; Lira, S.A.; Scadden, D.T.; Ma'ayan, A.; Enikolopov, G.N.; Frenette, P.S. Mesenchymal and haematopoietic stem cells form a unique bone marrow niche. *Nature* 2010, *466*, 829–834. [Google Scholar] [CrossRef]

25. McNiece, I.K.; Briddell, R.A. Stem cell factor. *J. Leukoc. Biol.* 1995, *58*, 14–22. [Google Scholar] [CrossRef]

26. Edling, C.E.; Hallberg, B. c-Kit--a hematopoietic cell essential receptor tyrosine kinase. *Int. J. Biochem. Cell Biol.* 2007, *39*, 1995–1998. [Google Scholar] [CrossRef]

27. Nakamura-Ishizu, A.; Takizawa, H.; Suda, T. The analysis, roles and regulation of quiescence in hematopoietic stem cells. *Development* 2014, *141*, 4656–4666. [Google Scholar] [CrossRef] [Green Version]

28. Solar, G.P.; Kerr, W.G.; Zeigler, F.C.; Hess, D.; Donahue, C.; de Sauvage, F.J.; Eaton, D.L. Role of c-mpl in early hematopoiesis. *Blood* 1998, *92*, 4–10. [Google Scholar] [CrossRef]

29. Mao, A.S.; Mooney, D.J. Regenerative medicine: Current therapies and future directions. *Proc. Natl. Acad. Sci. USA* 2015, *112*, 14452–14459. [Google Scholar] [CrossRef] [Green Version]

30. Duval, K.; Grover, H.; Han, L.H.; Mou, Y.; Pegoraro, A.F.; Fredberg, J.; Chen, Z. Modeling Physiological Events in 2D vs. 3D Cell Culture. *Physiology (Bethesda)* 2017, *32*, 266–277. [Google Scholar]

31. Lerescu, L.; Tucureanu, C.; Caras, I.; Neagu, S.; Melinceanu, L.; Salageanu, A. Primary cell culture of human adenocarcinomas--practical considerations. *Roum. Arch. Microbiol. Immunol.* 2008, *67*, 55–66. [Google Scholar]

32. Lopes, A.A.; Peranovich, T.M.; Maeda, N.Y.; Bydlowski, S.P. Differential effects of enzymatic treatments on the storage and secretion of von Willebrand factor by human endothelial cells. *Thromb. Res.* 2001, *101*, 291–297. [Google Scholar] [CrossRef]

33. Janz Fde, L.; Debes Ade, A.; Cavaglieri Rde, C.; Duarte, S.A.; Romao, C.M.; Moron, A.F.; Zugaib, M.; Bydlowski, S.P. Evaluation of distinct freezing methods and cryoprotectants for human amniotic fluid stem cells cryopreservation. *J. Biomed. Biotechnol.* 2012, *2012*, 649353. [Google Scholar]

34. Ruiz, J.L.; Fernandes, L.R.; Levy, D.; Bydlowski, S.P. Interrelationship between ATP-binding cassette transporters and oxysterols. *Biochem. Pharmacol.* 2013, *86*, 80–88. [Google Scholar] [CrossRef] [PubMed]

35. Kirchhoff, C.; Araki, Y.; Huhtaniemi, I.; Matusik, R.J.; Osterhoff, C.; Poutanen, M.; Samalecos, A.; Sipilä, P.; Suzuki, K.; Orgebin-Criste, M.C. Immortalization by large T-antigen of the adult epididymal duct epithelium. *Mol. Cell. Endocrinol.* 2004, *216*, 83–94. [Google Scholar] [CrossRef] [PubMed]

36. Kaur, G.; Dufour, J.M. Cell lines: Valuable tools or useless artifacts. *Spermatogenesis* 2012, *2*, 1–5. [Google Scholar] [CrossRef] [Green Version]

37. Rosa Fernandes, L.; Stern, A.C.; Cavaglieri, R.C.; Nogueira, F.C.; Domont, G.; Palmisano, G.; Bydlowskia, S.P. 7-Ketocholesterol overcomes drug resistance in chronic myeloid leukemia cell lines beyond MDR1 mechanism. *J. Proteomics* 2017, *151*, 12–23. [Google Scholar] [CrossRef] [PubMed]

38. Romano, P.; Manniello, A.; Aresu, O.; Armento, M.; Cesaro, M.; Parodi, B. Cell Line Data Base: Structure and recent improvements towards molecular authentication of human cell lines. *Nucleic Acids Res.* 2009, *37*, D925–D932. [Google Scholar] [CrossRef]

39. Miki, Y.; Ono, K.; Hata, S.; Suzuki, T.; Kumamoto, H.; Sasano, H. The advantages of co-culture over mono cell culture in simulating in vivo environment. *J. Steroid Biochem. Mol. Biol.* 2012, *131*, 68–75. [Google Scholar] [CrossRef]

40. Eridani, S.; Sgaramella, V.; Cova, L. Stem cells: From embryology to cellular therapy? An appraisal of the present state of art. *Cytotechnology* 2004, *44*, 125–141. [Google Scholar] [CrossRef] [Green Version]

41. Csaszar, E.; Kirouac, D.C.; Yu, M.; Wang, W.; Qiao, W.; Cooke, M.P.; Boitano, A.E.; Ito, C.; Zandstra, P. Rapid expansion of human hematopoietic stem cells by automated control of inhibitory feedback signaling. *Cell Stem Cell* 2012, *10*, 218–229. [Google Scholar] [CrossRef] [PubMed] [Green Version]

42. Le Blanc, K.; Frassoni, F.; Ball, L.; Locatelli, F.; Roelofs, H.; Lewis, I.; Lanino, E.; Sundberg, B.; Bernardo, B.M.; Remberger, M.; et al. Mesenchymal stem cells for treatment of steroid-resistant, severe, acute graft-versus-host disease: A phase II study. *Lancet* 2008, *371*, 1579–1586. [Google Scholar] [CrossRef]

43. Zon, L.I. Intrinsic and extrinsic control of haematopoietic stem-cell self-renewal. *Nature* 2008, *453*, 306–313. [Google Scholar] [CrossRef] [PubMed]

44. Heike, T.; Nakahata, T. Ex vivo expansion of hematopoietic stem cells by cytokines. *Biochim. Biophys. Acta* 2002, *1592*, 313–321. [Google Scholar] [CrossRef] [Green Version]

45. Ando, K.; Yahata, T.; Sato, T.; Miyatake, H.; Matsuzawa, H.; Oki, M.; Miyoshi, H.; Tsuji, T.; Kato, S.; Hotta, T. Direct evidence for ex vivo expansion of human hematopoietic stem cells. *Blood* 2006, *107*, 3371–3377. [Google Scholar] [CrossRef] [PubMed] [Green Version]

46. McNiece, I.K.; Stoney, G.B.; Kern, B.P.; Briddell, R.A. CD34+ cell selection from frozen cord blood products using the Isolex 300i and CliniMACS CD34 selection devices. *J. Hematother.* 1998, *7*, 457–461. [Google Scholar] [CrossRef] [PubMed]

47. Xie, J.; Zhang, C. Ex vivo expansion of hematopoietic stem cells. *Sci. China Life Sci.* 2015, *58*, 839–853. [Google Scholar] [CrossRef] [PubMed] [Green Version]

48. Vaidya, A.; Kale, V. Hematopoietic Stem Cells, Their Niche, and the Concept of Co-Culture Systems: A Critical Review. *J. Stem Cells* 2015, *10*, 13–31. [Google Scholar]

49. Breems, D.A.; Blokland, E.A.; Siebel, K.E.; Mayen, A.E.; Engels, L.J.; Ploemacher, R.E. Stroma-contact prevents loss of hematopoietic stem cell quality during ex vivo expansion of CD34+ mobilized peripheral blood stem cells. *Blood* 1998, *91*, 111–117. [Google Scholar] [CrossRef] [Green Version]

50. Walenda, T.; Bork, S.; Horn, P.; Wein, F.; Saffrich, R.; Diehlmann, A.; Eckstein, V.; Ho, A.D.; Wagner, W. Co-culture with mesenchymal stromal cells increases proliferation and maintenance of haematopoietic progenitor cells. *J. Cell Mol. Med.* 2010, *14*, 337–350. [Google Scholar]

51. Crisan, M.; Dzierzak, E. The many faces of hematopoietic stem cell heterogeneity. *Development* 2016, *143*, 4571–4581. [Google Scholar] [CrossRef] [PubMed] [Green Version]

52. Boulais, P.E.; Frenette, P.S. Making sense of hematopoietic stem cell niches. *Blood.* 2015, *125*, 2621–2629. [Google Scholar] [CrossRef] [PubMed] [Green Version]

53. Takano, T.; Li, Y.J.; Kukita, A.; Yamaza, T.; Ayukawa, Y.; Moriyama, K.; Uehara, N.; Nomiyama, H.; Koyano, K.; Kukita, T. Mesenchymal stem cells markedly suppress inflammatory bone destruction in rats with adjuvant-induced arthritis. *Lab. Invest.* 2014, *94*, 286–296. [Google Scholar] [CrossRef] [PubMed] [Green Version]

54. Haynesworth, S.E.; Baber, M.A.; Caplan, A.I. Cytokine expression by human marrow-derived mesenchymal progenitor cells in vitro: Effects of dexamethasone and IL-1 alpha. *J. Cell Physiol.* 1996, *166*, 585–592. [Google Scholar] [CrossRef]

55. Devine, S.M.; Hoffman, R. Role of mesenchymal stem cells in hematopoietic stem cell transplantation. *Curr. Opin. Hematol.* 2000, *7*, 358–363. [Google Scholar] [CrossRef] [PubMed]

56. Li, Z.; Qian, P.; Shao, W.; Shi, H.; He, X.C.; Gogol, M.; Yu, Z.; Wang, Y.; Qi, M.; Zhu, Y.; et al. Suppression of m(6)A reader Ythdf2 promotes hematopoietic stem cell expansion. *Cell Res.* 2018, *28*, 904–917. [Google Scholar] [CrossRef]

57. Ravi, M.; Paramesh, V.; Kaviya, S.R.; Anuradha, E.; Solomon, F.D. 3D cell culture systems: Advantages and applications. *J. Cell Physiol.* 2015, *230*, 16–26. [Google Scholar] [CrossRef]

58. Murray-Dunning, C.; McArthur, S.L.; Sun, T.; McKean, R.; Ryan, A.J.; Haycock, J.W. Three-dimensional alignment of schwann cells using hydrolysable microfiber scaffolds: Strategies for peripheral nerve repair. *Methods Mol. Biol.* 2011, *695*, 155–166. [Google Scholar]

59. Tee, D.E.H. Culture of Animal Cells: A Manual of Basic Technique. *J. R. Soc. Med.* 1984, *77*, 902–903. [Google Scholar]

60. Melissinaki, V.; Gill, A.A.; Ortega, I.; Vamvakaki, M.; Ranella, A.; Haycock, J.W.; Fotakis, C.; Farsari, M.; Claeyssens, F. Direct laser writing of 3D scaffolds for neural tissue engineering applications. *Biofabrication* 2011, *3*, 045005. [Google Scholar] [CrossRef] [PubMed]

61. Whitesides, G.M. The origins and the future of microfluidics. *Nature* 2006, *442*, 368–373. [Google Scholar] [CrossRef] [PubMed]

62. Mehling, M.; Tay, S. Microfluidic cell culture. *Curr. Opin. Biotechnol.* 2014, *25*, 95–102. [Google Scholar] [CrossRef] [PubMed]

63. El-Ali, J.; Sorger, P.K.; Jensen, K.F. Cells on chips. *Nature* 2006, *442*, 403–411. [Google Scholar] [CrossRef] [PubMed]

64. Dittrich, P.S.; Manz, A. Lab-on-a-chip: Microfluidics in drug discovery. *Nat. Rev. Drug Discov.* 2006, *5*, 210–218. [Google Scholar] [CrossRef] [PubMed]

65. Pampaloni, F.; Reynaud, E.G.; Stelzer, E.H. The third dimension bridges the gap between cell culture and live tissue. *Nat. Rev. Mol. Cell Biol.* 2007, *8*, 839–845. [Google Scholar] [CrossRef] [PubMed]

66. Haycock, J.W. 3D cell culture: A review of current approaches and techniques. *Methods Mol. Biol.* 2011, *695*, 1–15. [Google Scholar]

67. Toda, S.; Watanabe, K.; Yokoi, F.; Matsumura, S.; Suzuki, K.; Ootani, A.; Aoki, S.; Koike, N.; Sugihara, H. A new organotypic culture of thyroid tissue maintains three-dimensional follicles with C cells for a long term. *Biochem. Biophys. Res. Commun.* 2002, *294*, 906–911. [Google Scholar] [CrossRef]

68. Lancaster, M.A.; Huch, M. Disease modelling in human organoids. *Dis. Model Mech.* 2019, *12*. [Google Scholar] [CrossRef] [Green Version]

69. Lancaster, M.A.; Knoblich, J.A. Organogenesis in a dish: Modeling development and disease using organoid technologies. *Science* 2014, *345*, 1247125. [Google Scholar] [CrossRef]

70. Seet, C.S.; He, C.; Bethune, M.T.; Li, S.; Chick, B.; Gschweng, E.H.; Zhu, Y.; Kim, K.; Kohn, D.B.; Baltimore, D.; et al. Generation of mature T cells from human hematopoietic stem and progenitor cells in artificial thymic organoids. *Nat. Methods* 2017, *14*, 521–530. [Google Scholar] [CrossRef]

71. Yuhas, J.M.; Li, A.P.; Martinez, A.O.; Ladman, A.J. A simplified method for production and growth of multicellular tumor spheroids. *Cancer Res.* 1977, *37*, 3639–3643. [Google Scholar]

72. Fennema, E.; Rivron, N.; Rouwkema, J.; van Blitterswijk, C.; de Boer, J. Spheroid culture as a tool for creating 3D complex tissues. *Trends Biotechnol.* 2013, *31*, 108–115. [Google Scholar] [CrossRef] [PubMed]

73. Tanner, K.; Gottesman, M.M. Beyond 3D culture models of cancer. *Sci. Transl. Med.* 2015, *7*, 283ps9. [Google Scholar] [CrossRef] [PubMed] [Green Version]

74. Gillet, J.P.; Calcagno, A.M.; Varma, S.; Marino, M.; Green, L.J.; Vora, M.I.; Patel, C.; Orina, J.N.; Eliseeva, T.A.; Singal, V.; et al. Redefining the relevance of established cancer cell lines to the study of mechanisms of clinical anti-cancer drug resistance. *Proc. Natl. Acad. Sci. USA* 2011, *108*, 18708–18713. [Google Scholar] [CrossRef] [PubMed] [Green Version]

75. Li, Y.; Huang, G.; Li, M.; Wang, L.; Elson, E.L.; Jian Lu, T.; Genin, G.M.; Xu, F. An approach to quantifying 3D responses of cells to extreme strain. *Sci. Rep.* 2016, *6*, 19550. [Google Scholar] [CrossRef] [PubMed]

76. Polymeric Scaffolds in Tissue Engineering Application: A Review. *Int. J. Polymer Sci.* 2011, *2011*. [CrossRef]

77. Kleinman, H.K.; Philp, D.; Hoffman, M.P. Role of the extracellular matrix in morphogenesis. *Curr. Opin. Biotechnol.* 2003, *14*, 526–532. [Google Scholar] [CrossRef]

78. Raic, A.; Naolou, T.; Mohra, A.; Chatterjee, C.; Lee-Thedieck, C. 3D models of the bone marrow in health and disease: Yesterday, today and tomorrow. *MRS Commun.* 2019, *9*, 37–52. [Google Scholar] [CrossRef]

79. Llames, S.; Garcia, E.; Otero Hernandez, J.; Meana, A. Tissue bioengineering and artificial organs. *Adv. Exp. Med. Biol.* 2012, *741*, 314–336. [Google Scholar]

80. Futrega, K.; Atkinson, K.; Lott, W.B.; Doran, M.R. Spheroid Coculture of Hematopoietic Stem/Progenitor Cells and Monolayer Expanded Mesenchymal Stem/Stromal Cells in Polydimethylsiloxane Microwells Modestly Improves In Vitro Hematopoietic Stem/Progenitor Cell Expansion. *Tissue Eng. Part C Methods.* 2017, *23*, 200–218. [Google Scholar] [CrossRef] [Green Version]

81. Leisten, I.; Kramann, R.; Ventura Ferreira, M.S.; Bovi, M.; Neuss, S.; Ziegler, P.; Wagner, W.; Knüchel, R.; Schneider, R.K. 3D co-culture of hematopoietic stem and progenitor cells and mesenchymal stem cells in collagen scaffolds as a model of the hematopoietic niche. *Biomaterials* 2012, *33*, 1736–1747. [Google Scholar] [CrossRef] [PubMed]

82. Rodling, L.; Schwedhelm, I.; Kraus, S.; Bieback, K.; Hansmann, J.; Lee-Thedieck, C. 3D models of the hematopoietic stem cell niche under steady-state and active conditions. *Sci. Rep.* 2017, *7*, 4625. [Google Scholar] [CrossRef] [PubMed]

83. Reticker-Flynn, N.E.; Malta, D.F.; Winslow, M.M.; Lamar, J.M.; Xu, M.J.; Underhill, G.H.; Hynes, R.O.; Jacks, T.E.; Bhatia, S.N. A combinatorial extracellular matrix platform identifies cell-extracellular matrix interactions that correlate with metastasis. *Nat. Commun.* 2012, *3*, 1122. [Google Scholar] [CrossRef] [PubMed] [Green Version]

84. Chen, Y.; Gao, D.; Wang, Y.; Lin, S.; Jiang, Y. A novel 3D breast-cancer-on-chip platform for therapeutic evaluation of drug delivery systems. *Anal. Chim. Acta* 2018, *1036*, 97–106. [Google Scholar] [CrossRef] [PubMed]

85. Song, K.; Wang, Z.; Liu, R.; Chen, G.; Liu, L. Microfabrication-Based Three-Dimensional (3-D) Extracellular Matrix Microenvironments for Cancer and Other Diseases. *Int. J. Mol. Sci.* 2018, *19*, 935. [Google Scholar] [CrossRef] [PubMed] [Green Version]

86. Wu, J.; Xiao, Y.; Chen, A.; He, H.; He, C.; Shuai, X.; Li, X.; Chen, S.; Ren, B.; Zheng, J.; et al. Sulfated zwitterionic poly(sulfobetaine methacrylate) hydrogels promote complete skin regeneration. *Acta Biomater.* 2018, *71*, 293–305. [Google Scholar] [CrossRef] [PubMed]

87. Yi, H.G.; Lee, H.; Cho, D.W. 3D Printing of Organs-On-Chips. *Bioengineering* 2017, *4*, 10. [Google Scholar] [CrossRef]

88. Ozbolat, I.T. Bioprinting scale-up tissue and organ constructs for transplantation. *Trends Biotechnol.* 2015, *33*, 395–400. [Google Scholar] [CrossRef]

89. Novo, P.; Volpetti, F.; Chu, V.; Conde, J.P. Control of sequential fluid delivery in a fully autonomous capillary microfluidic device. *Lab. Chip.* 2013, *13*, 641–645. [Google Scholar] [CrossRef]

90. Ong, S.M.; Zhang, C.; Toh, Y.C.; Kim, S.H.; Foo, H.L.; Tan, C.H.; van Noort, D.; Park, S.; Yu, H. A gel-free 3D microfluidic cell culture system. *Biomaterials* 2008, *29*, 3237–3244. [Google Scholar] [CrossRef]

91. Zhang, Y.S.; Duchamp, M.; Oklu, R.; Ellisen, l.W.; Langer, R.; Khademhosseini, A. Bioprinting the Cancer Microenvironment. *ACS Biomater Sci. Eng.* 2016, *2*, 1710–1721. [Google Scholar] [CrossRef] [PubMed] [Green Version]

92. Shafiee, A.; Atala, A. Printing Technologies for Medical Applications. *Trends Mol. Med.* 2016, *22*, 254–265. [Google Scholar] [CrossRef] [PubMed]

93. Torisawa, Y.S.; Spina, C.S.; Mammoto, T.; Mammoto, A.; Weaver, J.C.; Tat, T.; Collins, J.J.; Ingber, D.E. Bone marrow-on-a-chip replicates hematopoietic niche physiology in vitro. *Nat. Method.* 2014, *11*, 663–669. [Google Scholar] [CrossRef] [PubMed] [Green Version]

94. Di Maggio, N.; Piccinini, E.; Jaworski, M.; Trumpp, A.; Wendt, D.J.; Martin, I. Toward modeling the bone marrow niche using scaffold-based 3D culture systems. *Biomaterials* 2011, *32*, 321–329. [Google Scholar] [CrossRef]

INDEX

A

Ability 84, 123, 201, 221

Absorbance 126

Acrylamide 66-67

Acrylate 124

Activation 9, 24, 58, 177, 194, 223

Agarose 157

Agonists 25

Albumin 98

Alignment 181

Amounts 180, 230

Animals 127, 202

Antibody 73, 96-97, 180

Anti-human 11

Apoptosis 36, 158, 160, 166-167, 169, 212, 227

Astrocytes 45, 54, 57

B

Biology 232

Bioreactor 94, 99, 104, 116

Bovine 203

Buffer 36-37, 179-180

C

Canine 154-155, 159-160, 164-169, 171

Carbon 98

Cellular 1, 8-9, 27, 49, 55, 71, 86, 175, 195, 223, 225

Chemicals 33-34, 55, 155, 221

Chimeric 209, 211-212

Co-culture 226, 236

Colchicine 67

Colitis 189

Collagen 13, 16, 19, 95-97, 102, 109, 111-113, 120, 229

Cortex 70, 74, 85

Culture 1, 3-5, 8, 10-11, 34-35, 40, 61, 68-70, 73, 75, 78, 81-82, 85-86, 90, 95-96, 99, 102-103, 105-109, 112, 123-126, 130, 132-133, 137-141, 143-144, 146-149, 153, 158, 160, 162, 164, 166-168, 170, 177, 181-186, 189, 203-204, 208, 212, 224-232, 234, 237-238, 240

Cyclic 94, 104-105, 112, 116-117

Cytokines 101, 106-107, 111-112

Cytoplasm 142

Cytotoxic 58

D

Density 25, 29, 41, 76-79

Dilution 11-12, 38

Dysplasia 178, 182-185, 189

E

Endocrine 172

Epiblast 123, 141, 205
Ethanol 99

F

Fibrin 95, 104-105, 107, 109
Fibroblast 72
Fibrosis 2, 7, 24, 27-29
Fluids 230

G

Gentamicin 212
Glutamine 35
Google 5-6, 27-31, 59-68, 85-91, 113-121, 144-152, 169-173, 195-199, 215-219, 232-240
Growth 27, 35, 40, 58, 69-73, 75-76, 78, 80, 82, 85, 87, 94-95, 117, 119, 124-127, 130-131, 135, 139-140, 143, 150, 154-155, 160, 164, 166-169, 177, 194, 213, 221, 224, 230

H

Hydrogels 140, 229

J

Jejunum 159

K

Kidney 201-204, 206-219

L

Landscapes 199
Ligaments 115
Ligands 193
Ligases 194
Lymphoid 222

M

Markers 41, 43, 95, 101, 106, 124, 132-138, 140-141, 143, 158, 160, 162, 167, 184, 186, 205-206, 222
Microscopy 59, 130, 157
Mycoplasma 35
Myocardial 27

N

Nephrons 206, 208, 213-214
Networks 87

O

Organs 4
Outgrowth 39, 51-52, 57-58, 68, 75, 87, 89

P

Parkinson 67
Patients 9, 24
Platform 26, 75, 84, 239
Polymers 125-126, 139, 143
Primers 38, 74
Promega 156, 158
Proteins 7, 12, 16, 134
Protocols 178, 213
P-value 192
Reversion 141
Rudiments 203

S

Serine 176
Signal 24, 108, 136
Silicon 2, 70-72, 75-85, 89-90
Software 10, 12, 36-38, 97, 100
Spheroids 28, 37, 39-43, 51-52, 54, 58
Stem-cell 199
Suitable 53, 57
Suppressor 194

Synergy 12

Systems 4, 8, 12, 33, 53, 58, 84, 93, 112, 153, 202

T

Tendons 94, 115

Teratomas 135

Threonine 176

Tissues v, 4, 69, 86, 112, 177, 213, 228

Toxicity 212

Troponin 12

T-test 20-21

Tyrosine 176, 196

V

Variations 162

Viability 38, 45-48, 58, 73, 78, 126, 139, 158

X

Xylene 179